Pills, Potions, and Poisons

Trevor Stone is Professor of Pharmacology at the University of Glasgow.

Gail Darlington is Consultant Physician and Rheumatologist at Epsom General Hospital.

Pills, Potions, and Poisons

How drugs work

TREVOR STONE

Professor of Pharmacology, University of Glasgow

and

GAIL DARLINGTON

Consultant Physician and Rheumatologist, Epsom General Hospital

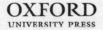
OXFORD
UNIVERSITY PRESS

OXFORD
UNIVERSITY PRESS

Great Clarendon Street, Oxford OX2 6DP

Oxford University Press is a department of the University of Oxford
and furthers the University's aim of excellence in research, scholarship,
and education by publishing worldwide in

Oxford New York

Auckland Bangkok Buenos Aires Cape Town Chennai Dar es Salaam Delhi
Hong Kong Istanbul Karachi Kolkata Kuala Lumpur Madrid Melbourne
Mexico City Mumbai Nairobi São Paulo Taipei Tokyo Toronto

Oxford is a registered trade mark of Oxford University Press

Published in the United States
by Oxford University Press Inc., New York

First published 2000

First published as an Oxford University Press paperback
(with corrections) 2004

A catalogue record for this book is available from the British Library

Library of Congress Cataloging-in-Publication Data
Data available

ISBN 0 19 860942 6

1

Typeset by
Footnote Graphics Limited, Warminster, Wilts

Printed in Great Britain
by Clays Ltd., St Ives plc

*Dedicated affectionately
to Tom and Alice
and
to Norman, Debbie, and Kelvin*

Foreword

Richard Wilson

Many of us read with horror the list of side-effects of drugs that comes with a bottle of pills. Even so, it is astonishing to realize that up to half of all the drugs prescribed by doctors are not taken according to the instructions, when the disease being treated—even a common one like blood pressure—is far more dangerous than the drugs. Of course, most people do not relish the idea of spending the rest of their lives depending on drugs, but this state of affairs represents an enormous waste of research and health workers' time and resources. Perhaps if people understood more about their medicines and how they are working to help them, there would be less waste and, overall, better health.

I met Professor Stone when I was Rector of Glasgow University (he is Professor of Pharmacology there) and, along with Gail Darlington, a consultant physician, they have cut through the medical and scientific jargon to present us with a summary of how drugs work in a language most of us non-scientists can understand. At the same time, they have liberally sprinkled the text with anecdotes and quotations, sometimes historical, sometimes humorous, and always providing fascinating insights into the people and human stories behind the discovery of drugs which we take for granted. I was fascinated to read whilst looking through ALCOHOL (I wonder why I was attracted to that section) that chemicals contained in it can interact with chemicals in the brain, like dopamine, to produce molecules which closely resemble morphine and its related drug heroin. Perhaps there is not such a difference between hard and soft drugs then! The book makes a fascinating, entertaining read. I am sure this book will find its rightful place among the growing number of books which contribute to the Public Understanding of Science.

November 1999   Richard Wilson

Preface

Normally we are almost unaware of the complexity of the human body. We take so much for granted about our bodies because they have evolved to a state in which a million different chemical reactions, some involving hormones, transmitters, receptors, and enzymes all function in a co-ordinated fashion, needing little or no deliberate help from us. Yet each component of our bodies is a marvellous and intricate machine, and it is only when something goes wrong that most of us become aware of our organs and tissues, and begin to seek information about how and why things work as they do.

The purpose of this book is to provide a basic understanding of drugs and how they work. It is written in an attempt to remove the mystery and, for some people, the fear, which surrounds the use of conventional medicines. It is hoped that it will be useful to a wide range of readers, whether or not they have any medical knowledge, and it has been written to provide a book which is both readable and enjoyable in its own right, and one which provides a source of facts and information about particular drugs when this is needed.

The book is neither a medical textbook nor a layman's guide to medicine and diagnosis, but explains some of the basic processes underlying diseases and the ways in which medicines act to combat those processes. Understandably, patients object to being expected to take, often without adequate explanation, the wide variety of pills, tablets, capsules, suppositories, ointments, and injections which their doctors prescribe. As a result, many patients worry about their drugs, particularly if they experience mild side-effects, and may stop a course of treatment far too early to produce the maximum benefit. Often the patient does not confess this to the doctor in case he or she might feel that the patient lacks confidence in them.

Ideally, doctors should always explain the medicines they prescribe, and patients should ask the questions that worry them about their treatment. How are these medicines working? Are they curing the disease or merely masking the symptoms? How are they reducing the symptoms of disease? What are the main side-effects to be expected and what causes them? Although it is not intended as a comprehensive guide to all the side-effects of drugs, the book does discuss the major ones and explains, where known, the reasons why those effects occur.

We have included most of the more common disorders for which useful drugs are available. In addition, chapters are included on conditions such as Alzheimer's disease for which few drugs have been available but for which the pharmaceutical industry is now able to offer hope since drugs are being developed which promise the possibility of real benefit to patients.

In addition we have taken a look at some of the drugs which are now widely used, not for the treatment of disease, but for recreation: drugs such as alcohol, nicotine, ecstasy, and marijuana. We also consider a few of the 'poisons' which may affect people on occasion, from bee stings to sheep dip, and glance at the enormous range of poisons found naturally in the plant and animal kingdoms. Finally, we have examined briefly the enormous complexity, costs, and ethical issues involved in drug development in the pharmaceutical industry, including the use of animals for medical research, the incidence of side-effects, and the issue of patient choice.

Although the book is intended primarily to explain the actions of the many drugs now used by doctors, a science called 'pharmacology', we have along the way provided a generous helping of 'physiology', the science of how the normal body works. We have included a glossary to help with terms which may be unfamiliar to some readers.

Acknowledgements

We are grateful to many people who have helped in the preparation of this book. Several colleagues and patients have kindly provided illustrations, or given permission for the use of illustrations including Professor Tony Payne (University of Glasgow), Professor Robert Anderson (National Heart and Lung Institute), Dr Chris George and Dr Louis Temple (Epsom General Hospital), Dr Dilip Murthy (International Centre for Health Sciences, Manipal), Mr and Mrs Thorp, and the staff of the Wellcome Photographic Library.

We thank Mr Gordon Smith and Mrs Marion Morrison in the Sally Howell Library at Epsom General Hospital for their untiring help in acquiring source materials and Mr Tom Stone, Dr Lewis Corina, Mrs Anne Corina, and Dr Kevin Browne for commenting on parts of the text. We are grateful to Dr Michael Rodgers and his team of reviewers, Mrs Claire Walker, and their colleagues at Oxford University Press for their frequent help and advice throughout the project, and to Mrs Alison Smith and Mrs Glenda Primarolo for their patience in typing sections of the text.

Finally, we reserve our most profound thanks for our spouses, Anne and Norman, who have read and commented on drafts of chapters and who have suffered long hours of neglect during the preparation of *Pills, Potions, and Poisons*.

Contents

How to use this book for reference

While we hope there will be many readers who enjoy this book from start to finish, there will undoubtedly be many who dip into it from time to time to find out about specific diseases or drugs. The drug names used may not at first seem to be the ones with which you are familiar. Drugs can have several names. Most drugs are complex chemicals and a full chemical name would often stretch over one or two lines in this book. When a drug enters animal or clinical testing, the chemical name is shortened to a more manageable size, such as diazepam.* This is known as the 'approved' or 'generic' name and this is the name we shall use in most cases in this book.

A company may take out a patent on a new drug in order to stop other companies stealing their hard-earned research results and making the same drug. After a few years, though, the patent will expire. At that time any company can make and sell the drug, which they will naturally want to advertise as their particular brand. Each company therefore gives the drug a 'brand' name, or proprietary name. Every drug may then be sold under its generic name or under a variety of brand or trade names in different countries or when used in combination with other drugs. So the drug propranolol is the main constituent of preparations known as Angilol, Apsolol, Berkolol, Inderal, Inderetic, Cardinol, Blocardyl, Avlocardyl, Dociton, Tonum, Caridol, Tesnol, Pranolol, and Pranovan. (The scientific name is spelled with a small initial letter; a trade or brand name is spelled with a capital letter.)

Similarly acetylsalicylic acid, or aspirin, is present in preparations called Alka-Seltzer, Anton, Aspirin, Anadin, Breoprin, Caprin, Claradin, Codis, Hypon, Safapryn, Solprin, Veganin, and about fifty others around the world. Of course, some of these preparations may contain other drugs as well, and some are specially formulated to give added qualities to the preparation: to be more readily soluble, or to have a longer-lasting effect.

To find *your* drug in this book, therefore, it will be necessary to find the approved drug name. This is normally on the label of a bottle of prescription medicine, or on the box or bottle of a medicine bought over the counter in a

---

* The chemical name of diazepam is 7-chloro-1,3-dihydro-1-methyl-5-phenyl-2H-1,4-benzodiazepin-2-one.

pharmacy, or on the information sheet inside the box. If in doubt, the doctor or pharmacist should be happy to give the correct name (and are obliged to do so if asked).

You are then in a position to look up your drug name in the index to this book, where you will find reference to your drug in the text of the book or in one of the tables. These tables list almost all the relevant drugs available in the UK or USA at the time of publication. Those indicated by (USA) in the tables are available *only* in the USA. The table will show you to which group your particular drug belongs, and you can then find the section of the chapter which describes that group and how it works.

CHAPTER 1

How do drugs work?

In the Middle Ages, drugs were believed to work according to *The Doctrine of Signatures*. The idea was that each potential remedy for disease could be recognized by some property or 'signature' on it. For example, rusty iron particles or red wine were supposed to be of value in restoring the colour of the blood in people who appeared pale due to anaemia; the saffron plant, because of its yellow colour was used to treat jaundice, while cyclamen plants were used to treat disorders of the ear because their leaves resembled the human ear. The mandrake plant (*Mandragora*) and ginseng have been used for a wide variety of ailments largely because their roots often resemble the shape of the human body.

Our knowledge of how drugs work—the study of pharmacology—has advanced beyond recognition since the days of the *Doctrine of Signatures*. We can now examine individually many of the thousands of chemical reactions occurring in the body, to isolate particular molecules and to study their structure and actions, and to examine the effects of diseases and drugs on the body in more detail than ever before. This enables us to understand many of the diseases affecting mankind, understand how the drugs we already have are working, and to 'design' new drugs at will.

In this book we shall explain what is now known about some of the major diseases and the drugs used to treat them, but we begin by introducing some fundamental ideas which will recur throughout the rest of the book.

What are drugs?

Drugs are chemicals: collections of atoms bound together to form molecules. A medicine—a pill, capsule, cream, or linctus, for example, contains drug molecules mixed together with inactive substances such as sugars and starches to make the tablet easy to handle or to make the linctus palatable. Mixtures of this sort are needed because the amounts of some drugs needed by humans are very small. A normal dose of morphine would fit onto a pin-head, and it would be extremely difficult to manufacture and to manipulate a tablet that small.

As we shall see in this book, some drugs such as aspirin and morphine have been extracted from plants, after crude preparations of those plants were used in folk and native medicine for centuries. Many other drugs have been synthesized by chemists who ingeniously stitch together groups of atoms to produce new variations on molecules present in plants, or molecules similar to those which occur in our own bodies. As a result, chemists produce thousands of molecules new to nature in an attempt to find ones which will cure a disease or a symptom without producing side-effects.

Their task is enormous. Most drug molecules contain between 10 and 100 atoms and the manner in which these can be combined is astronomical. A molecule consisting of 100 atoms could be put together in at least 1 million million different ways. The science of pharmacology is the science not only of trying to understand the basis of disease, but also of trying to design different configurations of these atoms in order to alleviate specific symptoms of a disease or, ideally, to cure the illness altogether.

Hormones and Receptors

Cells

The body is made up of millions of small units called cells which can be seen only under a microscope. About 10 000 cells would fit onto a pin-head. Cells are collected together to form larger units with a particular function. These large units are the tissues and organs such as the heart, kidneys, liver, pancreas, and brain. In order that the body and its organs may function smoothly, the different organs need to communicate with each other. They achieve this by producing chemicals called hormones. Each organ produces several hormones which enter the bloodstream and travel around the body to affect other organs.

Hormones and neurotransmitters

Hormones have very specific functions. Sex hormones produced by the female ovaries or the male testes are responsible for the development and maintenance of the genitals and secondary sex characteristics such as hairiness of the body and face, muscle size and the low pitch of the voice in men, and development of the breasts and menstruation in women. Insulin, a hormone produced by the pancreas, controls the body's use of sugar (glucose), while epinephrine (adrenaline*), produced by the adrenal glands, helps us to respond to stress.

The activities of many organs, including their production of hormones are

---

* The hormones which have been known as adrenaline and noradrenaline in the UK and much of Europe, are known as epinephrine and norepinephrine in North America. The Commission of the European Community has recently decided that the terms epinephrine and norepinephrine should be used universally.

controlled by nerves. Nerves affect the organs by secreting chemicals called neurotransmitters (because they 'transmit' information between nerves or from the nerves to the organs). These will be described in more detail later.

One feature of hormones and neurotransmitters is that their effects must be specific, producing effects only on those organs or cells where their action is needed and not everywhere in the body. How is this specificity achieved?

Drugs and dyes

The German chemist Paul Ehrlich (1854–1915) worked for a dye manufacturing company, *FarbenIndustrie*, and was fascinated by the way in which dyes attached so tightly to fabrics that they could not be removed by washing. He was also interested in why different bacteria produced very different diseases and suggested that the poisons produced by bacteria might produce their powerful effects by attaching tightly to specific sites in the cells of the body, just as dyes attached to clothing.

A British scientist, John Langley, proposed a similar idea in 1905, after testing a number of chemicals on animal tissues. Langley noticed that drugs such as atropine could prevent completely the effects of a few chemicals without affecting the responses to many others. He therefore proposed that animal cells possessed a 'receptive substance' to which only atropine, and the chemicals it would block, could attach. These ideas of Ehrlich and Langley are the forerunners of our present ideas that drugs often work via very specific molecules called 'receptors', often found on the surface of cells.

Receptors

Each of the millions of tiny cells has a wall or membrane around it, made of large and complicated molecules (collections of atoms). Within these membranes are special groups of molecules known as 'receptors', because they detect or 'receive' the molecules of hormones in the blood stream (Fig. 1.1). When a molecule of the hormone epinephrine, say, touches an epinephrine receptor in a cell membrane, it triggers a series of changes in the cell known as the response.

In the 1920s the American physiologist Walter Cannon was the first to describe the effects of epinephrine as preparing the body for 'fight or flight'. Epinephrine is produced by stress at times of fear or anxiety, fighting or anger, and the response to it includes a pounding heartbeat, twitching of the muscles, increased breathing, and a pale appearance of the face (as blood is diverted from the skin into muscles ready for action). These changes account for the fact that, when threatened, or when feeling nervous, we become very aware of our heartbeat and our faces may turn 'white with fear'.

There are different receptors for every hormone in the body—hormones like epinephrine, sex hormones (*see* Chapter 19), and insulin (*see* Chapter 3). Each

An organ such as the heart...

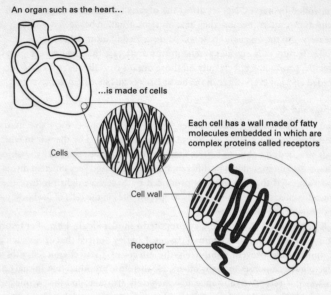

...is made of cells

Each cell has a wall made of fatty molecules embedded in which are complex proteins called receptors

Cells

Cell wall

Receptor

Receptors may be thought of as locks into which hormones and drugs fit like keys

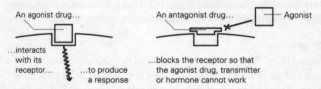

An agonist drug...

...interacts with its receptor...   ...to produce a response

An antagonist drug...   Agonist

...blocks the receptor so that the agonist drug, transmitter or hormone cannot work

Fig. 1.1 Cells, membranes, and receptors, and the effects of agonist and antagonist drugs.

hormone usually interacts with its own specific receptor or receptor family to trigger a unique set of events. Epinephrine, for example, produces the 'fight or flight' response by acting on receptors which respond only to epinephrine and the very similar hormone norepinephrine (noradrenaline). Other natural hormones are unable to act on these receptors. This specificity of hormone–receptor interaction is sometimes likened to a 'lock and key', since each hormone usually 'fits' only one type of receptor in just the same way that a key fits only one lock. Some hormones, however, can act on a family of several, similar receptors, each triggering a different set of responses. Epinephrine and norepinephrine, for example, can act on a family of about a dozen very similar receptors which allow these hormones to have a number of different effects.

Drug development

This simple idea of specificity—each hormone or neurotransmitter acting on its own receptors—is the basic concept underlying the development of new drugs, because it implies that drugs can be produced which, like the natural substances, will only act on one type of receptor to produce their desired effect. If a compound acts on several other types of receptor in addition, it is more likely to produce side-effects.

Nerves and receptors

At least as important as the effects of hormones are the effects of nerves. Almost every organ is connected to nerves which have two basic functions. Some of the nerves are 'sensory' which means that they detect, or sense, changes in an organ's blood supply, chemical environment, position, and temperature and signal that information to the brain. Some of the nerves are 'motor' and carry information from the brain to the organs, causing muscles to contract or glands to secrete hormones.

In the same way that different organs communicate with each other using hormones, nerve cells (neurons) also communicate with each other and the organs by releasing hormone-like chemicals known as 'transmitters' or 'neurotransmitters' because they 'transmit' information between nerves or from nerves to the tissues (Fig. 1.2). Transmitters are secreted by neurons very rapidly and their effects may be completed within a few thousandths of a second

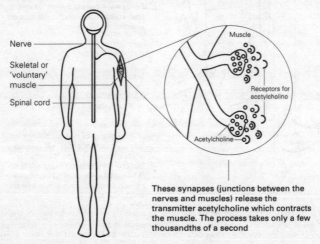

Nerve

Skeletal or 'voluntary' muscle

Spinal cord

Muscle

Receptors for acetylcholine

Acetylcholine

These synapses (junctions between the nerves and muscles) release the transmitter acetylcholine which contracts the muscle. The process takes only a few thousandths of a second

Fig. 1.2 The synapses (junctions) between nerves and muscle.

(milliseconds). This speed of transmission by nerves allows us to control our muscles quickly enough to type, play an instrument, or catch a ball.

Types of Receptor

Both hormones and transmitters produce their effects by acting on specific receptors. We shall need to refer to these frequently in this book and it will be helpful to describe some of them here (*see* Figs 1.3 and 1.4 and Table 1.1).

Norepinephrine receptors

There is a group of nerves known as the 'sympathetic' nerves which control our glands and involuntary muscles (those over which we have no conscious control such as those which make up the heart, stomach, and intestine). These sympathetic nerves release a neurotransmitter—norepinephrine—which can act on two families of receptors known as alpha (α) and beta (β) receptors.*

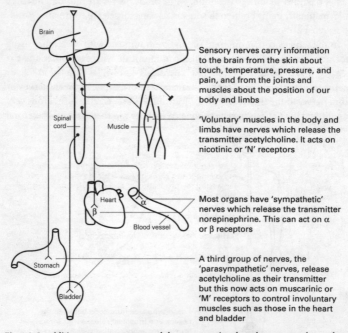

Sensory nerves carry information to the brain from the skin about touch, temperature, pressure, and pain, and from the joints and muscles about the position of our body and limbs

'Voluntary' muscles in the body and limbs have nerves which release the transmitter acetylcholine. It acts on nicotinic or 'N' receptors

Most organs have 'sympathetic' nerves which release the transmitter norepinephrine. This can act on α or β receptors

A third group of nerves, the 'parasympathetic' nerves, release acetylcholine as their transmitter but this now acts on muscarinic or 'M' receptors to control involuntary muscles such as those in the heart and bladder

Fig. 1.3 In addition to sensory nerves and those contracting the voluntary muscles, we have two types of involuntary (autonomic) nerves: the sympathetic and parasympathetic nerves.

* There are about eight members of the alpha family and three members of the beta family.

(a) Effects of the sympathetic nerves and the chemical transmitter they release (norepinephrine). The hormone epinephrine has similar effects

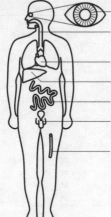

Contraction of muscles in the iris, which opens the pupil

Relaxation of muscles cells in the trachea (windpipe), allowing more air into the lungs

Increased heart rate and a stronger heartbeat

Release of glucose from the liver (to provide energy)

Reduced movements of the intestine

Contraction of the tubes from the testes (the vasa deferentia) producing ejaculation

Contraction of the blood vessels, raising the blood pressure

(b) Effects of the parasympathetic nerves and the chemical transmitter they release (acetylcholine)

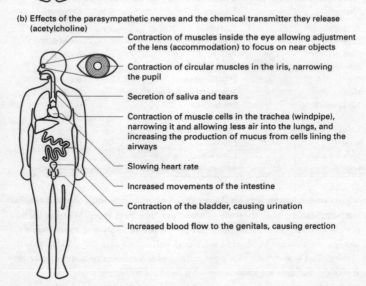

Contraction of muscles inside the eye allowing adjustment of the lens (accommodation) to focus on near objects

Contraction of circular muscles in the iris, narrowing the pupil

Secretion of saliva and tears

Contraction of muscle cells in the trachea (windpipe), narrowing it and allowing less air into the lungs, and increasing the production of mucus from cells lining the airways

Slowing heart rate

Increased movements of the intestine

Contraction of the bladder, causing urination

Increased blood flow to the genitals, causing erection

Fig. 1.4 The effects of the autonomic nerves.

Table 1.1 The effects of transmitters on body tissues

Transmitter: acetylcholine

Tissue	Effect	Receptor
Voluntary muscle	Contraction	N (Nicotinic)
Stomach	Contraction	M (Muscarinic)
	Acid secretion	M
Intestine	Contraction	M
Bladder	Contraction	M
Salivary glands	Secretion	M
Lachrymal glands	Secretion (tears)	M
Sweat glands	Secretion (sweating)	M
Eye	Constriction of pupil	M
	Accommodation for close vision	M
Heart	Slowing of heart beat	M
Airways	Contraction	M
	Secretion of mucus	M
Blood vessels in sex organs	Dilation (erection and swelling)	M
Blood vessels in the face	Dilation (blushing)	M

Transmitter: norepinephrine (noradrenaline) or the hormone epinephrine (adrenaline)

Tissue	Effect	Receptor
Stomach	Relaxation	α and β (β_2)
Intestine	Relaxation	α and β (β_2)
Bladder	Relaxation	α and β
Salivary glands	Secretion	α
Eye	Dilation of pupil	α
Heart	Increased rate and force	β (β_1)
Blood vessels	Contraction	α
	Relaxation	β (β_2)
Kidney	Renin secretion	β
Airways	Relaxation	β (β_2)
Male sex organs	Contraction of muscles (ejaculation)	α
Liver	Release of glucose	α and β

When norepinephrine acts on alpha receptors it makes the walls of blood vessels contract, leading to an increase of blood pressure. Beta receptors relax blood vessels, but they also make the heart beat more strongly and more rapidly, increase the amount of sugar in the blood, and reduce activity of the intestine (Table 1.1). Drugs which block the actions of epinephrine or norepinephrine at α or β -receptors are known as α or β-blockers respectively.

Acetylcholine receptor

A different group of nerves, known as 'parasympathetic' nerves, release a different transmitter, acetylcholine, onto glands and involuntary muscles.* Acetylcholine acts on receptors which are known as 'muscarinic' or M receptors (Figs 1.3 and 1.4) because they are also activated by the compound muscarine. Muscarine comes from the toadstool *Amanita muscaria*, the red mushroom with white spots often illustrated in children's stories and fairy tales.

Activation of muscarinic receptors stimulates the secretion of saliva when we eat, allows the eye to adjust, or accommodate, when we read or view nearby objects, and maintains activity of the intestine and stomach.

Table 1.1 is a list of some of these effects of acetylcholine in different organs of the body. Drugs which block the effects of acetylcholine are referred to as 'anticholinergic' and they may be used, for example, to reduce movements of the intestine in irritable bowel syndrome (*see* Chapter 4). They can also produce a dry mouth, blurred vision, and constipation by preventing the normal actions of acetylcholine to stimulate salivary secretion, cause accommodation of vision, and move food along the intestine. There are many drugs which have anticholinergic properties, so these symptoms occur quite commonly as side-effects.

Anticholinergic drugs in history

Two powerful anticholinergic chemicals in plants are hyoscine from henbane (*Hyoscyamus niger*) and atropine from deadly nightshade (*Atropa belladonna*). There is enough atropine in one berry from the deadly nightshade to kill an adult man, a fact which was often used in ancient Rome by the infamous Livia in her repeated and often successful attempts to gain power and influence by assassination.

The juice from belladonna berries was squeezed into the eyes of females intent on seduction as it blocks the acetylcholine receptors in the iris, causing the iris to dilate. Men are attracted to women with dilated pupils (and *vice versa*), normally without realizing that they feel this attraction.†

Voluntary muscles

The 'voluntary', or skeletal, muscles (because they are attached to the skeleton) allow us to move our body and limbs as we choose. Our movements of voluntary muscles are made by motor nerves which also release the transmitter acetylcholine. The receptors on the voluntary muscle which respond to acetylcholine are called 'nicotinic' or N receptors because in about 1900 the Cambridge physiologist John Langley discovered that they are also stimulated by nicotine. The amount of nicotine needed to stimulate these receptors is greater than that normally present in the bloodstream of smokers, but heavy smokers or people not used to smoking may experience muscle twitching when they smoke, from stimulation of their muscles by nicotine.

* Together the sympathetic and parasympathetic nerves, which control the involuntary muscles and glands, are known as the 'autonomic' nerves as they work automatically, without conscious control.
† A similar effect is obtained when dining by candlelight, as the dim light causes the pupils to dilate.

Receptors inside cells

A few hormones and drugs act on receptors which are not in the walls of the cells, but occur inside the cells. The steroid hormones and related drugs are an example. They bind to a molecule in the cell wall which transports them into the interior of the cell. There, they combine with their receptor molecule and the combination of steroid plus receptor then moves into the nucleus of the cell where it can modify the genetic machinery of the cell (the DNA, deoxyribonucleic acid). It is by changing the genetic machinery, or modifying the 'translation' of DNA into proteins, that steroids such as oestrogens and androgens determine our sex and, therefore, the formation of different organs and sex characteristics in males and females.

Agonism and Antagonism (Fig. 1.1)

A drug which has the same effect as a natural hormone or transmitter by activating the same receptor, is called an 'agonist' at that receptor. A drug which blocks or prevents the actions of the natural hormone or transmitter is known as an 'antagonist' or 'blocker' of that hormone or transmitter. Antagonism is usually the result of drug molecules interacting with receptors but sticking to them very tightly so that the natural hormone and transmitter cannot reach the receptor molecules to trigger a normal response.

Enzymes as drug targets

Some drugs do not affect receptors but act on a different set of targets called enzymes.

Every cell in the body carries out thousands of chemical reactions every second to produce energy, to grow, to repair damaged molecules or parts of the cell, to contract if it is a muscle cell, or to divide into two new cells. Many of these reactions are carried out by special molecules called 'enzymes', each enzyme being responsible for a different chemical reaction.

Enzymes are large proteins which assist and encourage a chemical reaction without becoming changed themselves. They are the biological equivalents of catalysts in chemistry. They allow reactions to occur very much more quickly than would occur naturally. For example, after the transmitter acetylcholine has been released by motor nerves to contract a voluntary muscle, it must be removed quickly in order that the muscle can relax ready to respond to another impulse in the nerve. The muscle cells carry the enzyme acetylcholinesterase in their walls; each molecule of this enzyme can destroy over 10 000 molecules of acetylcholine every second. By having a coating of enzyme molecules in their walls, the muscle cells can destroy the acetylcholine released by one nerve impulse in a few thousandths of a second, becoming rapidly prepared to respond to the next impulse.

In the course of this book we shall meet a range of enzymes which destroy transmitters or hormones in cells or in the blood. Other enzymes are called 'transporter' enzymes because they transport chemicals or hormones across cell walls.

Some drugs act by inhibiting enzymes, preventing them from carrying out their normal function. Just as drugs targeted at receptors need to be specific for the receptors of only one hormone or transmitter, those drugs acting on enzymes should ideally affect only one of the many thousands of different types in order to minimize side-effects.

Other drug targets: channels, transporters, and nucleic acids

In addition to receptors and enzymes, some drugs have a different set of targets. Some drugs act on pores in the walls of cells called channels. In order to live, all cells must have the correct balance of atoms and molecules inside and outside their walls. Atoms and molecules move across the walls through channels, which can be thought of as pores or holes in the wall. In fact, the channels are made by large proteins which change their shape to allow molecules through the wall. Some drugs act by increasing the 'size' of these channels, allowing molecules to flood into or out of the cells much more quickly than normal. Other drugs block the channels.

Many cells contain enzymes in their walls which actively push atoms or molecules across the wall. These are called 'transport enzymes', or simply 'transporters'. Drugs which are used in depression, for example, inhibit the molecules which transport amine transmitters into the nerve endings.

The molecules of DNA, which make up our genes, and of RNA (ribonucleic acid), which manufactures new proteins from the 'message' present in the DNA, can also be drug targets. The drugs which are used to treat cancer (see Chapter 18), for example, prevent the growth of cancer cells by interfering with these molecules of 'nucleic acids' (so called because they exist mainly in the nucleus of the cell). We shall encounter all these drug targets in more detail, in addition to a few less common ones, as we travel through this book.

Drugs of the future

It will soon be possible to target drugs to specific types of cell. The cells in every tissue or organ are 'labelled' with complex molecules on their surface, with names such as 'cell adhesion molecules' and 'histocompatibility antigens'. Cancer cells contain labelling molecules which are quite different from those of their parent tissue. Antibodies can be made to these molecules and attached to an anticancer drug. As the antibody sticks to a cancer cell label, it delivers a high dose of the drug directly to the cancer cells with little effect on the surrounding, normal cells.

The new science of genomics is also likely to lead to new drugs in the near future. Genomics involves identifying and studying the genetic differences and changes which are responsible for diseases. If a gene defect is found, the next stage of research is to identify the function of that gene, which might code for a receptor or enzyme. This knowledge in turn should allow chemists to design new drugs to act on the receptor or enzyme and correct the disease-causing defect.

Summary

- *Organs secrete hormones and nerves secrete transmitters which produce their effects on other tissues.*
- *Hormones, transmitters, and drugs act on receptor molecules in the walls of cells.*
- *Receptors can exist in several forms.*
- *Drugs which activate receptors are agonists; drugs which prevent the effects of hormones and transmitters are antagonists.*
- *Enzymes are proteins which facilitate chemical reactions in the cells. Some drugs inhibit enzyme activity.*
- *A major objective in developing a new drug is that it should only act on one member of a receptor family, or one enzyme, thus reducing side-effects.*

CHAPTER 2

Breathing: allergies, asthma, coughs, and colds

Lesley and Andrew were delighted to see their friends Joan and Keith, whom they had not seen for almost 15 years. After the initial greetings, Joan introduced her daughters Joanna, 10, and Sarah, 8, and everyone went in to the lounge and sat down. Within minutes, Sarah's eyes felt uncomfortable and she could feel tears running down her cheeks. The inside of her nose was also starting to itch, and she sneezed—once, twice, three times. Her nose began to run as well and her face became flushed because her body temperature had risen. Sarah was now breathing more quickly than when she had stepped out of the car. Her breathing was becoming noisier and wheezy and, as the adults' conversation paused for a moment, the sound of her wheezing was noticed by her mother. Joan took her coat, wrapped it around Sarah and took her outside. After Sarah had taken some breaths of fresh air, Joan sat with her in the warm car until a doctor arrived. Meanwhile Keith and his hosts soon discovered the cause of the problem: Lesley and Andrew had a pet cat. It had not been in the room with them, but Sarah was allergic to cats, and the fine particles of skin and fur from the cat's earlier presence had been enough to trigger the reactions. As soon as she was taken outside, Sarah started to recover and, within a couple of hours of leaving the house, Sarah was back to her normal self.

Allergies

Sarah was experiencing an allergic reaction—a set of bodily changes occurring when some people are exposed to agents in the environment to which they have become sensitive. The term 'allergy' was first used by the Austrian paediatrician Clemens Pirquet von Cesenatico in Vienna in 1906 and was coined from two Greek words—*allo* meaning 'other' and *ergon* meaning 'work'. The word allergy was meant to indicate that the symptoms were the result of the body working in response to external factors.

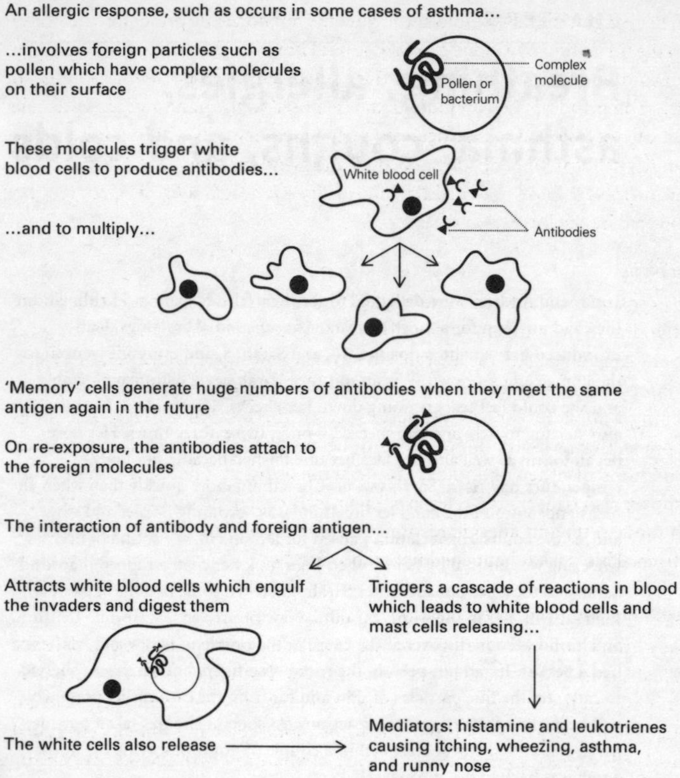

An allergic response, such as occurs in some cases of asthma...

...involves foreign particles such as pollen which have complex molecules on their surface

Pollen or bacterium

Complex molecule

These molecules trigger white blood cells to produce antibodies...

White blood cell

...and to multiply...

Antibodies

'Memory' cells generate huge numbers of antibodies when they meet the same antigen again in the future

On re-exposure, the antibodies attach to the foreign molecules

The interaction of antibody and foreign antigen...

Attracts white blood cells which engulf the invaders and digest them

Triggers a cascade of reactions in blood which leads to white blood cells and mast cells releasing...

The white cells also release ⟶

Mediators: histamine and leukotrienes causing itching, wheezing, asthma, and runny nose

Fig. 2.1 What causes an allergic response?

Antigens and Allergens*

Most particles of dust and pollen are filtered out or trapped by the hairs and mucus in our nose and airways, but if there is a large number of such foreign particles some of them may pass into the lungs and may even enter the bloodstream.

In the blood there are several million cells known as white cells or leucocytes, whose task it is to detect foreign molecules. These unfamiliar molecules are called 'antigens', When such a molecule has been detected, the white cell which found it begins to multiply, producing thousands of identical cells—clones— all of which can recognize the same 'antigen' (Fig. 2.1).

* An antigen which triggers an allergic reaction is sometimes known as an 'allergen'.

The recognition that a molecule is foreign (not normally present in the body) and the formation of a clone can take several hours or days when a new antigen is encountered. However, some of the cloned cells become 'memory cells' in the lymph glands. When an individual is exposed to the same antigen molecule on a later occasion, it will be detected by the memory cells within minutes. The memory cells can then divide to produce thousands of similar cells very quickly. This process is known as 'cellular immunity' since it is a form of protection produced by the formation of new cells.

Antibodies

On exposure to an antigen some of the white cells in the blood begin to produce antibodies to the antigen. Antibodies are large molecules which combine with the antigen and trigger the allergic reaction. Following exposure to many types of infection or antigen, some antibodies will remain in the bloodstream, keeping a lookout for any reappearance of the foreign antigen. If it does reappear, the antibody combines with the antigen and triggers the formation of millions of other antibodies to the same antigen. The antigen–antibody complex also triggers the release of chemicals called 'mediators' within a few minutes, so that an allergic response appears very quickly after exposure to antigen. This is what happened in Sarah's case.*

Mediators and the allergic reaction

The white blood cells are part of the immune system—the body's defence against invasion by bacteria and viruses. The immune system is extremely complex, but the main result of a person's being exposed to an antigen or an antigen–antibody complex is that the white blood cells, and similar cells called 'mast' cells present in the tissues, release mediators which include histamine and leukotrienes.†

The mediators are responsible for the signs of allergy:

1. They irritate the membranes lining the nose. They also dilate blood vessels in the nose and increase the leakiness of the walls of blood vessels. The increased blood flow through the vessels, together with the more permeable walls, results in some fluid being pushed out of the blood into the tissue lining the nose, causing congestion or a runny nose. Together, these effects produce the runny nose (rhinorrhoea) and sneezing of allergies, hay fever, and the common cold.

2. Mediators also relax blood vessels and activate sensory nerves in the skin (giving the redness and itching called 'urticaria').

* A rapid allergic reaction of this kind is also known as a 'Type I hypersensitivity reaction'.
† Other mediators include interleukins, platelet activating factor (PAF), and prostaglandins.

3. They increase the secretion of mucus by gland cells in the airways and contract the muscle cells in the airways. These two effects produce the wheezing, coughing, and shortness of breath seen in asthma.

4. The fever and feelings of tiredness associated with allergies, colds, and influenza are due to the effects of these mediators on the brain.

Why do allergies develop?

Why do allergies develop in the first place? Surveys suggest that more than 1 person in every 20 has suffered from asthma at some time in their lives and the incidence is increasing. In 1819 Dr John Bostock, a physician working at Guy's Hospital in London, first described to the Royal Society his own symptoms of what we now call 'hay fever'. He recorded only 28 other cases among his 5000 patients—an incidence of about 1 in 200. Today, about 1 in 10 people in industrialized societies show signs of hay fever. More than 1 child in 10 will show signs of asthma before the age of 10 years, although the condition will disappear again in about half of these children.

Most of us will have a few foreign particles in our bloodstream, but in such small quantities that they can be removed by an efficient immune system without our noticing. If a person is exposed to a large amount of antigen in the airways, or if some passes into the blood, it may trigger an allergic reaction. Alternatively, if a person is exposed to the same antigen on several different occasions the memory cells trigger a reaction in response to smaller amounts of antigen.

One possible reason for the increasing incidence of allergies is that chemical pollutants in the atmosphere and diet are acting as antigens to increase the sensitivity of the immune system as a whole so that more people show allergic reactions such as asthma in response to previously harmless stimuli. Asthma is virtually unknown among Eskimos and some remote Indian tribes where industrial and chemical pollution have not yet arrived. When inhabitants of New Guinea and Zimbabwe were introduced to the Western practice of sleeping indoors with blankets, the incidence of asthma rose dramatically.

Another popular idea is that allergies result from the accidental juxtaposition of harmless and dangerous stimuli. For example, a person's immune system may be very active in order to deal with an infection such as a cold or influenza. If at the same time, that person is exposed to other molecules, such as those found on cat hairs, the activated immune system may overreact to those normally innocent molecules and produce antibodies to these too. The stage is then set for an allergic reaction when the person is subsequently exposed only to the cat hairs. The increased incidence of allergies in modern society may, therefore, arise indirectly from an increased incidence of infections caused by the greater density of people.

Hay fever (seasonal or allergic rhinitis) and colds

The symptom which dominates at any one time is partly determined by the type of foreign protein (the antigen). In hay fever the symptoms are mainly confined to the nose as a result of the inhalation of pollen grains. Itching and/or dermatitis (inflammation of the skin) tend to occur after the skin has been in contact with an antigen such as a chemical constituent of a washing powder, soap, or cosmetic. Asthma is sometimes the result of inhaling house-dust mites (which live on shed skin scales) or their droppings, some pollens, or chemicals. These agents can pass into the lungs and trigger an allergic reaction there.

The symptoms of the common cold, such as coughing and sneezing, are due to the white cells producing mediators as they fight and digest invading bacteria and viruses.

Drug treatment

Decongestants

The runny nose and secretion of tears in colds and hay fever can be treated by drugs which prevent or oppose the effects of the mediators on blood vessels. There are two main groups of these drugs. One group contracts blood vessels by activating the alpha-receptors which normally respond to epinephrine and norepinephrine (*see* Chapter 1). Some of these drugs, such as phenylephrine, tramazoline, and xylometazoline act directly on the receptors to mimic the effect of epinephrine. Others, such as ephedrine, act on the sympathetic nerves, causing them to release their stores of norepinephrine which then act on the receptors. The contraction of blood vessels produced by these drugs opposes the immune system's attempts to dilate the vessels.

Antihistamines

The second group of decongestants are the antihistamines. When animals have an allergic reaction, the symptoms are different in different animals. Guinea-pigs, for example, show very intense constriction of the airways, whereas in dogs the blood vessels in the liver contract tightly, and in rabbits the blood vessels in the lungs contract. It was the British pharmacologist and later Nobel prize-winner Sir Henry Dale who first noticed in the 1920s that histamine had a variety of effects on the body, but the most marked effects were the same as those seen in response to antigenic challenge—constriction of the airways in guinea-pigs, contraction of liver blood vessels in dogs, and contraction of blood vessels to the lungs in rabbits. It was Dale who first proposed that histamine was an important mediator of the immune response.

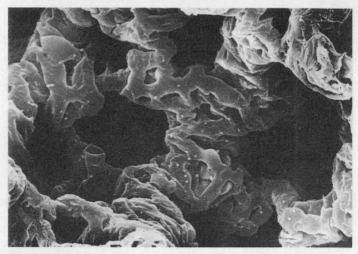

Fig. 2.2 A magnified view (more than 1000 times) of the air spaces (alveoli) in the lungs, surrounded by tiny blood vessels (capillaries). The life-giving exchange of oxygen and carbon dioxide occurs between the air spaces and the blood in the capillaries. (Professor A. P. Payne)

Histamine is one of the chemicals released into the bloodstream by white blood cells and mast cells when antibodies meet foreign antigens. In humans, histamine can cause narrowing of the airways, but it has a much greater effect on the blood vessels in the nose. Drugs which block the effects of histamine—antihistamine drugs—are, therefore, of more use in hay fever than in asthma.

In the nose, histamine relaxes the muscle cells in the small blood vessels so that more blood flows through them. Histamine also causes another type of cell, endothelial cells, to contract, creating gaps in the vessel wall through which fluid can leak out more easily than usual. The increased volume of blood in the vessels together with the easier movement of fluid across the vessel wall means that water is forced out of the blood into the nose, leading to a runny nose, irritation of the nasal lining, and sneezing. The antihistamine drugs (Table 2.1, p. 32) prevent all these changes.

Side-effects of antihistamines
The main problem with using antihistamines is that some of them, such as chlorpheniramine, cause drowsiness. This is because they enter the brain to some extent and block receptors for histamine and other transmitters which are involved in wakefulness and attention. Antihistamines should never be taken at the same time as alcohol as they increase each other's effects, making

it difficult for some people to stay alert and awake. The combination of some anthistamines and alcohol can even depress the brain enough to cause death.

Whenever possible one of the newer, although more expensive, non-sedating antihistamines should be used. These include acrivastine, a short-acting drug with effects lasting only a few hours, and astemizole, a long-lasting drug which needs several days to achieve its effects. Other non-sedative antihistamines include terfenadine and fexofenadine. There are, of course, occasions when sedation is a desirable feature, such as in people who cannot sleep well because of intense itching as a result of dermatitis.

All these drugs are usually taken by mouth, but nasal sprays containing antihistamines are being developed which should reduce the problems of sedation because the drugs will be delivered only to the nose and should not reach the brain in significant quantities.

Steroids

In more severe cases of hay fever, including those patients who have suffered from the problem for several years, the lining of the nose will show signs of long-term inflammation, and the best treatment is to administer anti-inflammatory steroids (*see* Chapter 19) directly into the nose using a spray. Steroids can reduce all the symptoms of hay fever, including the itching sensations, sneezing, runny nose, and nasal blockage because they prevent the mast cells from releasing any of the chemicals responsible for allergic symptoms, not just histamine.

The steroids take several days to become effective, but long-term sufferers could start treatment before the peak times of pollen production. The main problem with steroids is that, because they are preventing the immune system cells from releasing mediators, those cells can no longer attack and kill invading bacteria and viruses. The steroids, therefore, decrease the body's resistance to infection.

Cromoglycate

This drug was developed from a chemical called khellin, which occurs in the plant *Artemisia visnaga* and which had been reported to relieve symptoms of asthma in Middle Eastern people. Cromoglycate suppresses the release of all the irritant chemicals from mast cells after the antigen–antibody reaction, so it is just as useful for hay fever as for asthma. It is described more fully in the section on asthma. Cromoglycate should be used for some days or weeks before the pollen season in order for it to work fully.

Eye problems

Sufferers of hay fever know that the production of tears by reddened, itching eyes can be just as troublesome as problems with the nose. One of the most effective treatments for the eye problems is to use eye drops containing cromoglycate or the related drug nedocromil. By preventing the secretion of the chemicals responsible for the eye inflammation, they reduce these symptoms.

Ipratropium

Ipratropium is an antagonist at the receptors for acetylcholine. Some of the nasal problems in hay fever are partly due to the release of acetylcholine as well as histamine, and in a few patients the acetylcholine effects seem to be more important than histamine. If a sufferer does not obtain sufficient relief from antihistamines, the symptoms may still be reduced by blocking the acetyl-choline effects with ipratropium.

The release of acetylcholine from motor nerves to the trachea and bronchi contracts the airway muscles and increases the secretion of mucus. The release of acetylcholine is, therefore, responsible for some of the problems in asthma. Ipratropium can be delivered by an inhaler into the airways, blocking the acetylcholine receptors, and reducing the symptoms.

Drug allergies

White cells are best at detecting large molecules such as those released by, or present on the surface of, bacteria. However, in a few people, they may respond to the presence of much smaller molecules such as those found in a drug, thus provoking an allergic reaction to that drug and causing a skin rash or headache.

Coughs

Coughs are usually the result of irritation in the airways. Breathing through the mouth may allow particles of dirt and dust to enter into the windpipe (trachea) and these can stimulate receptors in the airway linings. When the immune system is fighting an invasion of bacteria or viruses the chemicals released by the white blood cells and mast cells can also activate those receptors and make them more sensitive to particles in the air. There is also usually an increased secretion of mucus in the airways during these reactions, which can itself cause local irritation. It is a combination of mucus and the chemicals produced by mast cells which triggers coughing in acute bronchitis and emphysema.

When the receptors in the airways are stimulated, the sensory nerves associated with them send impulses into the brain which responds with a reflex production of return messages back to the muscles of the chest and diaphragm where a co-ordinated contraction of the muscles produces the cough (Fig. 2.3).

Treatment

One approach to the treatment of a productive cough is to reduce the thickness of the mucus in the airways using either a mucolytic or an expectorant drug

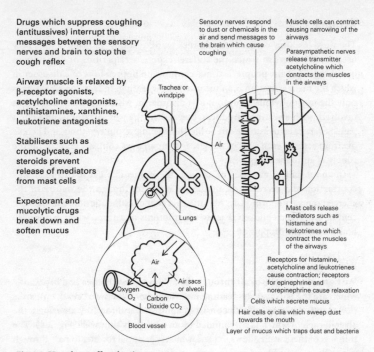

Drugs which suppress coughing (antitussives) interrupt the messages between the sensory nerves and brain to stop the cough reflex

Airway muscle is relaxed by β-receptor agonists, acetylcholine antagonists, antihistamines, xanthines, leukotriene antagonists

Stabilisers such as cromoglycate, and steroids prevent release of mediators from mast cells

Expectorant and mucolytic drugs break down and soften mucus

Sensory nerves respond to dust or chemicals in the air and send messages to the brain which cause coughing

Muscle cells can contract causing narrowing of the airways

Parasympathetic nerves release transmitter acetylcholine which contracts the muscles in the airways

Trachea or windpipe

Air

Lungs

Mast cells release mediators such as histamine and leukotrienes which contract the muscles of the airways

Receptors for histamine, acetylcholine and leukotrienes cause contraction; receptors for epinephrine and norepinephrine cause relaxation

Cells which secrete mucus

Hair cells or cilia which sweep dust towards the mouth

Layer of mucus which traps dust and bacteria

Air

Oxygen O_2

Air sacs or alveoli

Carbon Dioxide CO_2

Blood vessel

Fig. 2.3 How drugs affect the airways.

such as carbocisteine, methyl cysteine, or guaifenesin. These act on the gland cells in the airways to change the composition of the mucus so that it is thinner, less sticky, and more easily eliminated by coughing.

Non-productive coughs may be treated with antitussives—drugs which suppress coughing. They include several drugs related to morphine but which are much better at reducing coughing than reducing pain. Examples are codeine, dextromethorphan, and pholcodine. These drugs act on that part of the brain which is involved in the cough reflex just described. They depress the nerve cells in that area, so that nerve impulses arriving from the receptors in the airways are no longer able to set up a reflex cough (Fig. 2.3). These drugs are dangerous, however, when used with a cough which is producing significant amounts of sputum since the cough suppression may lead to the retention of these airway secretions. Those secretions may then cause blockage of some of the airways, allowing bacteria to become trapped and leading to infections such as pneumonia.

Asthma

The word 'asthma' comes from a Greek word meaning 'panting' and is now used for disorders in which the sufferer experiences periods of difficulty in breathing. To many people 'asthma' conjures up impressions of a disorder in which the main symptom is an inconvenient wheezing. In fact, the wheezing is only the most obvious symptom of a disorder in which most of the body is involved, with sweating, tiredness, bowel disturbances, dizziness, and chest pain. Severe cases of asthma can be life-threatening: about two thousand people die from asthma each year in the UK as their airways contract and cut off the supply of air to the lungs.

In about half of all cases of asthma, the immediate cause of the airway contraction and secretion is an allergic reaction, though the nature of the allergen can vary enormously. About 30 per cent of asthmatic adults and 80 per cent of asthmatic children react with symptoms of asthma when exposed to house-dust mite droppings.

Breathing

We normally breathe in air through the airways—the trachea and bronchi—which are the passageways leading into the lungs. When we breathe in, air is pulled into the lungs, which consist of about 300 million tiny air spaces, the alveoli, each of which is surrounded by an extremely thin wall (Fig. 2.4). The thinness of these walls allows oxygen, which is essential for life, to pass through the walls into the bloodstream very rapidly during each breath. At the same time carbon dioxide, which is a waste product of cell activity, passes from the blood in the opposite direction—through the walls of the alveoli into the air spaces, to be expelled when we breathe out.

The structure of the nose and its sticky mucous surfaces means that most solid particles in the air are filtered out, but if some breaths are taken through the mouth, or if there is a large number of particles in the air, some particles will pass into the lungs.

The airways have both sensory and motor nerves. The sensory nerves are stimulated by solid particles and produce the rapid, explosive exhalation which we call a cough (if triggered in the bronchi), or a sneeze (if triggered in the nose) and which blows the foreign particles out into the atmosphere.

Muscle cells are found throughout the trachea and bronchi. The nerves supplying these cells (motor nerves) release acetylcholine (*see* Chapter 1) which causes contraction of the muscle cells and produces narrowing of the airways. The motor nerves also increase the secretion of sticky mucus in the airways. The combination of muscle contraction and mucus traps bacteria, tiny insects, and particles of dust and stops them from passing into the lungs where they

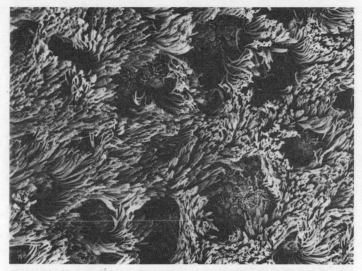

Fig. 2.4 A highly magnified view of the surface of the airways (bronchi) showing the hair-like cilia which trap dust and bacteria, sweeping them towards the mouth and nose and preventing them getting into the delicate tissues of the lungs. (Wellcome Picture Library, London)

could damage the delicate walls of the alveoli. The airways are also lined with cells possessing fine hairs, or cilia, which continuously sweep the mucus and its trapped contents towards the mouth and nose for elimination by spitting, sneezing, or swallowing.

In asthma the muscle cells of the airways contract abnormally, often with an oversecretion of mucus, which in asthmatic people is particularly thick and sticky and can block some of the airways. The contraction and secretion of mucus are often triggered by a chest infection, but other causes include allergies, stress, or anxiety, especially in children and adolescents. This narrowing of the airways reduces the supply of air and oxygen to the lungs and patients experience unpleasant sensations of fighting for breath, wheezing, and coughing. In extreme cases, and particularly if the airways do become plugged by mucus, patients may die from asphyxia unless the narrowing is treated quickly. Sometimes it is necessary to take over the process of ventilation for a very sick patient by putting them on to an artificial ventilator: such an action can be life-saving.

Chronic asthma

If exposure to foreign antigens continues for a long time, two things happen which make treatment of asthma much more difficult. The first is that the tissues of the bronchi become inflamed, with dilatation of blood vessels and leakage of fluid from the blood into the tissue. These changes cause further narrowing of the airways in addition to the effects of muscle contraction.

The second problem is that, largely because of the inflammation, the muscle cells become much more reactive to the natural chemicals causing contraction (the mediators discussed earlier), so that the doses of drugs which normally prevent contraction, and promote dilatation of the airways, become less effective. This over-reactivity means that asthmatic subjects are much more likely than normal people to react to events such as stress, exercise, or cold air, any of which may provoke an asthmatic attack. Four out of every five asthma sufferers will have an attack if they exercise in cold and dry conditions.

Phases of asthma

In many subjects, both the acute and chronic phases of asthma can be seen to some extent after each exposure to a triggering stimulus. The initial, early phase consists solely of constriction of the airways and secretion of mucus, and may last for only a few minutes. On average it reaches its peak of severity in about 15 minutes, and is over within about 90 minutes. This first phase is best treated with beta-receptor stimulants (*see* Chapter 1), xanthines, or anticholinergic drugs.

The early phase can be followed by the later, inflammatory, phase which appears only after several hours but which may last for a day or longer. The airways are much more sensitive than usual during this period. This may be the reason why patients are very vulnerable to further attacks of asthma in the days following an uncontrolled episode. Patients are advised to avoid anything which may trigger their asthma, such as exercise or cold, in the days immediately after an attack. This inflammatory phase can be prevented only by pretreating the patient with steroids or cromoglycate.

Chronic bronchitis and emphysema

Repeated bouts of airways infection or exposure to irritant chemicals and dust may lead to long-lasting (chronic) inflammation of the airways. The walls of the airways may become thinner than normal and the cells that line them produce more mucus than normal. The result is chronic bronchitis, often associated with shortness of breath, especially in cold weather, and the overproduction of mucus.

Emphysema, a disease which was first described in 1746 by Sir William Watson in a report entitled *An account of what appeared on opening the body of an asthmatic person,* is a related disorder in which the thin walls of the alveoli of the lungs have been damaged or destroyed, often by exposure to chemicals and dust particles. The most common cause of emphysema today is smoking.

People who have spent many years in mines, exposed to mineral dusts, may also develop lung diseases such as pneumoconiosis—a localized, inflammation of the lung with gradual destruction of the alveolar lining similar to emphysema.

Treatment for these conditions consists partly of increasing the amount of air getting into the lungs. The drugs used, therefore, are often the same drugs used to treat asthma and which relax the muscle cells of the airways and reduce mucus secretion.

Treatment of asthma

In trying to escape persecution in Spain the physician Maimonides sought refuge in the court of the Sultan Saladin. In return for his hospitality, the Sultan asked for advice to help his asthmatic son. The treatment recommended was to change city (to move from Cairo to Alexandria), to drink chicken soup every day, and to refrain from all sexual activity.

Fortunately modern remedies are more rational and easier to comply with than those of Maimonides. A Chinese scientist, Ko-Kui Chen noticed in 1923 that in one of the major Chinese catalogues of medicinal preparations, one particular plant, Ma Huang, occurred in several different remedies for asthma. Ma Huang is known outside China as *Ephedra vulgaris,* and when Chen succeeded in extracting from this plant the chemical responsible for its anti-asthma actions, he discovered that it was a chemical already isolated from the plant, called ephedrine. Ephedrine was soon introduced into medicine for the treatment of asthma (1926) and is still available today.*

Drugs used to prevent an acute asthma attack

Beta-receptor agonists

Among the most useful drugs for relieving the symptoms of asthma are the beta-receptor agonists. These are very similar to the natural compounds epinephrine and norepinephrine, and they reproduce its effects on beta-receptors (*see* Chapter 1). One effect of epinephrine via beta-receptors is to relax muscle cells of the airways. By inhaling a beta-receptor agonist from an aerosol, the constrictor effects of allergic mediators are partly counteracted by the dilator activity of the drug. Beta-receptors also reduce the secretion of

* Our debt to the Chinese Ma Huang does not end there. Supplies of the plant soon became limited and production of ephedrine from the plant became expensive. Attempts to produce a completely synthetic substitute then led Gordon Alles, a chemist working in the pharmacology department in the University of California, to produce amphetamine. Amphetamine was introduced in 1932 as Benzedrine, a drug which could be administered by an inhaler for the treatment of asthma. Amphetamine has also found valuable uses in the treatment of obesity, even though it is no longer used because of its serious side-effects and ability to cause addiction.

mucus by cells in the walls of the airways. Several drugs activate beta-receptors generally throughout the body. They include isoprenaline (isoproterenol), which acts directly on the receptors, and ephedrine and pseudoephedrine which activate the receptors both directly and indirectly by causing sympathetic nerves to release their stores of norepinephrine (*see* Chapter 1).

Selective beta-receptor agonists

When beta-receptors are activated, they can produce a number of physiological changes including stimulation of the rate and force of the heartbeat (*see* Chapter 1, Table 1.1). This is very undesirable in a drug being used to treat asthma, as it can raise blood pressure and increase irritability of the heart, which can in turn cause abnormal heart rhythms. These are thought to have been responsible for the deaths of many patients treated with non-selective beta-receptor agonists such as epinephrine and isoprenaline (isoproterenol in the USA). The pharmaceutical industry has been at the forefront of developing better drugs without these risks.

A major advance was made in the 1960s by the research team led by Sir James Black, a pharmacologist working in the research laboratories at ICI, a major pharmaceutical company in the UK (now Astra-Zeneca Pharmaceuticals). The discovery would lead to Black being awarded the Nobel Prize for Medicine in 1988. Black observed that the beta-receptors in the heart were slightly different from those in the bronchi, and could be activated and blocked by slightly different chemicals. The two types of beta-receptors were named beta-1 (in the heart), and beta-2 (in the airways). All the drugs listed in Table 2.2 (p. 33) are relatively selective for the latter. This means that, at the doses normally used for treatment, the drugs used for asthma should act only on the airways and should have little effect on the heart, particularly when breathed in as an aerosol directly into the airways. If taken by mouth, there may still be a small amount of heart activation and a few patients may also notice a slight tremor of the arms and hands, a side-effect of beta-receptor agonists which results from effects on the muscles. In addition to the direct effects of beta-agonists on the muscles of the bronchi, these drugs also suppress the release of the inflammatory mediators from the white cells and mast cells, which are largely responsible for causing the asthmatic symptoms. There are several popular selective beta-2-receptor agonist drugs, including salbutamol and terbutaline, (which are short-acting drugs used to abort an attack of asthma), and salmeterol and eformoterol which are long-lasting drugs reserved mainly for more severe cases (Table 2.2, p. 33).

Problems with beta-agonists

Despite being the most widespread and effective agents for treating asthma, the beta-receptor agonists have some drawbacks. In particular, it is important that

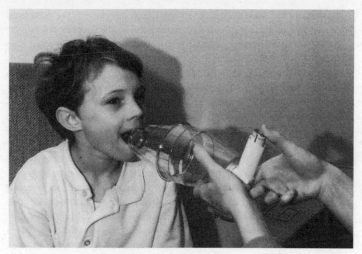

Fig. 2.5 A child using a spacer, specially designed to deal with the variations between children and their ability to time their breathing in relation to the dose of anti-asthmatic drug.

users do not greatly exceed the recommended doses. In too high a dose even the 'selective' beta-agonists can stimulate receptors in the heart and elsewhere, an action which can be dangerous and lead to abnormal heart rhythms and increased blood pressure.

If asthma is severe and patients take high doses of beta-agonist drugs for several years, the cells of the airways may try to adapt by reducing the number of beta-receptors. This can mean that the beta-agonist drugs and the body's own epinephrine can gradually become less able to prevent the effects of other chemical mediators involved in asthma. The patient's asthma may thus become, paradoxically, more severe.

Xanthines

Some of the earliest drugs used to treat asthma were xanthines—a group of compounds which includes caffeine, theophylline, and theobromine found in tea, coffee, cola beans, and chocolate. Theophylline is still sometimes used to treat asthma. Like the beta-receptor agonists, these drugs relax the bronchi and can be used to interrupt an attack of asthma. How they do so remains uncertain. One possibility is that they act on the same cellular processes as the beta-agonists but by-pass the beta-receptor. When beta-receptors are activated, they induce cells to produce more of a chemical known as cyclic AMP,* and it is this

* Cyclic AMP is an abbreviation for adenosine-3',5'-cyclic monophosphate.

which relaxes the muscle cells. The xanthine drugs prevent the cells from breaking down cyclic AMP, so that it accumulates inside the cells without any need to activate the receptors artificially by beta-agonist drugs. The result is an increase of cyclic AMP in the cells and relaxation of the airways.

An alternative idea is based on the finding by Stephen Holgate in Southampton, England, that a natural compound, adenosine, has no effect on the airways of normal subjects, but causes contraction in asthmatic subjects. The bronchial tissue of asthmatic subjects has become sensitive to adenosine. Several of the xanthines, including theophylline, are good antagonists of the effects of adenosine and may relax the airways by preventing the constrictor effects of adenosine in asthmatics. In addition to preventing muscle contraction in the walls of the bronchi, xanthines reduce the release of mediators from cells.

Of course, it is not necessarily the case that all drugs of one type act in exactly the same way, or act in only one way. It is quite likely that the various xanthines may act by a combination of these three mechanisms, as well as others still to be discovered. Xanthines are not, however, popular drugs for the treatment of asthma because they can cause a range of side-effects. For example, xanthines can stimulate the heart partly by blocking adenosine receptors and partly by preventing the breakdown of cyclic AMP, and they can act on the brain to produce tremor, anxiety, irritability, and insomnia (caffeine [see Chapter 24] is a xanthine!)

Anticholinergics

The nerves which supply the respiratory system release acetylcholine, which contracts the airway muscle and increases the secretion of mucus. Drugs which block the effects of acetylcholine—the anticholinergic drugs—can often reduce the severity of an asthmatic episode, especially if the attack has been triggered by chemical stimuli, exercise, or stress. Drugs such as atropine are effective, but will also block acetylcholine receptors in other parts of the body as well as the bronchi. This results in a number of unwanted effects including a reduction of salivary secretion leading to a dry mouth and difficulty in eating, paralysis of the muscles responsible for focusing the lens of the eye leading to blurred vision, and paralysis of the muscles of the intestine leading to constipation.

The unpleasantness of these side-effects has led to the development of drugs such as ipratropium. This is an anticholinergic drug which is normally administered as an aerosol, inhaled directly into the airways, and its chemical structure means that it is only poorly absorbed into the bloodstream. Ipratropium, therefore, has far fewer side-effects than other atropine-like drugs which are given as tablets.

Drugs used in chronic asthma

All the drugs described so far open the airways, and their actions are seen quite quickly so that they can be used to prevent, abort, or reduce the severity of an acute attack of asthma. There is in addition a group of drugs which are of no use during an asthmatic attack, but which help to reduce the inflammation of the bronchi, and so prevent attacks of asthma from starting. These drugs include cromoglycate and the steroids.

Cromoglycate and nedocromil

Cromoglycate was discovered accidentally by Roger Altounyan in the UK. He had been working for a small pharmaceutical company called Bengers* testing some of their potential anti-asthmatic compounds. This he did by precipitating an asthmatic attack in himself by breathing some animal hair and then observing whether the test compound would abort the attack. In 1964, the company thought it had found an effective drug, but when another batch was prepared, it was found to be inactive. It turned out the anti-asthmatic chemical in the original batch was an impurity. That was cromoglycate.

Both cromoglycate and nedocromil reduce the late, or inflammatory phase of an asthmatic attack, making the bronchi less reactive to stimuli. The most commonly used of these is sodium cromoglycate, a drug which is normally used as an aerosol. It acts partly on the white blood cells and mast cells, to suppress the production of those mediators which cause an asthmatic attack. It also probably interferes with the ability of some of those mediators, especially PAF, to contract the airways. Finally, it suppresses activity of the cholinergic nerves which contracts the airway muscle as a reflex response to irritation in the airway walls. Cromoglycate is less effective in adults than in children.

Ketotifen and lodoxamide suppress mediator release in a similar way to cromoglycate.

Steroids

The body's own steroids have very marked anti-inflammatory actions and a number of related compounds have been developed as drugs for use in chronic inflammatory conditions such as asthma and arthritis. Among those most frequently used in asthma are beclomethasone and betamethasone. Their mechanisms of action are discussed in more detail in Chapter 19, although in the treatment of asthma, they seem to have additional effects which suppress the production and release of mediators from mast cells.

These steroids are usually breathed directly into the lungs from an inhaler or nebuliser. This avoids most of the side-effects which can follow the use of high

* Later taken over by Fisons (now Astra-Zeneca Pharmaceuticals).

doses of steroids taken by mouth (*see* Chapter 19). However, they may cause the voice to sound huskier than normal, and the local suppression of the immune system may increase the possibility of infections around the mouth and throat. The steroids reduce inflammation of the airways, reduce the secretion of mucus, and increase the number of beta-receptors on the muscle cells, making them more sensitive to the relaxant effects of β-agonist drugs.

Leukotriene antagonists

The mediators produced by white cells and mast cells include chemicals called leukotrienes. These are fatty molecules which powerfully contract the muscle cells in the airways and promote mucus secretion. Two drugs have now been developed which are antagonists of the leukotrienes, preventing their effects in the airways. They are montelukast and zafirlukast. They cannot stop an asthmatic attack once it has begun but, if taken daily, they reduce the inflammation of the airways, reduce the secretion of mucus, and relax the muscle cells in the airway walls, decreasing the need for β-agonist drugs. They are especially useful in exercise-induced asthma, being more effective than salmeterol. Their effects in asthmatic patients are similar to those of steroids, but they should be much safer as they do not have the same range of side-effects of the steroids. One important aspect of these drugs is that patients do not become less sensitive to them with continued use, as can happen with some beta-antagonists.

Drugs of the future

Drugs such as montelukast have been introduced because of their ability to antagonize the effects of the leukotriene hormones in the airways. Another approach to this problem is to inhibit the enzyme which produces the leukotrienes, known as 5-lipoxygenase. This effect is shown by the drug zileuton which looks very promising in early clinical trials.

The chemicals released by cells in the airways also include hormones such as bradykinin and tachykinins. These are normally destroyed by an enzyme called neutral endopeptidase (NEP), and one approach to asthma and hay fever is to administer this enzyme directly to the airway or nasal linings in an aerosol. This molecule would then destroy the kinins as they were formed and prevent them affecting the airway muscles.

Platelet activating factor (PAF) is another, very powerful stimulant of bronchial muscle contraction. It has proved extremely difficult to produce drugs able to prevent the effects of PAF but one, bepafant, looks promising and is being tested in clinical trials.

The airway relaxation produced by beta-agonists such as salbutamol results from an increase in the amount of cyclic AMP inside the cells. An alternative strategy receiving intense research is to raise cyclic AMP levels by preventing its destruction by the enzyme phosphodiesterase (PDE). This effect is similar to that described for the xanthines. However, just as there are families of receptors, there are families of PDE enzymes. Many of the problems with xanthines arise because they affect all members of the PDE family throughout the body. A good anti-asthmatic drug with few side-effects would affect only one member of that family. This should still lead to relaxation of the airways but should not cause the changes in beta-receptors which have been described in this chapter and which may be dangerous in some patients. Several drugs of this type are being developed including zardaverine.

When the immune system is activated a number of substances called cytokines are produced, one of which, called interleukin-5, seems to be involved in triggering contraction of the airways. Several companies are developing drugs which interfere with the production or effects of interleukin-5 as a means of suppressing asthmatic reactions.

Chronic obstructive pulmonary disease (COPD)

This term describes several disorders such as emphysema, chronic bronchitis, and some cases of chronic asthma, all of which are characterized by chronic (long-lasting) restrictions to the flow of air into the lungs. In 90 per cent of such cases, the sole cause of the problem is smoking and, while stopping smoking can slow the rate of decline of lung function, the people concerned can never regain full, normal, lung function.

Treatment is essentially the same as for asthma, with beta-agonists, ipratropium, and steroids being useful.

Table 2.1 Drugs used in colds and hay fever

Sympathomimetics (α-receptor agonists)	Antihistamines
naphazoline	acrivastine
oxymetazoline	alimemazine
phenylephrine	antazoline
phenylpropanolamine	astemizole
tetrahydrozoline (USA)	azatadine
tramazoline	azelastine
xylometazoline	bromodiphenhydramine (USA)
	brompheniramine
Anticholinergics	cetirizine
ipratropium bromide	chlorcyclizine (USA)
	chlorphenamine
Steroids	chlorpheniramine
beclomethasone	clemastine
budesonide	cyproheptadine
flunisolide	diphenhydramine
fluticasone	diphenylpyraline
mometasone	doxylamine
triamcinolone	fexofenadine
	hydroxyzine
Mast cell stabilisers	ketotifen
lodoxamide	levocabastine
nedocromil	loratadine
sodium cromoglycate	mepyramine
	mequitazine
	mizolastine
	phenindamine
	pheniramine
	promethazine
	terfenadine
	trimeprazine
	triprolidine

Table 2.2 Drugs used in asthma

Beta-receptor agonists	Xanthines
albuterol	aminophylline
bambuterol	enprofylline
eformoterol	theophylline
fenoterol	
formoterol	**Steroids**
metaproterenol	beclomethasone
pirbuterol	betamethasone
reproterol	budesonide
rimiterol	fluticasone
salbutamol	
salmeterol	**Stabilisers**
terbutaline	cromoglycate
tulobuterol	ketotifen
	lodoxamide
Non-selective adrenoceptor agonists	nedocromil sodium
adrenaline / epinephrine	
ephedrine	**PAF antagonists**
isoetharine	bepafant
isoprenaline / isoproterenol	
orciprenaline	**Leukotriene antagonists**
pseudoephedrine	montelukast
	zafirlukast
Anticholinergics	
ipratropium	
oxitropium	

Summary

- *Antigens are usually foreign molecules which can trigger an allergic reaction.*
- *The symptoms of colds and hay fever are due to the release of 'mediators' such as histamine from white blood cells and the related 'mast' cells in tissues.*
- *Hay fever and cold symptoms can be treated by:*
  - *a) decongestant drugs, which contract blood vessels in the nose*
  - *b) antihistamines, which reduce the relaxation of blood vessels and reduce fluid secretion in the nose*
  - *c) ipratropium, which blocks the effects of acetylcholine in the nose*
  - *d) cromoglycate, which prevents mediator release and, therefore, the runny nose and production of tears*
  - *e) steroids (see Chapter 19).*
- *Asthma is often an allergic reaction to stress or pollutants.*
- *It may be controlled by:*
  - *a) drugs such as beta-receptor agonists or xanthines, which relax the airway muscle*
  - *b) ipratropium, which blocks the effects of acetylcholine on the airway muscle and mucus secretion*
  - *c) steroids*
  - *d) cromoglycate which prevents mediator release in the airways*
  - *e) antagonist drugs, which block the effects of leukotrienes on the airways.*

CHAPTER 3

Diabetes

A small girl called Jane was a typical, Canadian, fun-loving child with a great zest for life. One of her best friends was a boy called Fred Banting. When Jane was 14 years old, she began to lose a lot of weight, becoming extremely thin and almost constantly hungry. She was often very tired, and one day fell into a coma from which she never recovered. Fred was told that Jane had had diabetes, a disorder in which the body is not able to use sugar in the blood, even though the amounts present are far higher than in normal people. Jane died because at that time, around 1900, there was no treatment for diabetes.

About a decade before Jane's untimely death, a German scientist, Oscar Minkowski (1858–1931) working at the Universities of Strasbourg, Cologne, and Breslau, had noticed that when he removed the pancreas—a glandular organ lying in the abdomen—from dogs (to determine its role in digestion), the amount of sugar (glucose) in the blood and urine rose dramatically. As a similar change was known to occur in diabetes, he reasoned that damage to the pancreas might be involved in diabetes. In 1890 Georg Zuelzer, the Professor of Medicine at the University of Berlin showed that removing the pancreas from dogs caused a huge increase in the amount of sugar in the blood and urine, but that if the animals were given an injection of an extract of the pancreas, the blood and urine glucose levels in those 'diabetic' dogs were returned to normal. He then tried injecting the extracts into diabetic patients, but they were too impure and induced high fevers. Even more of a problem was that he soon ran out of extract since injections had to be given every day.

Fred Banting was so upset by the death of his friend Jane that he retained a strong desire to understand more about the disease and he graduated in medicine in 1916. Reading about the earlier experiments of Minkowski and Zuelzer, he wondered if part of the problem in purifying the active substance was that it was being destroyed by the enzymes in the pancreas which normally digest the proteins in food. In 1921, he went to the University of Toronto and persuaded Professor John Macleod to allow him to perform experiments to try to examine the function of the pancreas. Macleod agreed and asked another scientist in his laboratory, Charles Best, to help. In that same year, Banting and Best repeated Zuelzer's experiments and went on to perform some critical experiments of their own.

By tying off the duct leading from the pancreas to the intestine, Banting and Best caused the protein-destroying cells in the pancreas to die. The enzymes they produced by these cells could not escape into the intestine and began to kill the cells themselves. That left an almost pure population of the gland cells called beta-cells. They found that an extract of these beta-cells produced a powerful fall of blood glucose levels in the blood, and over the following year they gradually improved their extraction and purification procedure so that they would not run into the problems experienced by Zuelzer. By 1922, the group was ready to test their purified extracts in patients.

The first human patient to be given the injection was a seriously ill boy, Leonard Thompson, then aged 12. Leonard had exceptionally large amounts of glucose in his blood, and was losing huge amounts of water, about five litres per day, in his urine. The outlook was poor: Leonard was soon likely to be dead unless his diabetes could be controlled. Banting and Best began injecting their purified extracts of pancreas daily. After only two or three days, the boy was showing clear signs of recovery and was soon restored to a normal life. He lived a normal life for several years using daily injections from Banting and Best, until he was killed in a motor cycle accident.

Thus began a revolution in treating a previously untreatable and often fatal disorder, a revolution which was rewarded with the Nobel Prize for Banting and Macleod.* Their work was a key factor in the development of treatments for diabetes which affects around 30 million people worldwide.

Glucose

The body is very good at controlling the amounts of important substances such as sugar (glucose) in the blood. Maintaining the amount of sugar is necessary because it is one of the basic fuels which almost all cells need to survive. They use it to produce, among other things, a chemical called adenosine triphosphate (ATP) which acts as a 'reservoir' of energy within the cells. If the level of glucose in the blood falls too low we begin to feel tired, shaky, irritable, and hungry as we become aware of the need to eat something to raise the blood sugar again.

The organ most directly responsible for controlling blood glucose is the pancreas. When the pancreas is no longer able to control the storage and use of glucose, the condition of 'diabetes mellitus' occurs.

* Banting felt that Best should have been included in the prize and shared his portion with him. Macleod shared his half with the Canadian chemist James Collip (1892–1965) who had made some of the major contributions to purifying the crude extracts.

Diabetes mellitus

The symptoms of what we now call diabetes were recorded in an ancient Egyptian manuscript written about 1500BC and discovered in a tomb at Thebes by Georg Ebers in 1862 (and thereafter known as the Ebers papyrus). The word 'diabetes' itself was coined by Aretaeus of Capadokia, a Turkish physician, in AD20, and comes from the Greek word *diabaino* which means 'to pass through' or 'to siphon'. The increased quantity of sugar in the urine increases the osmotic pressure* of the urine, and stops water being reabsorbed into the bloodstream. This results in an increased loss of water in the urine (polyuria) and, as a result, a continual thirst. Water is, in a sense, passing straight through the body, being 'siphoned' through from the mouth to the urine.

The Latin word *mellitus* means honey-like or sweet and refers to the fact that the urine of diabetic patients tastes sweet because of the presence of sugar which has passed from the blood into the urine. This discovery is often credited to the British doctor Thomas Willis (1621–1675), but ancient Greek and Hindu physicians routinely tasted urine to help in their diagnoses, and were well aware of the sweet taste of urine from some of their patients. They also noticed that insects and ants were attracted towards such urine, and speculated that the sweetness might be due to the presence of honey or sugar. It was not until much later that the English doctor Matthew Dobson in Liverpool (in 1776) and the French chemist Michel Chevreul (in 1815) confirmed the presence of glucose in diabetic urine.

The symptoms of diabetes were first described by a Roman physician, Aulus Cornelius Celsus, in AD10. Celsus had made some of the earliest reliable and scientific observations about biology and medicine, publishing them in his book *De Medicina*. Although long forgotten, this text was one of the first and most influential medical books to be published (in 1478) after the invention of the printing press. In 1788, about a hundred years after the invention of powerful microscopes by the Dutchman Antoni van Leeuwenhoek, the British

---

* Osmosis is defined as 'the movement of water from a less concentrated to a more concentrated solution across a permeable membrane.' When a biological membrane exists between two compartments containing volumes of pure water, water molecules will pass freely across the membrane. If one of those volumes of water contains other molecules dissolved in it, those molecules will impede the free movement of water from that solution and there will be a net movement of water from the compartment with pure water (or a more dilute solution) across the membrane into the compartment with more dissolved molecules. This movement of water is called 'osmosis'. To make the concept clearer, imagine two groups of 100 men (equivalent to water molecules) on either side of a single gate in a wall. Each group is trying to pass to the other side of the wall. The rate at which men pass from side A to side B will be about the same as the rate from B to A. Suppose now that on side A we have a group of 50 men (water molecules) and 50 women (sugar molecules). Because women as well as men are now moving from A to B, more men will be passing from B to A than from A to B—there is a net movement of men from the more concentrated male group B to the less concentrated group A.

physician Thomas Cawley used a microscope to examine the pancreas. He described damage to the gland and a loss of pancreatic cells in patients suffering from diabetes. We now know that the cells which are lost belong to the special group called beta-cells which manufacture and secrete insulin in response to changes in the amount of glucose sugar in the blood.

Insulin

Insulin is a protein hormone which acts on most organs and tissues to promote the use or storage of glucose. For example, it causes cells in the liver to increase the conversion of glucose into glycogen and fats, forms of glucose which can then be stored until needed. Insulin acts on cells in several different tissues to increase the rate at which glucose passes into them from the blood, increasing the rate at which the glucose is broken down (metabolized) to produce ATP.

By regulating the movement of the essential fuel, glucose, into cells, and restraining the breakdown of protein and fats, insulin controls the growth and repair of tissues. In the absence of insulin, tissues are broken down at a more rapid, uncontrolled rate, so that diabetic subjects often become thin and lose muscle, with associated weakness as their fat and muscles are changed into sugar. The high rate of breakdown of fat produces chemicals called 'ketones'* which give the breath a sweet, fruity smell similar to that which follows alcohol consumption. These ketones can cause the cells of the brain to function incorrectly; as they accumulate without insulin treatment, diabetic patients may faint and fall into a coma during which the brain may be damaged permanently, or death may occur.

Type I and Type II diabetes mellitus

There are two distinct types of diabetes mellitus. About 90 per cent of patients with diabetes have the Type II disease.

Type I diabetes

Type I diabetes is also called insulin-dependent diabetes mellitus (IDDM) or juvenile-onset diabetes, as it usually begins before the age of 15 years. The term 'insulin-dependent' refers to the fact that the disorder is caused by a lack of insulin, and treatment is dependent on restoring the levels of insulin. The loss of the insulin-secreting beta-cells appears to be the result of the body's immune system attacking and destroying the pancreas (an autoimmune disease). Some destruction may occur after infection with viruses, especially those causing measles and mumps, leading to diabetes. There is, however, a strong hereditary influence, indicating some genetic susceptibility of the pancreatic cells.

* These include acetone, acetoacetic acid, and β-hydroxybutyric acid.

Type II diabetes mellitus

Type II or *non*-insulin dependent diabetes mellitus (NIDDM) is also known as 'maturity-onset' diabetes because it usually begins after the age of about 40 years. The symptoms are the same as for Type I—the presence of sugar in the urine, marked thirst, and weakness with a wasting of muscles. However, the problem is not usually a lack of insulin; patients often have normal or even raised amounts of insulin in their blood. The problem is partly that the cells of the body do not respond to the hormone—they are insulin-resistant. The reason why cells become resistant is not known, but it is usually associated with the patient's being overweight. In fact, diet and exercise are often sufficient to reduce the resistance to insulin and to allow patients to control their own glucose levels once again without the use of drugs.

Treatment

Insulin

Treatment of Type I diabetes often consists of replacing insulin using injections of the hormone: it cannot be given by mouth because it is a protein and would be rapidly destroyed by enzymes in the stomach. There is a range of different injections in which the insulin is present in crystals of different sizes: the larger the crystals, the slower the rate at which the insulin becomes absorbed, so that a single injection lasts longer. In some preparations, insulin is mixed with compounds which alter the rate of absorption into the bloodstream. As a result some of these injections work quickly and may be used in emergencies, while others work more slowly to provide a relatively constant level of insulin in the blood over many hours.

The insulin itself may be extracted from the pancreas of animals, usually pigs (porcine insulin). Human insulin is now produced from bacteria which have been genetically engineered to manufacture large amounts of the hormone. Although several other proteins can now be produced in this way, insulin was the first, a breakthrough made possible by the work of Sir Frederick Sanger, a British biochemist working in the University of Cambridge and who was awarded the Nobel Prize in 1958 for working out the complicated molecular structure of insulin. Once the structure of a protein is known, the structure of the gene which produces it can be worked out because there is a well-established genetic 'code' in which groups of three nucleotides—the basic building blocks of genes—are translated into the amino acids used to build the proteins (*see* Chapter 18). The gene can be made by chemists and inserted into bacteria which treat the new molecule as its own and generate the protein product. By cultivating these bacteria, insulin can almost literally be 'grown' at will. The insulin is then extracted from the bacteria and purified so that it is identical to the natural hormone.

Oral antidiabetic drugs

In 1942 Dr Michel Janbon, a French pharmacologist and head of the Medical Faculty at the University of Montpellier, noticed that an antibiotic drug reduced the level of sugar in the blood when given to animals. This effect was no longer seen if the pancreas was removed from the animals, suggesting that the drug was promoting the release of insulin from the pancreatic beta-cells. Janbon later noticed that patients treated with this drug showed signs of tiredness and dizziness that were associated with a drop in blood glucose and which could be prevented by giving them glucose.

The drug was one of a class of antibiotics called sulphonamides (see Chapter 17) and soon chemists had made many similar compounds which were called sulphonylureas. Patients with Type II diabetes mellitus can be treated with this group of drugs, which are known as the oral antidiabetic drugs because, as they are not proteins, they can be taken as tablets by mouth. They include glibenclamide and tolbutamide (Table 3.1, p. 44). These drugs act partly by increasing the release of insulin from the pancreatic beta-cells (so they can work only in patients in whom there are still some of these cells left in the pancreas) and partly by reducing the resistance of cells to the actions of insulin.

How do the oral antidiabetic drugs work?

To understand how the oral antidiabetic drugs work, consider the normal sequence of events leading to the secretion of insulin. Suppose the level of glucose in the blood rises. The cells of the pancreas are then able to produce plenty of their energy reservoir ATP, so the amount of ATP increases in the cells. As the ATP level increases, it closes a series of channels in the cell walls which normally allow potassium to pass through. There is a reciprocal movement of potassium and calcium across cell walls, so that as ATP reduces the movement of potassium, it increases the flow of calcium into the cells (Fig. 3.1). The secretion of all hormones is controlled by calcium, and the influx of calcium into pancreatic cells triggers the secretion of insulin. Conversely, as the level of blood glucose falls, ATP levels decrease and the potassium channels open so that calcium entry falls and insulin secretion is suppressed.

The oral antidiabetic drugs work directly on the potassium channels, causing them to close. This in turn allows calcium to flow into the cells and promote insulin secretion. These drugs also have a second action, which is to make cells increase the number of receptors for insulin in their walls. This makes the cells more sensitive to the normal amounts of insulin which are usually present in Type II patients.

Biguanides

There is a second type of oral antidiabetic drug which does not affect insulin release, but increases the sensitivity of cells to insulin and reduces the

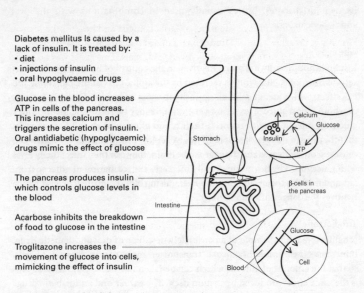

Diabetes mellitus is caused by a
lack of insulin. It is treated by:
• diet
• injections of insulin
• oral hypoglycaemic drugs

Glucose in the blood increases
ATP in cells of the pancreas.
This increases calcium and
triggers the secretion of insulin.
Oral antidiabetic (hypoglycaemic)
drugs mimic the effect of glucose

The pancreas produces insulin
which controls glucose levels in
the blood

Acarbose inhibits the breakdown
of food to glucose in the intestine

Troglitazone increases the
movement of glucose into cells,
mimicking the effect of insulin

Stomach

Intestine

Blood

Calcium
Glucose
Insulin
ATP

β-cells in
the pancreas

Glucose

Cell

Fig. 3.1 Drugs used in diabetes.

absorption of glucose from the intestine. This group of drugs—the
biguanides—includes metformin. We still do not know how these drugs modify
insulin sensitivity, but the overall effect is to increase the movement of glucose
into cells and to reduce the breakdown of muscle protein into glucose.

Because both types of oral antidiabetic drug decrease muscle and fat
breakdown, they may cause some patients to put on weight; careful control of
the diet is needed in these patients, since the development of obesity will make
their diabetic, insulin-resistant state, worse. The most worrying side-effect of
the sulphonylureas is that they can lower the level of glucose in the blood too
much, causing fainting and potential damage to the brain. The biguanides can
increase the amount of lactic acid in the body and should not be taken by
patients with liver or kidney damage.

Acarbose

α-glucosidase is one of the enzymes which helps to break down carbohydrates
in the food into smaller molecules of sugars, including glucose. Acarbose
inhibits this enzyme in the intestinal wall. By doing so, acarbose reduces the
amount of glucose produced from the food and, therefore, the amount of
glucose available for absorption into the bloodstream. It has a small effect on

its own in diabetes, but is usually used in combinations with the oral antidiabetic drugs.

Glucagon

Insulin is not the only hormone involved in the control of blood sugar levels. A second hormone, glucagon, is secreted by the alpha-cells of the pancreas, and has effects which are, in general, opposite to those of insulin. Diabetic patients in whom blood glucose levels are very variable may be recommended to carry glucagon injections with them. If their blood glucose levels fall to the extent that they are in danger of severe hypoglycaemia (low blood sugar) which can cause unconsciousness and damage to the brain, they can then inject themselves with glucagon. The hormone rapidly increases the formation of glucose from fats and from glycogen stored in the liver, raising blood glucose to a level which removes the danger of brain damage.

Troglitazone

Troglitazone is an example of a completely new type of oral antidiabetic drug. It increases the number of glucose 'transporter' molecules in the walls of cells, so that the amount of glucose which can be taken in by cells is increased. This is the same effect produced by insulin itself. The earlier oral antidiabetic drugs work best when the pancreas is not totally destroyed, leaving some insulin for them to release into the blood. Because troglitazone mimics insulin directly, it can work even in people who have no pancreatic cells left.

Complications of diabetes mellitus

The importance of treating diabetes correctly lies not only in the need to maintain the correct levels of glucose, but also in the fact that chronic diabetes is accompanied by degenerative changes in some tissues. For example, high levels of glucose in the blood for long periods changes the biochemistry of the lens of the eye (Fig. 3.2). This may result in clouding of the lens, i.e. a cataract.

The walls of blood vessels can become thickened in diabetic patients, reducing the movement of essential molecules from the blood into cells. Nerve cells may not function correctly, leading to changes in the sensitivity of patients to touch or temperature, and causing abnormal sensations such as 'pins and needles' in the skin. The retina of the eye may be damaged in a number of ways and blindness may occur unless the problem is treated correctly. Fatty substances are deposited on the thickened blood vessel walls, leading to atherosclerosis and an increased danger of heart disease and strokes. Most of these changes can be prevented or reduced by adequate and early treatment of the underlying diabetes and careful attention to the control of blood glucose levels.

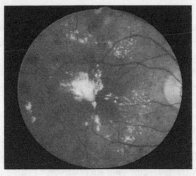

Fig. 3.2 Photographs of the retina in a patient with diabetes. The pale area is a region in which the cells of the retina have degenerated as a result of the diabetes, leading to partial irreversible blindness.

Over-secretion of insulin

The secretion of too much insulin by the pancreas is a very rare disorder, but may occur if there is a tumour of the beta-cells. The danger of patients becoming hypoglycaemic (too low a level of glucose in the blood) and suffering brain damage means that treatment is essential. The drug usually used, diazoxide, works at the same site as the oral antidiabetic drugs but with the opposite effect. In other words, it opens the special, ATP-sensitive potassium channels in the walls of the beta-cells. This reduces the inflow of calcium and slows the secretion of insulin.

Diabetes insipidus

There is a different and much rarer form of diabetes called 'diabetes insipidus'. The word 'diabetes' is still entirely appropriate because the most obvious symptom is a continuing loss of large amounts of water in the urine, resulting in severe thirst. The cause of diabetes insipidus is usually that the pituitary gland in the brain is unable to secrete antidiuretic hormone (ADH*). This hormone is important for reducing diuresis, that is, for reducing the loss of water into the urine. A lack of the hormone causes excessive water loss in the urine and severe thirst. Since this water loss has nothing to do with sugar, the urine definitely does not taste sweet, but rather 'insipid'.

---

* ADH is also called 'vasopressin' because it can cause contraction of blood vessels, leading to an increase in blood pressure.

Treatment

One way of treating diabetes insipidus is to replace the natural missing hormone, which can be given as an intramuscular injection. Another method is to use compounds which are very similar to ADH, such as lypressin or desmopressin and which the body does not break down as quickly as ADH itself. Although desmopressin can be taken as tablets, lypressin is taken in the more unusual form of a nasal spray. The protein drug can then be absorbed from the mucous membranes lining the nose without being broken down by the digestive enzymes in the stomach and intestine.

In a few cases of this rare disorder, the brain is producing ADH normally, but the kidney fails to respond, causing what is known as 'nephrogenic diabetes insipidus'. This is treated, somewhat surprisingly, by using diuretic drugs (*see* Chapter 5). Although these drugs normally increase the formation of urine, some of them have the opposite effect in patients with nephrogenic diabetes insipidus, although the reason is not understood.

Table 3.1 Oral antidiabetic drugs

Sulphonylureas	Biguanide
acetohexamide (USA)	metformin
chlorpropamide	
glibenclamide	**α-glucosidase inhibitor**
gliclazide	acarbose
glimepiride	
glipizide	**Glucose uptake enhancer**
gliquidone	troglitazone
tolbutamide	
tolazamide	**Drugs for diabetes insipidus**
	ADH (antidiuretic hormone, or vasopressin)
	desmopressin
	lypressin

Summary

- *Glucose sugar is an essential fuel for the body's cells. If the amount of glucose in the blood is too high or too low, the tissues cannot function correctly and coma and death may ensue.*
- *The level of glucose in blood is regulated by a protein hormone, insulin, produced by the pancreas.*
- *Type I diabetes mellitus ('juvenile' diabetes) occurs when the pancreas produces too little insulin. The symptoms include producing a large volume of urine and the presence of sugar in the urine.*
- *Type I diabetes is treated by injections of insulin or the oral antidiabetic drugs.*
- *Type II diabetes ('maturity-onset' diabetes) occurs when the tissues fail to respond to insulin in the blood. It is often associated with being overweight.*
- *Type II diabetes is treated by the oral antidiabetic drugs.*
- *Acarbose reduces the absorption of glucose from the intestine.*
- *Troglitazone increases the movement of glucose into cells.*
- *Diabetes insipidus is characterized by a large volume of urine but the sugar content is normal. It is due to a lack of antidiuretic hormone and is treated by drugs which act in the same way as the hormone.*

CHAPTER 4

Eating and digestion: ulcers, indigestion, diarrhoea, constipation, and vomiting

Until the early 1600s, people believed that 'digestion' involved simply the decomposition of food by the heat of the body. Johann van Helmont then showed that gastric juices could work even when taken out of the body and could even dissolve iron filings at room temperature.

On 6 June 1822 a 19-year-old Canadian, Alexis St Martin, received an accidental gunshot wound in the town of Michillimackinac, Michigan. An American army surgeon, William Beaumont* (1785–1853) was called from the nearby Fort Mackinac and, although he tended his patient as best he could, he reported that "The man will not live longer than 36 hours". He was wrong, and St Martin recovered gradually over the next two years with only one major reminder of his accident—a passageway that remained† between his skin and stomach. Beaumont took advantage of this and over several years he was able to add or remove materials from Alexis' stomach through this passage and make most of the earliest, scientifically meaningful studies of digestion. (St Martin, incidentally, later married, had 4 children and died at the age of 83 in 1886).

The gastrointestinal system

Eating can be one of the joys of life, and we perhaps underestimate the complex functions of the digestive system more than most of our organs. The digestive system breaks down the carbohydrates, fats, and proteins in food into their respective components of sugars, fatty acids, and amino acids. These can then be used to build new cells and repair damaged ones and supply the energy needed for cells to live.

---

* Beaumont never received any formal training in medicine but learned his trade through an apprenticeship.
† Such a passageway is called a fistula.

The stomach and intestine are dedicated to one purpose—the breakdown of food into a form which can be absorbed and used by the other tissues of the body to build, repair, and grow. Digestion begins in the mouth, where enzymes in the saliva start to break down starches and other molecules. The process continues in the stomach, where acid, produced by specialized 'parietal' cells in the stomach wall kill most bacteria and provide the conditions for a series of enzymes (see Chapter 1) to break down proteins into the amino acid building blocks of which they are made. After the partially digested food is pushed into the small intestine, a different set of enzymes set to work to complete the breakdown of proteins, and to begin the digestion of fats. Along the way, from the mouth to the anus, the products of digestion are absorbed across the intestinal wall into the bloodstream, for transport to the organs and tissues of the body.

This simple summary of the gastrointestinal system masks the enormous complexity involved. There is a large range of enzymes—proteins involved in breaking down the huge range of foodstuffs. The movement of food requires the co-ordinated activity of several different types of muscle cells in the walls of the intestines: food must be moved smoothly, at the correct rate to allow absorption and in the correct direction. The intestine also has elaborate systems for absorbing molecules across the wall of the intestine into the bloodstream, in which they can be transported to the various organs for use in repair and growth (Fig. 4.1). A system of this complexity is bound to have its share of medical problems.

Ulcers

An ulcer is an open sore in which the protective lining of the tissue has been broken. Ulcers can occur on the skin, tongue, or other tissue. Mouth ulcers (known as canker sores in the USA) are probably due to infection with some streptococcal bacteria. Cold sores are a form of ulcer caused by a Herpes virus. These oral ulcers are usually treated by a mildly antiseptic mouthwash together with an analgesic or local anaesthetic cream.

Peptic ulcers

A very common form of ulcer in the gut is the peptic ulcer, and at least one person in twenty is likely to have one at some time in their lives. The costs of treating ulcers accounts for around one tenth of the health budget in the UK.

Peptic ulcers were first described in about 1835 by Jean Cruveilhier, Professor of Anatomy and Pathology at the University of Paris. The term 'peptic' (from the Greek word *peptos*, meaning digested), simply indicates that the ulcer is surrounded by the digestive juices including acid and pepsin. These are

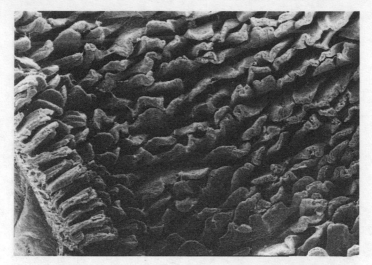

Fig. 4.1 A magnified view (about 1000 times) of the inner wall of the intestine, showing how the wall is folded to increase the surface area for the absorption of food. (Professor A Payne)

produced by the stomach, pepsin being one of the enzymes which breaks down proteins in the stomach into amino acids. Peptic ulcers are found in the stomach itself (Fig. 4.2), when they are sometimes called gastric ulcers, but may occur in the adjacent part of the small intestine—the duodenum—when they are called duodenal ulcers. Duodenal ulcers are more common than the gastric variety, largely because the stomach secretes a much more effective layer of mucus to protect itself against its own acid.

Peptic ulcers have long been thought to be produced by generalized stress, alcohol, eating spicy foods, and many other factors for which there is no convincing scientific evidence. Stress may be involved, particularly in situations in which the individual feels alone and isolated, with no one to share their problems, and in situations in which there appears to be no obvious solution to a problem. More recently, however, a particular type of bacterium has been shown to play a major role in peptic ulceration. It is called *Helicobacter pylori* and if eliminated with antibiotics many ulcers heal and do not recur (*see below*).

Whatever the cause, a major reason for the pain and discomfort of peptic ulcers is that the acid produced by the stomach irritates the exposed surfaces of the ulcer. This is why the pain from an ulcer is less in the morning (when there is no food at all in the stomach to cause acid secretion) and immediately after eating food, when the food absorbs the acid and stops it from reaching the ulcer.

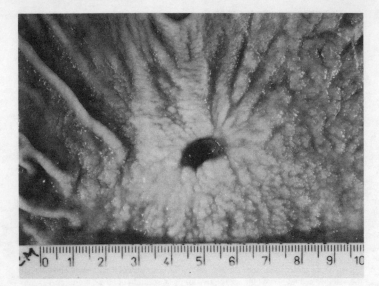

Fig. 4.2 A photograph of a stomach ulcer. The stomach has been cut open to reveal a large ulcer on the inner surface.

Treatment is aimed at reducing the amount of acid produced by the stomach, or protecting the ulcer against the effects of the acid.

Acid secretion

Acid is secreted by parietal cells, which produce their acid in response to several stimuli. Firstly, the presence of food in the stomach provokes the secretion of a hormone, gastrin, from cells in the stomach wall. Secondly, the act of eating (indeed, even the prospect of eating or the sight and smell of food) produces activity in parasympathetic nerves (*see* Chapter 1) which release acetylcholine as their transmitter. Both gastrin and acetylcholine can act on the parietal cells to secrete acid, but they can also act on a group of cells called paracrine cells which are found close to the parietal cells. Activation of the paracrine cells promotes the release of histamine which then stimulates the parietal cells to secrete acid (Fig. 4.3). This arrangement means that part of the acid secretion produced by acetylcholine or gastrin is mediated by histamine released from the paracrine cells. Drugs interfering with the actions of histamine are, therefore, more effective than those blocking either acetylcholine or gastrin. Histamine is also more powerful than acetylcholine or gastrin in stimulating the secretion of acid.

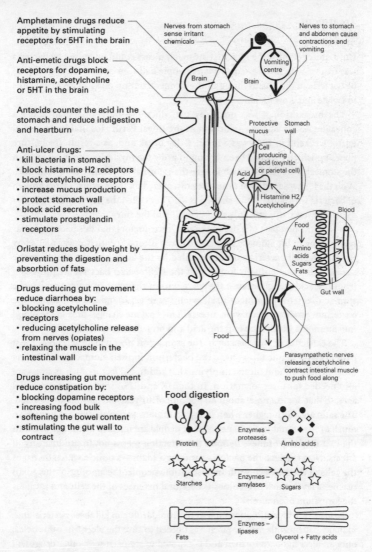

Amphetamine drugs reduce appetite by stimulating receptors for 5HT in the brain

Nerves from stomach sense irritant chemicals

Nerves to stomach and abdomen cause contractions and vomiting

Vomiting centre

Brain

Brain

Anti-emetic drugs block receptors for dopamine, histamine, acetylcholine or 5HT in the brain

Antacids counter the acid in the stomach and reduce indigestion and heartburn

Protective mucus   Stomach wall

Cell producing acid (oxynitic or parietal cell)

Acid

Anti-ulcer drugs:
• kill bacteria in stomach
• block histamine H2 receptors
• block acetylcholine receptors
• increase mucus production
• protect stomach wall
• block acid secretion
• stimulate prostaglandin receptors

Histamine H2
Acetylcholine

Blood

Food

Amino acids
Sugars
Fats

Orlistat reduces body weight by preventing the digestion and absorbtion of fats

Gut wall

Drugs reducing gut movement reduce diarrhoea by:
• blocking acetylcholine receptors
• reducing acetylcholine release from nerves (opiates)
• relaxing the muscle in the intestinal wall

Food

Parasympathetic nerves releasing acetylcholine contract intestinal muscle to push food along

Drugs increasing gut movement reduce constipation by:
• blocking dopamine receptors
• increasing food bulk
• softening the bowel content
• stimulating the gut wall to contract

Food digestion

Protein   Enzymes – proteases   Amino acids

Starches   Enzymes – amylases   Sugars

Fats   Enzymes – lipases   Glycerol + Fatty acids

Fig. 4.3 How drugs affect the stomach and intestine.

Treatment

Antibiotics

Until quite recently, the idea that stomach ulcers could be caused by bacteria was treated with intense scorn. Many people had seen cells which appeared to be bacteria in the mucus lining of the stomach but no one had ever been able to isolate and grow these.

The breakthrough was made by two doctors—Barry Marshall and his colleague Robin Warren—working at the Royal Perth Hospital in Australia. Easter weekend in 1983 was a long, 4-day break and, as a result, the culture plates on which they had been trying to grow the mysterious cells taken from the stomach were left for much longer than normal before they were examined. With the longer incubation time, they discovered on their return a large growth of bacteria with spiral, helix-shaped cells. They called the new bug *Helicobacter pylori*. However, this was only the beginning of the story.

It took the best part of a decade to convince doctors that this bacterium was really living in the stomach and could cause ulcers. Scepticism was fuelled by the fact that all bacteria should be killed by the large amount of acid in the stomach. It was eventually found that the *Helicobacter* bacteria are protected from the acid partly because they live within the layer of mucus which the stomach secretes to protect itself against the acid, and partly because the bacterium produces an enzyme, urease. This enzyme changes urea in the blood into ammonia which mops up the acid and protects the bacteria.

The existence of *Helicobacter* in the stomach is now widely accepted. Most patients with peptic ulcers have the bacterium in their stomach, as do many other people without ulcers, implying that additional factors such as stress are also needed for ulcer formation. In the UK and USA infection rates parallel ages, so that, for example, about 40 per cent of 40-year-old persons are infected. The rates are much higher when living conditions and sanitation are poorer: in much of Africa and India 80 per cent of people are infected by the age of 20. In the vast majority of these people, the infection seems not to produce any ill effects. Nevertheless, the bacteria produce a toxin—a poison which damages the cells of the stomach wall. In susceptible people, the amount of this toxin reaches a level which overcomes the natural defences of the cells and initiates the formation of an ulcer.

Treatment with antibiotics such as metronidazole can kill these bacteria and, in many patients this may be all that is needed to cure the ulcer.* In some cases, once an ulcer has been formed and is exposed to stomach acid, other drugs will be needed to reduce acid formation or protect the stomach wall, until the

* *Helicobacter* also seem to be associated with a rare form of stomach cancer called mucosa associated lymphoid tissue lymphoma. This cancer can be treated with antibiotics which kill *Helicobacter pylori*.

stomach lining is healed. Nevertheless, the realization that antibiotics can effectively cure stomach ulcers may be one of the most significant medical breakthroughs this century, and represents a triumph of scientific detective work against conservative scepticism.

Helicobacter, cancer, and other problems

Since the discovery of the relationship between *Helicobacter* and ulcers, Martin Glaser and his colleagues at Vanderbilt University, USA, have found a strong association between the bacterium and stomach cancer. From a sample of almost 6000 men, Glaser showed that those who developed stomach cancer were six times more likely to have infection by *Helicobacter*.

Even more strangely, there is a correlation between the existence of *Helicobacter* in people and the occurrence of phenomena as different as cot deaths in babies and heart disease in adults. It was Barry Marshall again who first noted that an unusually high proportion of cot death babies were infected by *Helicobacter*. Perhaps the toxins produced by these bacteria have a hand in far more illnesses than just ulcers.

H2 antihistamines

An alternative approach to reducing acid secretion is to block the effects of the histamine released by the paracrine cells (Fig. 4.3). The drugs available include cimetidine and ranitidine, which are simple antagonists, competing with histamine for the same site on the receptor molecule in the cell walls. Although histamine produces a variety of effects throughout the body, including changes of blood pressure (*see* Chapter 15) and contraction of the airways (*see* Chapter 2), none of the antihistamine drugs which prevented those effects was able to prevent acid secretion in the stomach. The reason for this difference was a mystery until the work of Sir James Black and his team, then working at the Smith Kline French Research Institute at Welwyn, England. This team found that histamine was acting on a different type of receptor in the stomach from those found elsewhere in the body. The histamine receptors in the blood vessels and airways were called H1 receptors. The histamine receptors in the stomach were labelled H2 receptors. The important result of this difference is that the drugs which have been developed to suppress acid secretion have no effect on blood pressure or breathing.

Side-effects of H2 receptor antagonists are very rare, although cimetidine can interact with the receptors for the sex hormones. One result of this is that, if high doses of cimetidine are used, men become impotent and may show enlargement of their breasts, a condition known as 'gynaecomastia'. Both these effects should disappear when the drug is stopped and treatment to cure an ulcer usually takes only about six weeks.

Pump inhibitors

A different type of drug inhibits the mechanism by which the acid is produced in the stomach. The walls of the parietal cells contain an enzyme which pumps acid (in the form of hydrogen ions or protons, H^+) into the stomach. This proton pump can be inhibited by drugs such as omeprazole, thereby stopping the secretion of acid.

Anticholinergic drugs

Since acetylcholine is partly responsible for promoting the secretion of histamine and acid from the stomach wall, an alternative approach is to use drugs which block the receptors for acetylcholine on the parietal and paracrine cells. One such drug is pirenzepine, which does not produce the array of side-effects—dry mouth, blurred vision, and constipation, which can be produced by other acetylcholine antagonists (*see* Chapter 1). The reason is that the receptors for acetylcholine in the stomach are different from those in the mouth, eye, and intestine. The stomach receptors are M1 muscarinic receptors, whereas most other effects of acetylcholine involve M2 and M3 muscarinic receptors. Pirenzepine is, therefore, quite selective in its actions on the stomach. Although available until recently, pirenzepine has now been withdrawn, largely because the use of antibiotics and histamine antagonists is much more effective.

One of the dangers with any drug which reduces the formation of acid in the stomach is that, in addition to beginning the process of digestion, acid is an important protective mechanism. The acid normally kills most of the bacteria taken in with food, so if the stomach contains less acid, there is a greater possibility of bacteria surviving to cause infections. There is also a possibility that if stomach acid is suppressed for a long time, the growth of stomach cancer may be encouraged.

Protective drugs

The stomach wall is normally protected against damage by its own acid by a layer of mucus—a gel-like material which lines the stomach wall. Cells in the stomach wall (different from those which secrete acid) secrete bicarbonate into this layer so that, as acid diffuses into it from the stomach contents, it will be neutralized before it comes into contact with the stomach wall.

Sucralfate

Sucralfate is a drug which consists of a complex between aluminium hydroxide and sucrose. The molecules of sucralfate polymerize (i.e. combine to form much larger molecules) in the acid medium of the stomach. The result is a gel which sticks tightly to the exposed surfaces of ulcers, enhancing the effect of natural mucus and protecting the ulcer until it heals. Sucralfate also increases the secretion of the stomach's natural mucus.

Carbenoxolone

During the 1940s it was noticed that the Dutch developed very few ulcers, a situation which might be related to their eating large amounts of liquorice. A scientific study of liquorice then confirmed that this was the case. Liquorice contains many chemicals, one of which is glycyrrhizinic acid, and from it the drug carbenoxolone was produced by chemists. Carbenoxolone increases the secretion of mucus in the stomach and also causes it to become thicker and more sticky, so that it offers an ulcer more protection against acid. Carbenoxolone used alone is not usually enough to allow ulcers to heal fully but it can be used in combination with other anti-ulcer drugs.

Bismuth

Bismuth salts act in a similar way to sucralfate, but also have some antibiotic activity and increase the secretion of mucus and bicarbonate. One of these drugs, best known by its trade-name De Nol,* is proving exceptionally good at treating peptic ulcers, and prevents a recurrence of ulcers more effectively than many other treatments. Unfortunately there is a risk of bismuth being absorbed in the body where it can damage the brain, so the use of bismuth compounds is generally discouraged.

Misoprostol

Misoprostol has both of the effects described so far—it reduces acid secretion *and* it increases the production of protective mucus. Normally, the production of acid and mucus is regulated by a series of chemicals called prostaglandins. Some of these promote the formation and secretion of mucus, and restrict the secretion of acid. Misoprostol is an agonist at the receptors for prostaglandins and therefore shares these effects, reducing acid and increasing mucus secretion and helping ulcers to heal.

Misoprostol is particularly useful in people who have to take large doses of aspirin and similar anti-inflammatory drugs for the relief of arthritis (*see* Chapters 6 and 20). These drugs block the body's manufacture of prostaglandins, so that the stomach secretes more acid and less mucus. These effects explain why aspirin irritates the stomach and can induce the formation of ulcers (*see* Chapter 6). By substituting for the missing prostaglandins, misoprostol helps to prevent the irritation and ulceration. The main side-effect of misoprostol is diarrhoea, which occurs because activation of prostaglandin receptors increases the movements of the bowel.

* Tripotassium dicitratobismuthate.

The drug cannot be used in pregnant women because it can produce abortion.

Antacids

Several drugs neutralize the acid present in the stomach and help the ulcerated stomach wall to heal. These compounds, the antacids, include sodium bicarbonate, calcium carbonate, magnesium hydroxide, magnesium carbonate, magnesium trisilicate, and aluminium hydroxide, which can be given by doctors on prescription. These drugs are discussed in more detail in the section on indigestion.

Drugs of the future

Two of the hormones which stimulate acid secretion in the stomach are cholecystokinin (CCK) and gastrin. Several companies are trying to make new drugs to block the receptors for these hormones, in the belief that this will be an alternative way to treat peptic ulcers. They should work in cases where these hormones are acting in addition to acetylcholine and histamine to increase acid production. Some disorders are known in which the primary fault is an increase in the body's production of CCK or gastrin (such as the Zollinger-Ellison syndrome caused by a tumour or the gastin-producing cells in the stomach), leading to ulcers which cannot be treated easily by the antihistamine drugs.

Indigestion, heartburn, dyspepsia, colic, and gripes

If the stomach secretes too much acid, it can give rise to the pain known as indigestion or heartburn. The medical term for indigestion—dyspepsia*—reflects the cause as an abnormal secretion of acid. Heartburn occurs when a little of the acid in the stomach is pushed into the base of the oesophagus (the gullet, taking food from the mouth into the stomach). As this area is situated just below the heart, the burning pain produced often seems to come from the heart. If the stomach acid frequently comes into contact with the oesophagus, it can cause irritation and inflammation.[†] By neutralizing the acid, the antacid drugs such as sodium bicarbonate, calcium carbonate, magnesium hydroxide, magnesium carbonate, magnesium trisilicate, and aluminium hydroxide, reduce the pain and discomfort of heartburn.

There is not much to choose between the different antacid preparations. Magnesium compounds tend to cause increased intestinal movements leading to diarrhoea, partly because magnesium salts remain in the gut and increase

---

* The word 'dyspepsia' comes from the Greek *dus-* meaning bad, and *peptos*, meaning digested.
[†] A condition known as reflux oesophagitis.

the bulk being moved along the intestine, and partly because magnesium increases the secretion of the hormone CCK, which increases activity of the intestine. Aluminium compounds, on the other hand, tend to relax the intestine, causing slower movements and constipation. If preparations contain a combination of magnesium and aluminium, their effects tend to cancel out, leaving intestinal activity largely unchanged.

Despite the ease with which these various indigestion treatments are available from pharmacies, they must be used only when necessary, and not regularly as a habit. Firstly, the presence of alkaline substances in the stomach increases the secretion of acid, so that the stomach may then become even more acidic than usual after the alkaline antacid has disappeared. Repeated use of antacids, therefore, could paradoxically make the dyspepsia worse. The fluctuations of gastric acidity also seem to allow the growth of some bacteria which would be killed by the normally continuous acidity of the stomach.

Secondly, reducing the acidity in the stomach can reduce the absorption of iron, aspirin, and some vitamins and antibiotics.

Thirdly, the absorption of antacid molecules will reduce the acidity of the urine as it is formed in the kidney. This favours the formation of kidney stones.

Antacids should never be used by anyone with kidney problems, or on renal dialysis, as the absorption of ions from the antacid can disturb the delicate balance of ions in the blood which is normally controlled by healthy kidneys but is not always controlled in kidney disease.

Finally, some antacid preparations contain bismuth salts. As noted earlier, these are not generally recommended because if any of the bismuth is absorbed into the blood, it can cause damage to the nervous system. There has also been concern among doctors and scientists that repeated use of aluminium salts could lead to the accumulation of aluminium in the brain, a situation which may lead to Alzheimer's disease. This theory is still unproven.

Colic

Feelings of discomfort can arise from the build up of gas in the stomach, the discomfort and pain being called colic, or gripe. The noisy results of colic in a small child will be familiar to most mothers. The problem is helped, in children or adults, by giving dimethicone or simethicone. This is an anti-foaming agent which reduces the surface tension of gas bubbles, allowing them to coalesce and to be expelled continually in small quantities, without the build up of gas which causes the painful colic and the sudden eruption of wind.

Food poisoning

Food poisoning can be caused by many different types of bacteria (*see* Chapter 17), the most common being *Escherichia coli* (*e. Coli*), *Campylobacter, Salmonella,*

Shigella, and *Listeria*. It can also be caused by some viruses. Most of the estimated one million cases in the UK and four million in the USA each year are not serious enough to need medical attention. More severe cases, needing hospital admission in 1998, were usually due to *Campylobacter* (58 059 cases in the UK), with fewer cases due to *Salmonella* (23 420), *E. coli* (887), or viruses (1964).

There are dozens of different strains of these organisms, only some of which cause food poisoning, and some cause other diseases (*see* Chapter 17). Bacteria enter the stomach in food which has not been properly handled, stored, or cooked. Good food hygiene is important, and thorough cooking should kill these bacteria. Symptoms of food poisoning—abdominal pain and cramps, nausea, vomiting, and diarrhoea, are due to the bacteria secreting chemical poisons (toxins) which irritate the nerve endings in the intestine wall. They also reduce the absorption of water from the intestine, so that very soft faeces are produced (diarrhoea). Traveller's diarrhoea is usually caused by *E. coli* picked up in poorly cooked or reheated food.

The more severe cases of food poisoning occur when the number of bacteria eaten is high, and some burrow into the walls of the intestine, causing intense pain and inflammation. Unless treated, these cases can be fatal. Although the problem of resistance to drugs is growing, most cases can be treated easily with antibiotics (*see* Chapter 17).

Because so many bacteria are becoming resistant to antibiotics, alternative strategies to deal with food poisoning are being studied. One approach being pursued by Rob Aitken and his team at Glasgow University is to make vaccines. The toxins produced by some bacteria consist of molecules large enough to stimulate the immune system, so antibodies can be produced against them (*see* Chapter 2). These antibodies can then be used as a vaccine which, when injected into people suffering from food poisoning, combine with the toxins and inactivate them.

Drugs altering intestinal movements

Occasional bouts of diarrhoea or constipation occur in most people and are often due to slight changes in the diet, or minor instances of food poisoning.

Diarrhoea

The safest method of reducing some types of minor, non-infective diarrhoea is to increase the bulk of the food contents in the gut, preferably with materials which will absorb some of the excess fluid. This can be achieved either by eating more fibre in the diet, or by taking prescribed doses of bran, methylcellulose, ispaghula husk, or sterculia fibre.

A very different method of control is to use drugs such as opiates. These include morphine (*see* Chapter 6), codeine, diphenoxylate, and loperamide.

These drugs all reduce the release of acetylcholine from parasympathetic nerves and thereby block the stimulant effect of these nerves on movements of the intestine.

Irritable bowel syndrome (IBS)

In some people the intestine changes activity with no apparent cause or explanation. These changes may be accompanied by considerable abdominal discomfort or pain, and are referred to as the 'irritable bowel syndrome'. The intestinal activity may sometimes increase, causing diarrhoea, and sometimes decrease causing constipation. The cause or causes are not fully understood and are controversial, though some cases are believed to be due to 'food intolerance': eating foods which are not well tolerated by some individuals even though most people find them harmless. These cases of IBS can, therefore, be controlled by suitable changes to the diet.

Unfortunately drug treatments for IBS are limited because it is such an unpredictable disorder. The movements of the intestine are regulated by acetylcholine, released from parasympathetic nerves (see Chapter 1), which increases activity, and by norepinephrine, released from sympathetic nerves, which decreases activity.

One approach to treating diarrhoeal phases of IBS is to use drugs which block the receptors for acetylcholine. These include atropine, hyoscine, dicyclomine, poldine, and propantheline. Since all these drugs block muscarinic receptors for acetylcholine, they will all produce side-effects due to blocking receptors in organs other than the gut. Patients may experience reduced salivation and dry mouth, together with blurred vision and difficulty in adjusting their focus to close objects (see Chapter 1).

Another anticholinergic drug is darifenacin. It has a more selective effect on the muscle cells of the intestine with much less effect on the stomach or heart, because it only blocks a type of muscarinic acetylcholine receptor known as M3. It should have fewer side-effects than the other drugs available at present. Since M3 receptors are involved in contractions of the bladder produced by acetylcholine, darifenacin is also useful to reduce incontinence and to reduce the frequency of urination in patients in whom the bladder is overactive.

There are also several drugs which act directly on the muscles of the intestinal wall to cause relaxation, slowing the transport of food and reducing the diarrhoea. These include alverine and mebeverine. Peppermint oil has a similar effect, and may be used in mild cases.

Intestinal stimulants

In some cases, it may be desirable to increase the movement of food or drugs through the gut. For example, after surgical operations the gut may be very sluggish for several days, and may require a little prompting to improve the transport and absorption of food. The intestine may also be rather inactive in diabetes.

Speeding up the movement of food from the stomach into the duodenum will reduce the possibility of stomach contents and acid coming into contact with the oesophagus. Gastric stimulants are, therefore, useful in the treatment of heartburn and inflammation of the oesophagus. They are also useful in increasing the movement out of the stomach of drugs which irritate the stomach wall and cause bleeding or vomiting (such as some of the anticancer drugs). The drugs used for this purpose are metoclopramide, domperidone, and cisapride.

Metoclopramide and domperidone both block receptors for the neuro-transmitter dopamine. Normally dopamine is released by nerve cells in the wall of the stomach and duodenum, where it inhibits movement of the intestine. By blocking the receptors, metoclopramide and domperidone increase the movements of the stomach and duodenum. Metoclopramide also increases the release of acetylcholine from the parasympathetic nerves and, since the normal action of acetylcholine is to stimulate intestinal muscle contractions, gut movements are increased. Cisapride works entirely by this last action—increasing acetylcholine release to mimic the bowel stimulant effects of parasympathetic nerves.

A new word was introduced recently into English—undigestion. This simply refers to a lack of movement of food in the stomach and small intestine and responds to treatment with domperidone.

Laxatives

Drugs which are used specifically to reduce constipation are known as laxatives or cathartics. Many laxative preparations are easily available from pharmacies, and as a group they are undoubtedly used by many people when it is quite unnecessary to do so. It is not unusual, for example, for a person to have two or three days without evacuating their bowels, yet many people would consider themselves constipated in this situation and resort to drugs quite unnecessarily.

Laxatives fall into three categories. Firstly, there are materials which simply increase the bulk volume of the gut contents, so that the intestinal muscles have more solid matter to push along. These include bran, methylcellulose, ispaghula, and sterculia fibre. There are also several substances which are not absorbed from the gut and which cause fluid to be retained in the lumen of the gut. They are known as 'osmotic laxatives'* and include magnesium hydroxide, other magnesium salts, and sugars such as lactulose and lactitol. Their overall effect is the same as that of the bran-like compounds, increasing the volume of intestinal contents while keeping them soft.

* See footnote on p. 37.

Secondly, there are compounds which soften and lubricate the gut contents, easing their passage along the intestine. These include liquid paraffin, arachis oil, and docusate sodium.

Finally, there are drugs known as 'stimulant' laxatives because they act on the muscular walls of the intestine to increase the movement of food along it. The oldest of these, having been used for many centuries, are Senna extracts prepared from the dried leaves or seed pods of Senna plants, or Cascara extracts prepared from the bark of the buckthorn tree. The active chemicals* in these extracts act on the last part of the large bowel, the colon, to increase its movements and facilitate evacuation. They do this by activating the nerve cells which lie in the wall of the bowel and which control the speed and frequency of contractions.

Bisacodyl is a chemical which was produced in an attempt to find a safer replacement for the laxative phenolphthalein. Both bisacodyl and a related drug, oxyphenisatin, also activate nerve cells in the colon to increase its movements and aid evacuation.

Changes in bowel habits

Any person who notices a change in their bowel habits lasting more than a few days should see their doctor. Prolonged constipation, for example, must not be treated simply by taking laxative drugs for weeks or months. A change of bowel habit may signal a serious underlying disorder such as cancer and, since cancer of the colon is becoming ever more frequent in developed societies, rapid diagnosis and treatment are essential.

Haemorrhoids

Also known as 'piles', haemorrhoids are engorged and swollen veins around the anus. They are often the result of pressure around the anus, and can occur during pregnancy or in a sedentary occupation. The usual treatment is to apply creams or ointments which make the passage of the faeces past the affected areas easier, and less painful. Some of these preparations also contain a local anaesthetic to reduce the pain in more severe cases and many contain a steroid such as hydrocortisone or prednisolone (*see* Chapter 19) to reduce inflammation. In some cases, however, haemorrhoids need to be injected with phenol to harden the skin and make them less sensitive, or removed surgically.

Control of feeding

Obesity is a growing problem in affluent countries. In the UK in 1994, 58 per cent of men and 49 per cent of women weighed more than the ideal, while

* Chemically, they are derivatives of 1,8-dihydroxyanthraquinone, also known as Danthron.

almost 1 in 5 Americans are more than 20 per cent over their recommended weight. Being overweight increases the chance of developing diabetes, high blood pressure, and heart disease. Obesity is partly a result of excessive eating and of a high-carbohydrate, high-fat diet, but in many people it is also partly the result of abnormal chemistry in the brain.

Feeding is controlled by a region of the brain called the hypothalamus and this in turn responds to the amount of a protein called leptin in the blood. The brain seems to modify metabolism and food intake so that the amount of leptin in the blood is maintained at a constant level. Leptin is secreted by cells in the fat tissue of the body: as the amount of fat increases, the amount of leptin produced will increase and this increases body metabolism so that some of the fat is used up. Leptin also acts on the hypothalamus to reduce appetite and the amount of food eaten.

Conversely, as the amount of fat in the body falls, the level of leptin also falls. Body metabolism is then reduced and food intake increased so that fat stores are restored. In obese people it appears that something has gone wrong with this control mechanism so that the leptin is no longer able to control the body weight, perhaps because the brain is no longer sensitive to it.

Anti-obesity drugs

Drugs which reduce feeding are known as appetite suppressants. The simplest drugs in this category are those which increase the bulk of material in the stomach, generating a feeling of 'fullness' which stops further eating. These drugs include methylcellulose.

Drugs may also work directly on the brain to suppress appetite. The first drugs to be used clinically were amphetamines, such as dexamphetamine, which worked by increasing the amounts of the neurotransmitters norepinephrine and 5HT* produced by cells in the brain. The hypothalamus controls food intake by balancing the activities of these and the amphetamines shift the balance between them in the direction which reduces feeding. The amphetamines are no longer used for this purpose because of their tendency to stimulate the brain and cause addiction. Related drugs used more recently were fenfluramine and dexfenfluramine, but both have now been withdrawn because they disturbed the functioning of the valves in the heart which might lead to heart failure after several years of use.

The main drug recommended for obesity in the UK is phentermine, which stimulates the release of norepinephrine and seems able to reduce appetite without producing addiction. Combinations of phentermine and fenfluramine are still obtainable illegally and are known as Phen/Fen drugs.

* 5-hydroxytryptamine.

Orlistat

This drug has been introduced only very recently. In the intestine fatty substances (lipids) are broken down by enzymes called lipases into smaller molecules which can then be absorbed across the intestine wall. Orlistat inhibits the activity of these enzymes, reducing the breakdown of fat and, therefore, its absorption. The result is a reduced caloric intake, especially of fats, leading to a gradual loss of weight.

The main problem with the drug is that some vitamins are dissolved in fat, so that a reduction of fat absorption could lead to a deficiency of fat-soluble vitamins unless a supplement is taken (*see* Chapter 22). Other side-effects include the production of soft, fatty stools, flatus (wind), and incontinence.

Drugs of the future

One of the brain transmitters involved in the regulation of feeding is known as neuropeptide Y (NPY). Leptin, for example, reduces the formation of NPY in the brain. Several pharmaceutical companies are hoping to develop drugs which can block the receptors for NPY in order to regulate feeding and, therefore, body weight.

Cholecystokinin in the brain is also involved in the control of feeding, and drugs are being developed which can activate CCK receptors to reduce appetite and turn off feeding. Finally, there is a type of beta-receptor for epinephrine— the beta-3 receptor, which exists on fat cells. The activation of these receptors increases the breakdown of the fat so that it can be used as a fuel or changed into glucose for use as fuel. Drugs which stimulate these receptors without affecting beta-receptors on other cells are showing promise as anti-obesity drugs.

Nausea and vomiting

Nausea, the unpleasant feeling which often precedes vomiting, and vomiting itself (emesis) are common symptoms of both disease and side-effects of drugs. They are a protective mechanism which has probably evolved to remove foreign chemicals as soon as possible after they enter the body. They are also often associated with situations such as early pregnancy and travelling (motion sickness). Vomiting is a reflex triggered by a combination of factors, usually involving receptors for several chemicals such as dopamine, 5HT and peptides in the stomach and intestine, together with activation of similar receptors in the brain. Vomiting is controlled by a region of brain called the vomiting centre. When this senses the presence of unusual chemicals in the blood (or large amounts of substances such as oestrogen during early pregnancy) it triggers the co-ordinated contraction of the stomach and abdominal muscles which we call vomiting.

Anti-emetic drugs

Several drugs reduce vomiting by blocking the receptors for dopamine. These drugs include metoclopramide and a group of phenothiazines (Table 4.1, p. 67). The main problem with these drugs is that they also block dopamine receptors in other parts of the brain. This can cause abnormal involuntary muscle movements and spasms which sometimes resemble the symptoms of Parkinson's disease (*see* Chapter 9). Domperidone blocks the dopamine receptors in the gut but does not pass into the brain. It is less effective than the above drugs but does not produce parkinsonian symptoms.

There are also several antihistamine and anticholinergic drugs available (Table 4.1) which reduce nausea and vomiting by blocking histamine and acetylcholine receptors in the brain's vomiting centre.

Anticancer drug and radiation-induced vomiting

Treatment with anticancer drugs and radiation therapy often causes nausea and vomiting which can be very difficult to control with single drugs. Patients are often prescribed a combination of drugs such as metoclopramide, anti-histamines, and dopamine antagonists. However, several drugs are much more effective against anticancer drug vomiting. They include drugs which block a special type of receptor for 5HT—the 5HT3 receptors. These drugs, such as ondansetron, block 5HT3 receptors near the vomiting centre and interrupt the vomiting reflex. They also reduce the activation of 5HT receptors by anticancer drugs in the gut.

Nabilone

Another drug with great promise is nabilone. It was developed after reports from women in the 1960s that smoking marijuana during pregnancy reduced their morning sickness. Nabilone was made from one of the chemicals in marijuana and has proved to be one of the best drugs for suppressing vomiting induced by anticancer drugs. It must be used under supervision as it may cause drowsiness as well as visual hallucinations, changes of mood, confusion, and poor concentration if the dose used is high—these are some of the effects obtained with marijuana (*see* Chapter 24).

Motion sickness

The idea that drugs might be able to prevent the sickness associated with travelling was born in 1947. Antihistamines were known to reduce the itching caused by allergies in some people and one of them, diphenhydramine, was given to a female patient in early 1947 by Leslie Gay at the Johns Hopkins University in Baltimore. The patient had suffered for many years from travel sickness which caused her to feel ill when travelling on buses, but while taking the antihistamine she found this was no longer the case. The drug was tested on several other patients with motion sickness with a similar beneficial result. A larger trial followed using soldiers on a troop ship, with the result that 4 per cent of those receiving diphenhydramine felt ill, whereas 25 per cent of those receiving a dummy placebo tablet were sick. The drug was marketed as Dramamine* and has remained popular as a travel remedy ever since.

Parts of the brain concerned with movement and position of the body in space (the vestibular areas) monitor the correspondence between the appearance of the world seen through the eyes and the sense of body position detected by receptors in the ear, skin, muscles, and joints. If we are standing on a boat, for example, the eyes signal that the floor is flat and we are standing firmly on it. The vestibular nerves and those from the muscles and joints, however, may be signalling that the body is moving from side to side or backwards and forwards as the ship rolls. This confusion of information can trigger feelings of nausea and vomiting in some people. One of the most effective treatments for the condition is to lie down with the eyes closed, because the brain no longer receives part of the conflicting information from the eyes.

The messages between nerve cells in these parts of the brain involve the transmitters acetylcholine and histamine, and motion sickness is best stopped by drugs which block receptors for these in the brain. Hyoscine, an acetylcholine antagonist, is one of the most effective, but its blockade of muscarinic receptors (*see* Chapter 1) causes a dry mouth, blurred vision, and constipation if used repeatedly.

Several antihistamines are also available to treat motion sickness, although they also affect receptors for acetylcholine. They include cyclizine, cinnarizine, promethazine, and dimenhydrinate; the latter two can produce sedation and sleep in some people. This is because there are some nerve cells which use histamine or acetylcholine as their transmitter in an area called the reticular formation which is responsible for keeping us awake.

Menière's disease

The middle portion of the ear apparatus contains three canals organized at right angles to each other. These are also part of the vestibular apparatus which feed information to the brain about their position in space. If there is a middle ear infection the signals from these canals become confused, causing dizziness (vertigo), nausea, and vomiting. These can be controlled to some extent by the

---

* The active ingredient is a combination of diphenhydramine and 8-chloroethyltheophylline, called dimenhydrinate.

anticholinergic and antihistamine drugs. In a disease called Menière's disease, named after Prosper Menière, who first described the symptoms and cause in 1861, the pressure of fluid in the canals increases and again disrupts the nerve signals from the position–sensitive cells, causing dizziness, nausea, and vomiting. The increased fluid pressure in other parts of the middle ear cause hearing loss.

These conditions can usually be helped by the antihistamine drugs, but Menière's disease also needs treatment to reduce the pressure of fluid, either by surgery or by using diuretic drugs (*see* Chapter 5) which can reduce the amount of fluid produced.

Morning sickness

The high levels of oestrogens in the blood during early pregnancy stimulate the vomiting centre and cause 'morning sickness'. This does not need treatment unless very severe. Doctors avoid prescribing any drugs during pregnancy if at all possible, in case they should cause damage to the development of the unborn baby. If absolutely necessary to reduce nausea and vomiting, antihistamine or phenothiazine drugs may be used for short periods of time.

Table 4.1 Eating and digestion.

Antacids for indigestion	Anti-ulcer drugs	Anti-diarrhoeal drugs	Gut motility stimulants	Anti-emetics
aluminium hydroxide	**Antacids**	atropine	metoclopramide	**Antihistamines**
calcium carbonate	aluminium hydroxide	alverine	domperidone	buclizine
hydrotalcite*	calcium carbonate	codeine	cisapride	cinnarizine
magnesium carbonate	magnesium carbonate	darifenacin†		cyclizine
magnesium hydroxide	magnesium hydroxide	dicyclomine		dimenhydrinate
magnesium trisilicate	magnesium trisilicate	dicycloverine		meclozine
sodium bicarbonate	sodium bicarbonate	diphenoxylate		promethazine
		hyoscine		propiomazine (USA)
	Histamine H2 antagonists	loperamide		thiethylperazine (USA)
	cimetidine	mebeverine		trimethobenzamide (USA)
	famotidine	morphine		
	nizatidine	poldine		**Phenothiazines**
	ranitidine	propantheline		chlorpromazine
				perphenazine
	Proton pump inhibitors			prochlorperazine
	lansoprazole			trifluoperazine
	omeprazole			
	pantoprazole			**5HT3 antagonists**
	rabeprazole			granisetron
				ondansetron
	Prostaglandin receptor agonist			tropisetron
	misoprostol			
				Miscellaneous
				betahistine
				domperidone
				hyoscine
				metoclopramide
				nabilone

* This is a compound of aluminium hydroxide and magnesium carbonate.
† Currently undergoing clinical trials and should be available in 2000.

Summary

- *Ulcers in the stomach (gastric ulcers) or intestine (duodenal ulcers) are sometimes known as peptic ulcers. The pain associated with them arises from the action of acid on a damaged group of cells.*
- *Peptic ulcers are often due to infection by the bacterium* Helicobacter pylori. *Ulcers can often be treated by killing the bacteria with antibiotics.*
- *Other drugs which reduce acid secretion also help to cure an ulcer. These include drugs which block H2 receptors for histamine, acetylcholine receptors, or the acid pump enzyme in the stomach.*
- *Drugs such as sucralfate and carbenoxolone increase the amount or effectiveness of the protective layer of mucus lining the stomach wall.*
- *Misoprostol activates receptors for the prostaglandin hormones, which reduce acid secretion and increase mucus formation.*
- *Antacids nullify the presence of acid and reduce the pain caused by excess acid in indigestion and heartburn.*
- *Diarrhoea can be controlled by fibres which increase the bulk of the intestinal contents, or by opiate-like drugs which slow the movements of the intestine.*
- *Irritable bowel syndrome is difficult to treat because it involves periods of constipation and periods of diarrhoea. It is often treated with drugs which slow the movements of the gut such as dicyclomine (an acetylcholine antagonist) and mebeverine (which relaxes the intestinal muscles).*
- *Metoclopramide increases the movements of the stomach and intestine when this is reduced after operations.*
- *Laxatives increase the bulk of food or lubricate movement along the intestine, but include drugs such as bisacodyl which stimulates bowel movement.*
- *Appetite and feeding can be suppressed by amphetamine-like drugs and drugs which inhibit 5HT removal from receptors. Orlistat reduces the absorption of fats from the intestine resulting in weight loss in obese people.*
- *Drugs which block acetylcholine or histamine receptors suppress nausea and vomiting due to pregnancy and travelling.*
- *Antagonists at 5HT3 receptors, or drugs derived from cannabis, reduce the vomiting caused by drugs used in the treatment of cancer.*

CHAPTER 5

The kidney

The two kidneys are mainly excretory organs. Unwanted chemicals in the body, coming either from the food we eat or produced by the body itself, are passed out in the urine. It is the function of the kidneys to make urine.

How is urine produced?

After blood has entered the kidneys, it passes through a dense network of tiny blood vessels (capillaries). The pressure of the blood in these capillaries is sufficient to force some of the fluid from the blood through the thin capillary walls. These walls act rather like a sieve and the blood is filtered through them so that only water, with small molecules dissolved in it, can normally pass through. This filtered fluid is collected into one end of a long, coiled tube called a nephron, or kidney tubule (Fig. 5.1). These are so thin that there are about a million of them in each of our two kidneys. The filtered fluid in the tubule contains ions such as sodium, potassium, calcium, chloride, and bicarbonate, small molecules such as sugars and amino acids, some of the body's waste products, such as uric acid, and unwanted chemicals from the diet. But this is only the beginning of the formation of urine.

So much water and salts (ions) are filtered that, if the first filtrate were excreted as urine, we should rapidly die from dehydration unless we drank gallons of salty water every day. The amount of urine formed in the kidney is about 180 litres, or 50 gallons, per day. However, as the fluid passes along the tubule, the kidney cells reabsorb most of the salt and water so that only about 2 litres (3 pints) of urine reaches the bladder.

There are several mechanisms for reabsorbing all this salt and water but all are based on the same principle. The kidney cells contain, in their walls, 'transporter' molecules which pick up sodium ions and transport them out of the tubule and push them back into the blood. The positively charged sodium ions are followed by negatively charged chloride ions (since oppositely charged particles, like the poles of magnets, are attracted to each other) and by water. The overall result is that the kidney reabsorbs about 99 per cent of the sodium,

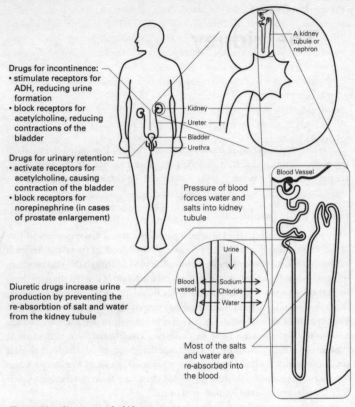

Drugs for incontinence:
• stimulate receptors for ADH, reducing urine formation
• block receptors for acetylcholine, reducing contractions of the bladder

Drugs for urinary retention:
• activate receptors for acetylcholine, causing contraction of the bladder
• block receptors for norepinephrine (in cases of prostate enlargement)

Diuretic drugs increase urine production by preventing the re-absorbtion of salt and water from the kidney tubule

A kidney tubule or nephron

Kidney
Ureter
Bladder
Urethra

Blood Vessel

Pressure of blood forces water and salts into kidney tubule

Urine

Blood vessel — Sodium — Chloride — Water

Most of the salts and water are re-absorbed into the blood

Fig. 5.1 How drugs act on the kidneys.

chloride, and water which had been filtered out of the capillaries. The urine which eventually reaches the bladder is left as a solution containing a little sodium and chloride, together with the unwanted, waste chemicals. The conservation of water means that we can continue for many hours without needing to drink. In some desert-living animals, so much water is reabsorbed by the kidneys that they excrete, not liquid urine but solid crystals of waste uric acid.

Why use drugs to change urine formation?

The word diuresis means the formation of urine, and a diuretic drug is one which increases the amount of urine produced. Because the water lost in the urine originally came from the blood, the volume of blood in the body will be correspondingly reduced. This can have two beneficial effects in some people. Firstly, the smaller volume of blood means that the blood pressure will often be less. Diuretic drugs are often, therefore, used to reduce high blood pressure in people with hypertension (*see* Chapter 15).

Secondly, the smaller blood volume and blood pressure reduce the amount of work that the heart has to do in pumping blood around the body. Diuretics are, therefore, useful in patients with weak hearts. When the pumping efficiency of the heart is reduced, water can accumulate in the lungs, reducing the amount of oxygen which can pass from the air into the blood and causing breathlessness and feelings of tightness in the chest. By reducing blood volume and pressure, diuretics help to eliminate such excess water from tissues and restore normal breathing.

Diuretics can also be used to reduce the amount of water which accumulates in the tissues of some women in the premenstrual phase of their hormonal cycle.

How do diuretic drugs work?

There are several types of diuretic drug. Among the most commonly used are those known as thiazides (Table 5.1, p. 77) and the loop diuretics, frusemide, and bumetanide. These all work in a very similar way, by inhibiting the transporter enzymes which reabsorb sodium from the kidney tubules. As a result sodium, chloride, and water are lost into the urine—a diuresis.

Thiazides

The thiazides are relatively mild drugs. The blood pressure may fall sufficiently quickly with the first few doses that the patient may feel faint, but this effect is not seen after the first few doses.

In addition to their actions on the kidney, the thiazides relax the walls of the blood vessels and change their sensitivity to neurotransmitters and hormones. This effect helps to lower blood pressure in people with hypertension (*see* Chapter 15) and explains why these are often the first drugs to be tried in this condition.

Loop diuretics

Frusemide and bumetanide also inhibit the sodium transporters, but they are sometimes called 'loop' diuretics, because they act on a specialized part of the kidney tubule where there is a hairpin-like bend or loop (Fig. 5.1). They are powerful drugs, able to increase the volume of urine several-fold in a couple of hours, and can be of great value in treating people with weak hearts, and in increasing the elimination of a drug taken in overdose. They are so strong, though, that the dose must be carefully controlled or too much salt and water may be excreted, blood pressure will fall too low, and the patient may faint.

Problems

One of the difficulties with these diuretics is that the increased loss of sodium in the urine is essential for their effects. If a person increases their salt intake in the diet, the effect of the drugs can be cancelled and they will be less effective. On the other hand, if a person cuts down on their salt intake at the same time as taking diuretics, the effect of the drugs will be increased, with a greater risk of fainting.

The main problem with all these drugs stems from the fact that some of the sodium reabsorbed from the tubule is exchanged for potassium ions. As diuretics increase the amount of sodium in the urine, there is a greater exchange for potassium, with the result that potassium levels in the blood may fall. When this happens, muscles contract less well, so that people may have feelings of weakness in their muscles, and may experience constipation as the movements of the intestine are reduced. The most serious risk is that a fall in blood potassium can cause changes in the rhythm of the heartbeat. If patients notice changes in their heartbeat, they should see their doctor immediately. Most of these problems can be corrected by the doctor's prescribing additional tablets containing potassium to replace that which has been lost in the urine.

Thiazides increase the loss of magnesium from the body, and decrease the loss of calcium. The loss of magnesium may cause increased activity of nerves and muscles, leading to twitching and cramps. The decreased loss of calcium can cause the opposite effect, namely weakness in the muscles. The loop diuretics increase the loss of both calcium and magnesium from the body. Whether a particular patient experiences no side-effects, weakness, or twitching, will depend on their individual balance of sodium, potassium, magnesium, and calcium in the body.

Finally, the thiazide drugs can reduce the kidney's excretion of uric acid, one of the body's waste products. In most people this is not a problem, but in people with gout (which is caused by the formation of uric acid crystals in the joints; (*see* Chapter 20), this condition may be made worse.

Alternative diuretics

If a person loses too much potassium with the drugs just described, they can be given a different type of drug known as a 'potassium-sparing' diuretic. These include spironolactone, amiloride, and triamterene.

Spironolactone works by preventing the actions of a hormone called aldosterone. Aldosterone is a steroid hormone, produced by the adrenal glands, which increases the exchange of sodium for potassium (Fig. 5.1). By blocking this hormone's effects, spironolactone can prevent this exchange and thus prevent the depletion of potassium from the body.

Amiloride and triamterene work by reducing the movement of sodium from the kidney tubules into cells where it would be exchanged for potassium. These potassium-sparing drugs can be used on their own as diuretics, but are most often used together with the thiazides and loop diuretics to reduce the loss of potassium produced by these drugs.

Xanthines

Diuretic drugs such as caffeine and theophylline are also present in tea, coffee, chocolate, and cola drinks and cause the diuretic effects of these foods. They have several effects on the kidney, including inhibition of sodium absorption (like the thiazides). They also increase blood flow through the kidney, partly by blocking the blood vessel contraction produced by a local hormone, adenosine, and partly by increasing the force of contraction of the heart. The inhibition of sodium absorption, together with the increased blood flow in the kidney available for filtration, increases the volume of urine produced.

Osmotic diuretics

Mannitol is an 'osmotic diuretic'. It is filtered into the urine in the kidney tubule in large enough amounts to change the osmotic pressure* of the tubule fluid. The effect of this is simply to reduce the amount of water which the kidney cells can reabsorb into the blood. The volume of urine in the kidney tubules remains higher than normal, producing a diuresis. Mannitol is sometimes used to maintain urine production and kidney function when the kidney has been damaged, for example by a poison or drug overdose, because it will help urine formation even though the kidney cells may not be working properly.

Incontinence

Normally urine passes from the kidney into the bladder where it is stored. As the urine expands the bladder, sensory nerves in the bladder wall begin to become active, signalling to the brain and making us aware that the bladder is filling and that we need to urinate. Normally the muscles at the neck of the bladder remain tightly closed until we relax them voluntarily to urinate. Then the parasympathetic nerves (*see* Chapter 1) become active, secreting acetylcholine and causing the bladder to contract and eliminate the urine.

A troubling complaint of some patients, especially the more elderly, is that

---

* See Footnote on p. 37. Osmotic pressure is a measure of the amount of water moving across cell walls by osmosis.

they need to urinate very often, or they lose control of the bladder so that urine leaks out even when they are not ready to urinate and may not be conscious of a full bladder. These problems are together known as incontinence and may be particularly troublesome at night, as urination may occur while the patient is asleep, a condition known as 'nocturnal enuresis'.

Incontinence is due to the fact that the wall of the bladder becomes stiffer with age and can hold a smaller volume of urine before the sensory nerves in the bladder wall initiate the desire to urinate, or trigger urination reflexly in situations where voluntary control is lost (e.g. during sleep).

Treatment

One treatment for nocturnal enuresis is the drug desmopressin. This is related to the natural hormone called antidiuretic hormone (ADH which is so called because it increases the amount of water re-absorbed in the kidney, reducing the production of urine). Desmopressin is usually taken at night so that less urine is produced while asleep, the bladder does not fill as much as usual, and there is less chance of enuresis.

The most widely used drugs for incontinence are the anticholinergic drugs such as oxybutynin and tolterodine. Acetylcholine is the neurotransmitter produced by the parasympathetic nerves which contracts the bladder to cause urination. The anticholinergic drugs block the receptors for acetylcholine and so stop the nerves causing contraction of the bladder. They also tend to have other effects such as reduced salivation, blurred vision, and constipation (*see* Chapter 1) since they block receptors for acetylcholine in all tissues, not just the bladder.

One drug which is currently being tested in clinical trials is darifenacin (made by Pfizer). This has a more selective action on the acetylcholine receptors on the muscles cells, with much less effect on the heart, stomach, and nerves. It should have fewer side-effects than current anticholinergic drugs.

Urinary retention

Conversely, some patients find it difficult to urinate, leading to what is called urinary retention. This problem may occur after some surgical operations in the abdomen or when the passage of urine along the urethra is obstructed by enlargement of the prostate glands in men. The prostate glands secrete part of the seminal fluid which is formed during ejaculation. With ageing, these glands may become enlarged* sufficiently to press on and partially block the adjacent

---

* The enlargement is often harmless, a condition known as benign prostatic hypertrophy, but it may sometimes be associated with the development of cancer of the prostate. Cancer of the prostate is discussed in Chapter 18.

urethra (the tube taking urine from the bladder through the penis or vulva to the exterior) impeding the flow of urine. Patients may experience frequent urges to urinate, since the bladder is never emptied as completely as in a normal person, or problems with urination such as hesitancy (a marked delay between preparing to urinate and the beginning of urine flow), and a weak or slow flow of urine. The symptoms of urinary retention just described can occur at as early as 30 years of age. One in every five men aged 40–64, and two of every five aged 65–80 have problems with urinary retention due to prostate enlargement.

What causes prostate enlargement?

The male hormone, testosterone, is changed in the prostate glands into a similar chemical (dihydrotestosterone) which increases the growth of the prostate cells, leading to its enlargement.

Treatment

Treatment depends on the cause of the problem. Retention following an operation is best treated using drugs which activate the receptors for acetylcholine, mimicking the normal effects of the parasympathetic nerves and producing contraction of the bladder. These drugs include those which act on the receptors directly such as bethanechol. Other drugs prevent the breakdown of acetylcholine by the enzyme acetylcholinesterase (*see* Chapter 1). These drugs, such as distigmine, prolong the effects of acetylcholine released from the nerves and increase contraction of the bladder.

Retention caused by prostate enlargement is best treated with drugs which reduce the contraction of the muscle cells around the prostate gland and aorta. Contraction is produced by norepinephrine (noradrenaline) released from sympathetic nerves and acting on alpha-receptors (*see* Chapter 1). The drugs used block these alpha-receptors (Table 5.1, p. 77), allowing the muscle cells to relax and relieving the urinary obstruction.

The side-effects of these drugs are a result of the blockade of alpha-receptors in other parts of the body. Blood vessels in the head relax, for example, causing headaches and the blood pressure may fall when standing quickly, causing fainting.

Finasteride

Finasteride blocks the enzyme which causes the conversion of testosterone to dihydrotestosterone. As a result, the levels of dihydrotestosterone fall, the prostate shrinks, and the retention of urine is improved. To reach this stage may need treatment for at least six months, during which the patient has to cope with side-effects such as failure of ejaculation and impotence due to the change in the balance of the sex hormones.

(Dihydrotestosterone is believed to be the chemical partly responsible for male pattern baldness. Because it prevents the formation of this hormone, finasteride is likely to be available soon on prescription for the treatment of baldness.)

Kidney stones

If the amount of calcium in the urine is too high, calcium salts may form crystals which grow into 'stones' in the bladder. These can cause pain and discomfort. If they are passed out in the urine they can also cause pain as they travel through the urethra. Patients susceptible to the formation of stones can be treated with sodium cellulose phosphate. Calcium interacts with this compound to form other chemicals which are more soluble in water and are less likely to form crystals and stones.

Table 5.1 Drugs affecting the kidney and bladder

Thiazides	Osmotic diuretic	Drugs for urinary retention
althiazide	mannitol	Cholinergic drugs
bemetizide		bethanecol
bendrofluazide		
bendroflumethiazide	**Drugs for incontinence**	
benzthiazide	ADH analogue	**Anticholinesterase drugs**
buthiazide	desmopressin	distigmine
chlorothiazide		
chlorthalidone*	**Anticholinergic drugs**	**Adrenoceptor blockers**
clopamide*	amitriptyline	alfuzosin
clorexolone	darifenacin†	doxazosin
cyclopenthiazide	flavoxate	indoramin
hydrochlorothiazide	imipramine	prazosin
hydroflumethiazide	nortriptyline	tamsulosin
indapamide*	oxybutynin	terazosin
mefruside*	tolterodine	
methylclothiazide (USA)		
meticrane		
metolazone		
polythiazide		
quinethazone (USA)		
trichlormethiazide (USA)		
xipamide		

Loop diuretics
azosemide
bumetanide
ethacrynic acid
etozolin
frusemide
furosemide
muzolimine
piretanide
torasemide

Potassium-sparing diuretics
amiloride
canrenoate
triamterene
potassium canrenoate
spironolactone

---

* These drugs are not chemically thiazide compounds, but their actions are very similar.
† Darifenacin is in advanced clinical trials and should be available in 2000.

Summary

- The kidneys produce urine by filtering blood and then reabsorbing water and salts from the kidney tubules.
- Over 99 per cent of the water and salt are reabsorbed into the blood so that only waste chemicals are lost into the urine.
- Drugs which increase urine formation are diuretics. They are used to help to lower blood pressure in patients with high blood pressure or weak hearts.
- Diuretics prevent salt and water from being reabsorbed from the urine into the bloodstream.
- Some diuretics increase the loss of potassium from the body and this may need to be replaced by supplements.
- Xanthine drugs such as caffeine inhibit water reabsorption and increase blood flow to the kidney.
- Incontinence occurs when the bladder is contracted by nerves releasing the transmitter acetylcholine after loss of conscious control.
- Drugs to treat incontinence block the receptors for acetylcholine.
- In cases of urinary retention, the bladder contractions can be increased by drugs which activate receptors for acetylcholine.
- If urinary obstruction is due to enlargement of the prostate gland, drugs can be used to relax the muscles of the urethra and to facilitate urination.
- Kidney stones are caused by the crystallization of calcium salts in the kidney, ureters and bladder. They can be prevented by substances which interact with calcium to form compounds which are more easily dissolved in water and are less likely to form stones.

CHAPTER 6

Painkillers

The *spongia somnifera* (or sleep-inducing sponge) was the means of lessening
the pain and horror of mediaeval surgery. The recipe called for a sponge to
be steeped in a water and wine mixture of opium, lettuce, hemlock,
hyoscyamus, mulberry juice, mandragora, and ivy. Once prepared the sponge
was dried and kept until it was needed; it was then moistened so that the
juice could be drunk.*

Pain

The word 'pain' comes from the Latin *poena* meaning punishment, since pain
was once believed to represent punishment from the gods. Although it has a
major impact on the lives of many people, pain is still extremely difficult to
study. Consider how you would explain pain, and the feeling of hurting to one
of those rare people who is born without any sense of pain. It is very, very
difficult to describe pain and to explain its unpleasantness and what it is about
pain that brings with it the associated feelings of fear, anxiety, and worry.

Yet pain is necessary for survival. People born without the sensation of pain
frequently damage their skin by banging, scraping, or burning it, or damage
their muscles and joints by stretching, twisting, or bending them without being
aware of the harm that they are doing. They damage their bodies so much, in
fact, that few of these patients live to middle age.

Pain protects us from our environment. It is the extremely uncomfortable
feeling which we experience when the body begins to be damaged, and it thus
warns us to try to remove the cause of the damage. In fact, pain is often
accompanied by a protective reflex (a rapid movement which is beyond our
voluntary control) which may be sufficient to remove us from the source of
damage. Examples of protective reflexes are the rapid removal of a hand from a
hot surface or raising a foot from a pin on the floor. Unfortunately, few of us
escape feeling pain at some time in our lives, and it is hardly surprising that,
since the earliest signs of civilization, humans have tried to devise methods of

* From *Modern drug use* by R. D. Mann, 1984, p.168.

reducing pain. Medicinal preparations to reduce pain—analgesics*—are among the oldest remedies known to mankind.

What causes pain?

Usually pain is the result of an event which either damages cells or is likely to do so in time. For example, a heavy object placed on the skin may be enough to crush and damage some cells and may threaten others by reducing their blood supply. The pain produced is the result of two different factors. Firstly the damaging object, whether it is heavy, sharp, hot, or very cold, will slightly deform the endings of sensory nerves in the skin—the nerves which send signals to the brain about the state of the skin and its temperature. The deformation causes these nerves to increase the rate at which they send impulses into the spinal cord and brain where this increase causes us to experience pain.

The second factor is that as cells are damaged, the chemicals they contain spill out and act on the nerve endings to increase their rate of signalling even further. The list of chemicals is large, but the ones we shall meet several times in this book include histamine, kinins (a group of proteins), prostaglandins, and leukotrienes. Prostaglandins are a group of unsaturated fatty acids similar to those found in oils and margarines, and are called prostaglandins because they were first found in secretions from prostate glands. Leukotrienes are very similar.

First and second pain

Events or objects which cause tissue damage trigger two types of pain. If a finger is trapped in a door, there is an immediate stabbing pain, associated with a shout of pain and removal of the finger from the door. This pain can be identified as coming from the precise point of entrapment. This is called 'first pain'. The finger may be rubbed or shaken and the pain disappears very quickly. After a few seconds there is then a delayed, slowly developing, duller, aching type of pain which feels as if it comes from the whole area in and around the point of damage. This is 'second pain'.

The difference between first and second pain lies in the nerves carrying the signals to the brain. When the finger is first trapped, impulses are triggered in nerves called 'A-delta fibres' which conduct their signals quickly, at about 10 metres per second, into the spinal cord. These cause first pain. Another group of nerves—the 'C fibres' are more sluggish, sending information at a speed of less than 1 metre per second. The two types of pain have different functions. First pain prompts us to remove the source of damage as quickly as possible. Second pain ensures that we continue to pay attention to the wound for some minutes afterwards, providing treatment such as licking, rubbing, or staunching

* The Greek and Latin word 'analgesia' means absence of pain.

any bleeding. Rubbing or shaking a wound has a sound physiological basis, since these manoeuvres activate the ordinary sensory nerves in the skin which respond to touch. The impulses from these nerves are able to reduce the flow of signals from the pain-carrying A-delta and C fibres in the spinal cord, reducing the sensation of pain.

Aches and pains

During an infection by bacteria or viruses, aches and pains arise mainly as a result of the body's efforts to fight the invading organisms. The immune system produces antibodies to the viruses or fragments of bacteria (*see* Chapter 2). Before killing the viruses or bacteria, the antibodies attach to them and trigger the release of chemicals such as histamine and prostaglandins from various types of cell around the body, including white cells in the blood and mast cells (these are similar to white blood cells but exist in the tissues). Together these various chemicals stimulate nerve endings throughout the body which give rise to the sensation of aches and pains we experience during an infection. They also relax blood vessels, and increase blood flow to the head. This puts pressure on nerve endings in the vessel walls, increasing their activation and causing a headache.

Dysmenorrhoea is a form of pain experienced by some women during menstruation. It is caused by prostaglandins which cause painful contractions of the uterus and it can usually be treated with mild pain-killers.

Pain arising from damage to nerves themselves can occur after amputation of a limb (phantom limb pain), as a result of long-standing diabetes (diabetic neuropathy), after surgical operations, or after a stroke. These forms of pain may be difficult to treat with conventional painkillers, but they may be controlled by other drugs such as antidepressants and antiepileptic drugs which reduce the abnormal activity of the damaged nerves.

Mild analgesics

Aspirin

The chemical name for aspirin is acetylsalicylic acid, and a glance at the contents of most cold, headache, and influenza remedies bought at the pharmacy or supermarket will reveal that many contain this drug. Aspirin is certainly a useful drug for reducing pain produced by small amounts of tissue damage and for the aches (including headaches) and fever caused by colds, influenza, and other infections (Fig. 6.1). As we shall see later, however, there are much safer drugs now available, such as paracetamol (acetaminophen) and ibuprofen, and these should always be used in preference to aspirin for mild aches and pains.

Aspirin itself is not a new drug. In their own way, the ancient Greeks knew

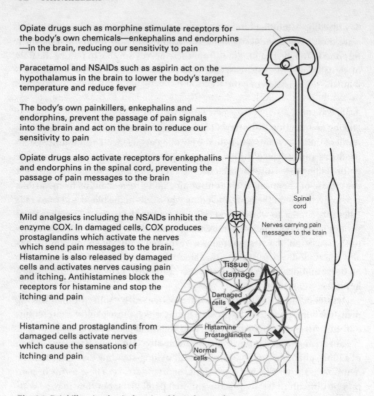

Opiate drugs such as morphine stimulate receptors for the body's own chemicals—enkephalins and endorphins—in the brain, reducing our sensitivity to pain

Paracetamol and NSAIDs such as aspirin act on the hypothalamus in the brain to lower the body's target temperature and reduce fever

The body's own painkillers, enkephalins and endorphins, prevent the passage of pain signals into the brain and act on the brain to reduce our sensitivity to pain

Opiate drugs also activate receptors for enkephalins and endorphins in the spinal cord, preventing the passage of pain messages to the brain

Mild analgesics including the NSAIDs inhibit the enzyme COX. In damaged cells, COX produces prostaglandins which activate the nerves which send pain messages to the brain. Histamine is also released by damaged cells and activates nerves causing pain and itching. Antihistamines block the receptors for histamine and stop the itching and pain

Histamine and prostaglandins from damaged cells activate nerves which cause the sensations of itching and pain

Spinal cord

Nerves carrying pain messages to the brain

Tissue damage

Damaged cells

Histamine
Prostaglandins

Normal cells

Fig. 6.1 Painkillers (analgesic drugs) and how they work.

of aspirin 3000 years before its 'rediscovery' in modern times. The bones of mummified bodies show that some types of arthritis were not uncommon among the ancients, and one method of treating them was to crush the bark and leaves of the willow tree (*Salix alba*) in oil, and apply the preparation to the painful joints and muscles. Hippocrates recommended willow bark for the treatment of gout and the removal of warts.

In 1763 an English cleric, the Reverend Edmund Stone, noticed that some rural workers in Chipping Norton would treat aches, pains, and fevers by making preparations of the bark of the white willow tree, and he observed that similar preparations lowered the temperature of patients with fever. About 1830 an Italian chemist, Raffaele Piria, isolated a compound which he called salicin (after the willow, *Salix alba*) from willow bark, but it was soon shown that salicylic acid could readily be obtained from it and that it was this which caused the relief from pain and inflammation. Salicylic acid proved to be a valuable drug with which to treat disorders such as gout and arthritis as well as diseases like colds in which fever was prominent. However, salicylic acid was not the most pleasant drug for patients to take, with marked stomach upsets and nausea, so the German pharmaceutical company Bayer initiated a programme to synthesize chemicals similar to salicylic acid. One of these, acetylsalicylic acid, was produced by Charles Frederick von Gerhardt (1816–1856), Professor of Chemistry at the University of Strasbourg, France, in 1853. However, since it was so similar to salicylic acid and would be changed in the body to salicylic acid, it was left on the shelf untested for almost fifty years.

In 1899 Felix Hoffman, a chemist working for the Bayer company in Germany, tried several of the company's compounds on his arthritic father who could no longer tolerate the stomach upsets and intense nausea produced by taking salicylic acid. The acetyl compound proved to be more effective as well as a more pleasant drug and, after more extensive tests, it was soon marketed by Bayer under the trade name 'Aspirin' (because early samples of salicylic acid had been obtained from the meadow-sweet plant *Spiraea*, so the name was coined from the letter 'a' for acetyl and 'spiraea'). Today around fifty tons of aspirin are consumed every day in the USA.

Aspirin is one of a group of drugs known as non-steroidal anti-inflammatory drugs (NSAIDs) because, while they are good at reducing inflammation, they are quite different chemically from the steroid substances discussed in Chapter 19. NSAIDs also reduce the increased body temperature we call 'fever'.

Fever

The clinical thermometer was invented by Sanctorius of Padua (1561–1636) and by the late 1700s the measurement of body temperature had become a standard feature of the medical examination. When encountered, fever was reduced either by giving quinine, since this was known to reduce the fever of malarial infection, or (since this usually did not work for non-malarial fever) by physical measures such as immersion in a cold bath. In 1875, Carl Buss reported an observation he had made on typhoid patients in Switzerland. He had administered salicylic acid to help suppress the aches and general discomfort of the condition, but noticed that the high, feverish body temperature also declined. When chemical derivatives of salicylic acid were later produced, such as aspirin, it was found that these too were generally fever reducing.

During the course of an infection, prostaglandin production increases in the brain. In the case of bacterial infections, a group of substances called lipopolysaccharides, produced by the bacteria, trigger the synthesis of prostaglandins in the brain. This happens mainly in an area of brain called the hypothalamus, one function of which is to control our body temperature.

Normally, body temperature is maintained at a remarkably constant 37 °C (98.4 °F), although it fluctuates by around 1 °C above and below this every 24 hours, and throughout the menstrual cycle in women. This control is achieved by the hypothalamus which receives information from the skin about its temperature, and has cells which detect the temperature of the blood. The hypothalamus is able to adjust the body's activities to maintain body temperature at 37 °C—the 'set point'. If blood temperature increases, the hypothalamus causes blood vessels in the skin to relax, a change which increases the loss of heat from the body surface to the air, and which increases the production of sweat. As the sweat evaporates it cools the skin and the blood flowing through it.

Conversely, if blood temperature falls, sweating is reduced and blood vessels in the skin contract, making the skin cold and white in appearance. The hypothalamus also triggers shivering, which generates heat in the muscles and helps to warm the body.

One of the consequences of infection is that those prostaglandins produced in the hypothalamus alter the 'set-point' to a new, higher value. The hypothalamus, therefore, tries to raise blood temperature to meet this value, producing fever by closing skin blood vessels, making us feel cold, and triggering shivering, even though it may be a hot summer's day. Body temperature may rise to 40 or 41 °C (103 to 105 °F), a change which may have evolved to increase the activity of the body's defence systems and fight the infection more quickly. If a serious infection develops rapidly, however, the hypothalamus may try to raise body temperature too much and too quickly. With the rise in temperature, cells need more oxygen and blood. Since there is not enough blood to increase the supply to every cell in the body, the increased demand for blood can result in some cells becoming starved of oxygen and dying. As they die, they may release, or cause the release of, more histamine and prostaglandins. This initiates a vicious cycle which can lead to the death of the patient. This is why doctors are happy not to interfere too much if body temperature increases only by 2 or 3 °C, but may use drugs to reduce temperature if it rises more than this.

What has all this to do with aspirin?

The prostaglandins are produced by an enzyme called cyclo-oxygenase (COX). In 1971 Sir John Vane, working at the British drug company Wellcome (recently merged into GlaxoWellcome), discovered that COX was inhibited by aspirin, which chemically alters part of the enzyme molecule so that it can no longer work. (Vane later received the Nobel Prize for this discovery.) In the presence of aspirin, prostaglandins can no longer be generated. In the various tissues of the body, this means less stimulation of the pain-sensitive nerve endings, and less aching of muscles and joints, and explains the pain-killing action of aspirin. There is also less relaxation of blood vessels in the head and this, together with the analgesic action, means fewer headaches. Finally, it means fewer prostaglandins in the hypothalamus, so that the set-point will not be changed, and no fever will be induced: this is the fever-reducing or 'antipyretic' action of aspirin.

Inflammation

Some of these bodily changes can also occur in response to localized infection. Suppose that you cut yourself while gardening, and some bacteria enter the wound. Several things will happen. Firstly, blood from the cut will clot. As it does so, some blood cells and some of the damaged skin cells release chemicals called 'chemotactic factors', which attract many thousands of white blood cells into the area. These transform into aggressive cells (phagocytes) which engulf bacteria and kill them. The phagocytes, along with cells called 'mast cells' and cells damaged directly by the cut release histamine, prostaglandins, and kinins. These cause the localized pain and tenderness we feel around a wound and, by relaxing local blood vessels, cause the associated redness, swelling, and warmth which we call 'inflammation'. By impairing prostaglandin formation, aspirin can reduce all of these signs of damage. Because histamine release contributes to the pain and swelling of this local inflammatory response, some antihistamine creams and ointments can also be used to reduce the symptoms of mild infections. (A cream is water-based and can be washed off easily by water; an ointment is oil-based and should be water-resistant.)

Of course, drugs such as aspirin and antihistamines do nothing to kill or hinder the infecting bacteria. In severe cases of infection, it may be necessary to administer antibiotics (see Chapter 17) to kill the bacteria.

What are the main side-effects of aspirin?

Stomach

Since aspirin is an acidic compound it is absorbed well in the acid contents of the stomach. When it has passed into the cells it changes into an ionized form which means that it cannot easily escape from the cells. In other words, the aspirin tends to become trapped, and to accumulate in the cells lining the stomach.

In a normal person, prostaglandins are secreted by the stomach wall and tend to limit the amount of acid produced. They also promote the formation of a thick layer of mucus which helps to protect the stomach from being damaged by its own acid and they facilitate the repair of cells when damaged (see Chapter 4). Since aspirin reduces the production of prostaglandins there will be fewer of these hormones in the stomach of a person taking frequent doses of aspirin.

As a result, the stomach produces more acid but less protective mucus. Together, these effects irritate the stomach wall, perhaps with bleeding and ulcer formation. As a rule, aspirin should not be taken by anyone with a history of stomach or duodenal ulcers unless under close medical supervision, and it should always be taken with food.

In fact severe or even fatal bleeding from the stomach can occur in occasional, unfortunate people after only one or two aspirin tablets, particularly if these are taken when the stomach lining is already irritated by alcohol. This is a particular danger in people over 65. As noted earlier, the newer analgesics such as paracetamol (acetaminophen) and ibuprofen are much safer and should always be used in preference to aspirin for minor aches and pains.

Salicylism

If a person takes aspirin in high doses, or regularly over a long period of several months or years in doses which gradually accumulate in the tissues of the body, a number of symptoms may develop due to salicylate poisoning. The condition is known as salicylism. The symptoms include severe headaches, ringing in the ears (tinnitus), and a tremor of the hands. Care must be taken with the size of aspirin doses taken, since the highest doses needed for some disorders, such as arthritis, are close to those which produce salicylism in some people.

Blood clotting

This section could be called 'When is a side-effect not a side-effect ?' The answer might be 'When aspirin is used to prevent blood clotting'. Aspirin slows the rate at which blood clots and this may be a nuisance in most people taking aspirin to treat a headache, toothache, or arthritis. However, this anticlotting effect can be useful in people liable to have heart attacks, and aspirin may be taken in *small* daily doses to reduce the risk of a second or subsequent heart attack.

We all take for granted the ability of blood to clot and close a wound after injury. However, many different chemicals in the blood are involved in clotting, including two members of the prostaglandin family—prostacyclin and thromboxane. If a blood vessel is damaged, a group of cell fragments in the blood called platelets begin to release histamine, thromboxane, and other compounds which initiate clotting. The platelets clump together, cause red cells to do the same, and trigger the formation of sticky protein clots around the clumps. Because aspirin prevents the formation of thromboxane, along with all other prostaglandins, it slows the clotting process so that blood takes considerably longer than normal to clot. Anyone taking large or frequent doses of aspirin should be careful to avoid injury since they may lose more blood than a person free from aspirin.

Aspirin prevents the formation, not only of thromboxane, but also of prostacyclin, a prostaglandin released by the blood vessels themselves and which prevents blood clotting. In other words thromboxane and prostacyclin have opposite effects and clotting occurs only when the amounts of thromboxane and other clotting activators exceed the amounts of prostacyclin and other clotting inhibitors. Because aspirin blocks the formation of both thromboxane and prostacyclin, high doses will have rather unpredictable effects on clotting.

Fortunately, blood vessels are continually making new COX enzyme and, thus, prostacyclin. In contrast, platelets are not complete cells (since they have no nucleus to generate new enzymes), and they cannot produce new COX and thromboxane. It is possible, therefore, to find doses of aspirin which abolish thromboxane production with much less effect on prostacyclin formation, and thus shift the balance between these different prostaglandins in such a way that clotting is inhibited and not encouraged.

This ability of aspirin to inhibit blood clotting has received a great deal of attention in recent years because of the high incidence of deaths from coronary thromboses. If a blood clot (thrombosis) occurs in a coronary blood vessel (which carries blood to the heart), then a heart attack may occur—the heart can no longer pump blood efficiently and the patient may die. Several large clinical trials have now shown that aspirin can reduce both the chance of dying from a heart attack and the likelihood of a second one. One report analysed results from 17 187 patients in 417 hospitals and concluded that giving aspirin within 24 hours of a heart attack reduced the chance of death by one quarter. Put another way, for every four people who died from their heart attack, one could have been saved if they had taken aspirin immediately. For long-term use in this situation to prevent the occurrence of a second heart attack, the dose of aspirin is around 75 mg per day, or about one quarter of the amount found in a single aspirin tablet bought as a cold or headache remedy.

While aspirin clearly reduces the likelihood of a second or later heart attack, its effects on a first attack are less certain. Nevertheless, some doctors believe that regular low dose aspirin (75 milligrams per day) can reduce the probability of a first heart attack. This view, together with the ability of aspirin to reduce the chance of dying from a first attack means that many doctors now recommend patients at risk to carry around an aspirin tablet so that it can be swallowed at the first sign of a heart attack.

Dangers

Strokes

The use of aspirin is complicated when 'strokes' are considered. Most strokes are due to a clot or thrombosis in blood vessels supplying the brain. A smaller number are due to a haemorrhage from a weak vesssel in the brain. In either case, the blood supply to part of the brain is cut off and many nerve cells in that region will die. The result can be a loss of the ability to speak or a paralysis over part of the body. Since aspirin reduces blood clotting, people who take aspirin regularly are less likely to develop thromboses in these vessels and to have a stroke than people not taking the drug. The danger, of course, is that if bleeding occurs from a weak blood vessel, clotting will not occur as quickly as normal and the stroke may be made worse by the aspirin. Since most strokes are the result of thromboses, not bleeding, the benefit is in favour of taking aspirin. If a patient suffers a stroke, however, a brain scan will be needed to confirm that the cause is not a haemorrhage before aspirin can be given safely.

Reye's syndrome in children
Aspirin should not be given to a child under twelve years of age. If given to some children to treat the symptoms of a viral infection, such as influenza and chickenpox, they may develop a disorder known as Reye's syndrome. The mechanism by which aspirin does this is not known, but the disorder involves serious liver problems and brain damage and can be fatal. Since it is not always obvious when children are infected by some of these viruses, either because the infection is at a very early, pre-symptomatic stage, or because they have already acquired some immunity, it is safest not to use aspirin at all in children under twelve.

What are the alternatives to aspirin?

Paracetamol (acetaminophen)
One of the major alternatives to aspirin is paracetamol (also called aceta-minophen). The introduction of paracetamol was unnecessarily delayed for 50 years. It was made and tested by the Bayer company in 1893 but, although it was clearly an effective analgesic and antipyretic drug, it appeared to damage haemoglobin and was not developed further. In fact paracetamol has no such effect on haemoglobin and the damage seen by Bayer must have been due to a chemical contaminant. It was not until about 1950 that two chemists—F. B. Flinn and Bernard Brodie—at Yale and Columbia Universities re-examined paracetamol and discovered that it was not responsible for the damage.

Their interest in paracetamol arose from the fact that a related drug, phenacetin, had been in use as an analgesic for several decades but evidence was emerging that long-term use could cause liver and kidney damage. Flinn and Brodie showed that whereas the tissue damage was due to the phenacetin molecule, the analgesic and antipyretic properties were due to paracetamol which was produced from phenacetin in the body. The result of their work was that paracetamol was first marketed under the trade name 'Panadol' by the Sterling-Winthrop company in 1953 and as 'Tylenol' in the USA.

Paracetamol has less effect on the body's COX enzymes than aspirin and so does not reduce inflammation, and it does not stop the activation of pain-sensitive nerve endings to the same extent as aspirin. It does inhibit COX in the brain, though, and this gives it most of its ability to block pain, and to prevent fever.

Safety of paracetamol

Paracetamol is much safer than aspirin since it does not accumulate in the stomach wall, does not inhibit COX in the stomach, and can be given to children. It is the best drug to use in the home to reduce the unpleasant symptoms of viral illnesses and to deal with minor aches and pains, headaches, and hangovers. Its main danger is that if taken in large overdoses it can cause permanent, life-threatening damage to the kidneys. Since it is so readily available, a number of suicide attempts occur every year by people taking paracetamol. Most of these people do not die but have to live the rest of their lives with seriously damaged liver or kidneys.

The reason why paracetamol is dangerous in overdose is that it causes the liver to use up its supply of a protective chemical called glutathione. Damaging chemicals produced from paracetamol are then free to attack the liver and kidney. This damage can be minimized by injecting the patients with acetyl-cysteine, a compound which replaces the lost glutathione and protects the liver from damage. Some drug companies are now considering including another natural chemical, methionine, in paracetamol tablets since this increases the liver's supply of glutathione and reduces the formation of the toxic chemicals responsible for kidney damage: it should be harmless to people taking recommended doses but would prevent the organ damage produced by overdoses.

Ibuprofen

The second alternative is ibuprofen. This is a different type of chemical from aspirin and paracetamol, but has many of the same characteristics: it is an effective painkiller with mild anti-inflammatory activity and can lower body temperature (antipyretic activity). Ibuprofen is the painkiller often recommended for use with children who have aches and pains associated with fever. There are a number of related drugs which are used mainly for their anti-inflammatory activity and are discussed in more detail in Chapter 20. They should not be taken by elderly people, in particular, who are at risk from their side-effects such as bleeding from the stomach. They should not be used simply as painkillers since paracetamol is much safer.

Capsaicin

Capsaicin is the chemical which gives chilli peppers their hot, spicy taste. It first stimulates the nerves in the mouth to give the spicy sensation but, if eaten regularly, it damages those same nerves so that we become less sensitive to the spices. This is one reason why people who eat a lot of 'hot' foods make them more and more spicy as time goes on. This property of capsaicin has now been put to medical use by making it available as a cream, which can be applied to painful areas of skin, for example over chronically aching muscles and joints. The cream stings slightly at first as it stimulates the nerves but, as these become desensitized and weaker over several weeks of use, they are less able to send information to the brain, so muscle or joint aches and pains become less.

Combinations

If stronger painkillers are needed, there are several preparations in which two analgesic drugs, such as paracetamol and codeine, are combined in the same tablet. These can be used for moderate or severe pain when prescribed and used under medical supervision.

Two types of COX

In the last few years scientists have found that the enzyme which produces prostaglandins, COX, exists in two distinct forms—COX-1 and COX-2. COX-1 exists normally in the body, producing the prostaglandins which protect the stomach, as described above, and the kidney. COX-2 is produced by cells only when they are involved in inflammation, such as in the joints of patients with arthritis. It is COX-2 which is responsible for producing the prostaglandins which sensitize nerve endings and give rise to the pain associated with inflammation.

The discovery of these two forms of COX explains some previously mysterious properties of the non-steroidal anti-inflammatory drugs (NSAIDs). Scientists had never fully understood, for example, why some drugs such as aspirin irritate the stomach so seriously, while others, such as ibuprofen, had much less effect, at doses which produced similar degrees of pain relief. We now realize that aspirin had a far greater effect on COX-1 in the stomach (it inhibits COX-1 about 150 times more than COX-2), whereas ibuprofen is more active on COX-2.

The existence of these two forms of COX means that it should be possible to develop drugs which inhibit only COX-2 and not COX-1. Such a drug should only prevent the formation of pain-producing prostaglandins, and would not affect those affording protection of the stomach. This would be good news for the one patient in every five who cannot take NSAID drugs because of the stomach pain and cramps they produce.

Such was the enthusiasm of the pharmaceutical industry for this idea of COX-2 inhibitors that several drugs are already in various stages of testing in animals or humans, and one is already available. This is meloxicam. So far, meloxicam has proved to have very few side-effects on the stomach or kidney. Another of these selective COX-2 inhibitors soon to become available is celecoxib (Celebrex®), developed by the Searle Company.

As a bonus to this story, there is a growing belief that COX-2 may be involved in causing cancers of the colon. Drugs such as meloxicam and celecoxib are, therefore, being tested for possible use in treating or preventing this increasingly common form of cancer. The evidence so far suggests that COX-2 inhibitors stop the growth of blood vessels into the tumours and intitiate the killing of the tumour cells. Ari Ristimaki, a scientist working at the University of Helsinki, and others have begun to find effects of COX-2 in other types of cancer too. These include cancers of the stomach and the lung, which might also be treatable using COX-2 inhibitors.

Kidney damage (analgesic nephropathy)

Several of these NSAIDs and paracetamol can produce kidney damage. This is most likely to occur when these drugs are taken in combinations with each other for several days or weeks, especially if taken together with a high amount of caffeine (in tea and coffee). All painkillers, however harmless they may seem, should only be used alone, for as short a time as possible and only when really necessary.

The reason for this damage seems to be that prostaglandins help to protect kidney cells, probably by controlling their blood supply. Since the NSAIDSs and paracetamol all inhibit the synthesis of prostaglandins, this protection is lost.

Rheumatoid arthritis

Arthritis is usually treated by NSAIDs, many of which have strong anti-inflammatory activity combined with some analgesic activity. These drugs will be discussed in Chapter 20.

Strong 'narcotic' analgesics

The NSAIDs and paracetamol are useful for pain which is relatively mild and easily controlled, usually resulting from a minor injury, cold, or influenza. Larger, more extensive or serious injuries such as those arising from road accidents, surgery, war, or the growth of cancers within the body, need treating with much more powerful analgesics. Most of these have been developed from opium.

Opium

When the seed capsule of the tropical poppy plant, *Papaver somniferum* is cut in several places, the sap or juice oozes out and dries on the outside of the capsule. This dried sap has for centuries been called opium from the Greek word *opos* meaning juice. Crude preparations such as opium and laudanum have been popular for centuries to reduce pain. The German–Swiss physician and alchemist Paracelsus (1493–1541) produced a preparation he called laudanum, by dissolving opium in alcohol—a rather powerful concoction—which was widely used in the Middle Ages by those who could afford it and by many well-known individuals such as Samuel Johnson, to produce relief from the pain of everything from toothaches and broken bones to gout and cancers. The effectiveness of laudanum was no doubt a result not only of the ability of opium and alcohol to reduce pain, but also the additional calming effect of a drunken sleep.

As the twenty-first century opens, there is a great threat to young people in the West from opium which is smuggled in from sources in Asia. Until the end of the nineteenth century, however, the British East India company was responsible for supplying thousands of tons of opium to countries such as China, making huge profits in the process. When China tried to stop the import of opium, the British military blockaded several Chinese trading ports in the First Opium War (1839–1842). When the British eventually won this dispute, the Chinese were forced to hand over Hong Kong to the British as part of the settlement deal. Only in 1997 was this returned to Chinese hands.

In the middle of the nineteenth century, opium was so freely available that people used it as people today use alcohol or nicotine. Around 1850, the annual consumption of opium averaged 5 grammes per person, and it could be bought openly from almost any grocery shop in the country. In 1868 the first laws were made to restrict its use and to limit its availability to licensed premises (the Pharmacy Act), but these were largely ignored until greater penalties and more serious enforcement were introduced in 1908. Nevertheless, opium remained popular with soldiers during military campaigns. Until about 1916 it was still possible to purchase, from ordinary shops, kits containing morphine with syringes and needles for injection as 'a useful present for friends at the front'. This easy availability of opium ended in 1920 when, in the UK, the Dangerous Drugs Act meant that opium, morphine, and several other drugs such as cocaine, could be obtained only with a doctor's prescription and only from a registered pharmacy.

How did modern painkillers first develop?

Friedrich Serturner (1783–1841) was born in Neuhaus, near Paderborn in Germany. In 1799, when 16 years old, he heard doctors complaining that some samples of opium were more effective than others in stopping pain in their patients. It occurred to Serturner that there might be only one active substance in opium, and that the different activities could be due to different amounts of this unknown substance. Over the next few years, this young man managed to extract from opium a white powder which he then tested on himself and three friends. They all suffered severe nausea and vomiting, and slept for over 24 hours. No-one took much notice of this until 1806. In that year Serturner developed a toothache so intense that opium was unable to stop it. He took some of his powder—not as much this time as in 1799—and found that the pain disappeared. Now scientists paid attention. The chemical isolated by young Friedrich was given the name 'morphine' after the Greek god Morpheus, the god of sleep, in recognition of Serturner's original experience. Today morphine is available as a pure chemical, unadulterated by the thousands of substances which are also present in crude preparations of opium; crude opium is not now used, but pure morphine is still used as an 'analgesic' drug.

The fact that morphine and related drugs in high doses do produce sedation and sleep led to their being called 'narcotics' (narcosis means sleep). In some countries, however, the term narcotic has come to refer to any drug which may be abused or which can cause addiction.

In 1874 a team led by Frederick Pierce at St. Mary's Hospital in London made and tested a drug related to morphine. It was one of the first drugs ever produced by modifying a natural molecule. Twenty years later Heinrich Dreser (1860–1924), Director of Research for the Bayer company at Eberfeld in Germany, was seeking more powerful morphine-like drugs which would still work in patients who no longer responded to morphine. The drug he selected was the same one studied at St Mary's and which Bayer eventually marketed under the brand name 'Heroin',* the name reflecting the feeling that this was a heroic drug, or perhaps a drug for heroes. Heroin certainly is a more powerful painkiller but, as we now know, it is also much more likely than morphine to produce addiction. Within four years of heroin's introduction to medicine in 1898 it was the subject of laws in many countries prohibiting its use.

Heroin is certainly a painkiller, and produces psychological and physical dependence, as does morphine. In fact, most of the effects of heroin are due to its being changed into morphine in the brain. The difference is that heroin passes into the brain much more quickly than morphine so that it produces a much more dramatic and intense euphoria, or 'high' feeling, with more rapid

* The generic name is diacetylmorphine.

and much more severe withdrawal symptoms than morphine. It is, therefore, much more likely to produce dependence (addiction). Much of the danger of heroin is that it produces pleasant sensations which can lead to an individual developing a strong desire, or craving, to experience more. The effects of heroin have been described by Philip Robson* as follows:

> The modern chaser or injector of heroin is likely to report a powerful rush of pleasure, perhaps amounting to ecstasy, as the drug abruptly washes over the brain. This subsides into a delicious relaxed, dreamy, cocooned feeling as anxieties and fear melt away. The user's head may droop and his eyes close as he goes 'on the nod'. The body feels heavy, warm. If problems come into the mind at all, they are suffused with optimism and confidence that all will turn out well.

What exactly is meant by 'addiction' and tolerance?

Addictus was a Roman who built up huge debts which he was unable to repay. He was, therefore, sentenced to slavery under those to whom he was in debt. The word addiction has, as a result, come to refer to the state in which an individual has succumbed to the pleasures of a drug and, in order partly to avoid the effects of withdrawal, has become enslaved by its effects.

Addiction, or dependence, is a term which is often misunderstood. It is not the case that anyone who takes a dose of morphine will become instantly dependent on it for life. Some individuals, certainly, will find the sensations of warmth, satisfaction and well-being produced by a single injection so over-whelming that they will come back for more. Most people, however, may not become addicted until after several doses, the euphoria which the drug produces becoming stronger each time, until they become dependent on it— they may feel that they cannot live without the pleasurable sensations given by the drug. Some people, on the other hand, may have many doses of morphine and enjoy the feelings it induces, but do not feel the need for it when it is not necessary for medical purposes.

(Unfortunately not all addictive drugs have this useful time interval before a patient becomes hopelessly dependent on them. Drugs such as 'crack', a potent variant of cocaine (*see* Chapter 24) may make users dependent on them after only one or two doses. They are, therefore, of great danger to people who try to experiment with taking drugs for fun: after a single trial people may find themselves unable to give up the drug.)

When taken by mouth, morphine is absorbed sufficiently slowly that any feeling of well-being, or euphoria, is relatively mild, and addiction occurs only if the drug is consumed in large quantities. Dependence became a major problem only in the nineteenth century after the invention of the hypodermic syringe

* From *Forbidden drugs*, 1995, Oxford University Press, p. 142.

and needle by a Scotsman, Alexander Wood, working in Edinburgh in 1855. This allowed drugs to be given rapidly and directly into the bloodstream. The rush of morphine into the brain gives a feeling of pleasure, relaxation, and emotional warmth which causes some people to become addicted. Morphine gets into the brain almost as quickly after smoking opium, as the drug passes rapidly across the lungs into the bloodstream and then into the brain. Opium addiction is, therefore, quite common in countries which permit opium smoking.

Since sudden withdrawal from morphine or heroin causes withdrawal symptoms, which can be extremely severe and unpleasant, modern treatment aims to achieve a more gradual withdrawal from the drugs. This is achieved by replacing it with another drug which leaves the body more slowly. The body is thus allowed to adapt to the falling levels of drug gradually over several weeks rather than over a few days. The drug usually used for this substitution therapy is methadone, developed in Germany to compensate for reduced supplies of morphine during the second World War. It was originally called Dolophine, after Adolf Hitler.

Tolerance

Related to addiction is the problem of tolerance. After the first few doses, the body starts to become used to the morphine so that, for the same amount of pain relief (analgesia), the dose needed has to be progressively increased. After regular daily treatment for a few weeks, a patient may need more than one hundred times more morphine than at the start of treatment. Unfortunately, patients become tolerant to its pain-relieving action more easily than to its euphoric activity, so increasing the dose to achieve the same reduction of pain may cause a proportionately greater degree of euphoria. The longer treatment is continued, therefore, the more likely it is that a person will become addicted.

Physical and psychological dependence

Addiction, or dependence as it is known scientifically, is a two-headed monster. On the one hand there is the psychological driving force of desire for the beautiful feelings of euphoria, much as sexual activity is driven by desire for the feelings of pleasure and orgasm. This is known as 'psychological dependence'. On the other hand there are exceedingly unpleasant consequences if the craving for morphine is not fulfilled. A person experiences very strong 'withdrawal symptoms' within about two days of the last dose. These symptoms are very unpleasant but not usually life-threatening, sometimes being likened to a severe bout of influenza—restlessness, runny nose (rhinorrhoea), fever, intense sweating, nausea and vomiting, cramps, depression, trembling, aches and pains, dehydration, diarrhoea, insomnia, and irritability. They also include pilo-erection, the scientific word for 'goose pimples' or 'gooseflesh', the symptom which is thought to account for the expression 'going cold turkey' to describe addicts undergoing withdrawal from drugs. These, therefore, are the signs and symptoms of 'physical dependence' and they are a major factor in keeping people addicted to a drug. However, the main reason for addiction does not seem to be the desire to avoid this physical unpleasantness, but the desire to enjoy the psychological effects. If an addict is helped through the withdrawal phase (which lasts about ten days) he or she still feels a strong feeling of need— a craving—for the drug which lasts for several months and is often the reason people return to their addiction.

Another reason for believing that the psychological aspects of taking morphine are of major importance in causing dependence is that dependence is far more likely to occur among people taking drugs for social or 'recreational' reasons, than in patients receiving morphine to relieve pain. Patients should be reassured that addiction is rarely seen when drugs are given for pain relief, unless very high doses are given for a long time. The importance of the situation in which drugs are taken is also illustrated by the fact that 90 per cent of American soldiers who used heroin regularly while serving in the Vietnam war have never used it since returning home.

What causes tolerance and dependence?

This question can be answered at two levels. Firstly, there are areas of the brain which seem to make up a 'reward' system. When these are stimulated by drugs, they generate the feelings of craving which drive us to obtain and consume more drugs. The reward system is described more fully in Chapter 24.

Secondly, single cells adapt to the presence of addictive drugs. Suppose a drug such as morphine occupies a receptor R in the cell walls which usually responds to a transmitter (T) (Fig. 6.2); the cells then adapt by increasing the number of receptors they produce so that some are available to combine with T, even in the continued presence of morphine. Because morphine now occupies only a fraction of the available receptors, its effects will be less than before, so a higher dose will be needed to achieve the same effect. This sequence will be repeated as long as morphine is being taken, with ever-increasing doses needed to produce effects. This is the development of tolerance.

If, after several doses, morphine is withdrawn suddenly, the cells will find that they have a very large number of receptors for which there is no morphine to interact, but which the transmitter T can stimulate. This abnormal degree of activation by T causes the effects we call 'withdrawal' symptoms.

Other problems with opiate drugs

In addition to causing addiction, morphine, heroin, and several other opiate drugs (those present in opium) may cause nausea and vomiting. This may even suppress the activity of those parts of the brain responsible for breathing.

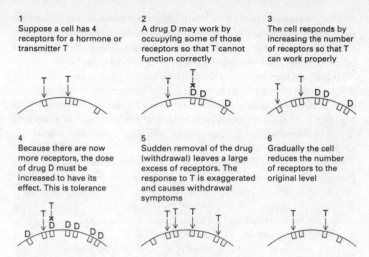

1
Suppose a cell has 4 receptors for a hormone or transmitter T

2
A drug D may work by occupying some of those receptors so that T cannot function correctly

3
The cell responds by increasing the number of receptors so that T can work properly

4
Because there are now more receptors, the dose of drug D must be increased to have its effect. This is tolerance

5
Sudden removal of the drug (withdrawal) leaves a large excess of receptors. The response to T is exaggerated and causes withdrawal symptoms

6
Gradually the cell reduces the number of receptors to the original level

Fig. 6.2 How our cells become tolerant to a drug and dependent upon it (the basis of drug dependence or addiction).

Breathing is normally controlled by a part of the brain known as the 'respiratory centre', towards the back of the brain. This sends electrical messages out along the nerves to the diaphragm and to the muscles which move the ribs to make us breathe in. When these messages stop a few seconds later, the muscles of breathing, or respiration, relax and the elasticity of the chest tissues squeeze air out of the lungs. The cycle is then repeated for the next breath. The cells which make up the respiratory centre of the brain are sensitive to the level of carbon dioxide in the blood. It is the gradual rise in carbon dioxide level which helps to start a new breath cycle. This is partly why we breathe more quickly when we exercise, as active muscles generate much more carbon dioxide than resting ones. One effect of morphine is to reduce the sensitivity of the respiratory centre to carbon dioxide and to depress the automatic activity of this region, so that breathing becomes slower and may stop completely during sleep, resulting in death.

Since patients become tolerant to the pain-relieving effects of morphine more rapidly than to the respiratory depressant effects, there is a real danger that increasing the dose to achieve satisfactory pain relief may cause so great a depression of breathing that the patient dies. Doctors are, of course, well aware of this problem and are able to avoid it, but drug addicts are frequently at risk of dying from the suppression of breathing.

It is particularly important that drugs such as morphine, which have a generally depressant effect on the brain, should not be taken at the same time as other depressants such as alcohol. Generally speaking, two such depressants will enhance each other's effects, producing a much greater effect than either substance alone, and increasing the risk of coma or even death.

Fortunately, there are several drugs which are morphine antagonists, that is they block the effects of morphine and similar compounds on their receptors in the cells. One of these is naloxone. If this is administered to a patient who has taken or received too much morphine, it will displace morphine from its receptors and reverse most of its effects, including those of pain relief and suppression of breathing.

Another problem with morphine is that it causes several groups of cells around the body, known as mast cells,* to release histamine into the bloodstream. Histamine can lower blood pressure, sometimes leading to fainting. It also contracts the muscles in the walls of the airways—the trachea and bronchi —reducing the flow of air into the lungs. Morphine may sometimes, therefore, precipitate an attack of asthma in susceptible subjects.

Finally, morphine inhibits the action of muscles in the stomach and intestine, reducing the movement of food along the gut and thereby causing constipation. It does this by blocking the release from nerves of acetylcholine, which normally maintains movement of food through the gut by contracting the muscles of the intestine.

What about more modern opiate-like drugs?

Because morphine and heroin produce so many problems, the pharmaceutical industry has spent billions (in any currency) developing pain-killing drugs which provide a better and safer alternative: drugs which do not inhibit breathing, do not trigger asthma, and do not cause addiction. The industry's chemists have synthesized thousands of chemicals differing from morphine by a few atoms here and there, and many alternative drugs are now available (Table 6.1, p. 103). Some of these are important improvements on morphine. There have been many successful attempts to produce drugs such as pethidine (meperidine) which are chemically quite unlike opiates, but those which have good pain-killing activity still produce some dependence.

Other drugs, although largely free from some of the dangers of morphine, bring their own particular risks and side-effects. Pentazocine, butorphanol, and nalbuphine may provoke vivid dreams or even hallucinations in some people.

The two most promising drugs are meptazinol and tramadol. Both act on the brain to produce analgesia, but have only weak actions at the mu-receptors (*see below*) which are involved in the analgesic and respiratory effects and the

* Mast cells are similar to white blood cells but are found within the tissues of the body.

addictive properties of drugs. As a result, both drugs produce analgesia without any depression of breathing and they do not seem to be addictive.

How do morphine-like painkillers work?

This question needs to be answered at two levels—that of the whole animal* and that of the cell. At the level of the whole animal opiates work by suppressing the brain's reaction to pain. If a person has an injury which causes great pain, they are usually given opiate drugs. These work on what are called the 'higher' levels of the brain, such as the cerebral cortex, so that patients report that they can still feel the pain, but that they are much less worried about it. It is as though the opiates eliminate the anxiety, fear, and concern about pain, rather than the pain itself. This action is quite different from the effects of drugs which reduce anxiety about life in general (such as the benzodiazepines, Chapter 13) as these do not alter patients' reactions to pain.

At the cellular level, we need to consider the cell walls and their receptors. Like most other drugs discussed in this book, morphine acts on receptors in the walls of cells. For a long time it was a great puzzle that the brains of animals (including humans) should respond to small amounts of morphine when there was no evidence that those same animals produced morphine. Why should the brain have receptors to respond to morphine produced by poppies? In the early 1970s several pharmacologists including Candace Pert and Solomon Snyder at Johns Hopkins University in the USA demonstrated that there were receptors for morphine in the brain, suggesting that animals might be able to produce chemicals related to morphine and which could act on the morphine receptor. The biological activity of morphine might simply be an accident in which the morphine molecule was able to fit onto a receptor intended for a different substance.†

The hunt then began by research groups throughout the world to find the animal equivalent of morphine. The winners were a group of pharmacologists in Aberdeen, Scotland, which included Hans Kosterlitz (1900–1996) and John Hughes. Hughes processed extracts of cattle brains from the local abattoir, separating out individual chemicals and then testing them to see whether their effects were similar to those of morphine. After about three years work, Hughes had isolated two substances which he called 'enkephalins'. These were quite

---

* Human beings are animals.

† No-one knows whether chemicals such as morphine (and others discussed later in this book such as strychnine, cocaine, and caffeine) are produced by plants for some biological purpose. Some of these chemicals may be waste by-products of normal biochemical reactions in the plants. Others may help to determine the growth, shape, size, and colour of the plant, while others may have evolved by protecting the plant from unwanted attackers. An animal which eats a few nuts of *Nux vomica*, for example, will soon die or at least feel rather unwell from strychnine poisoning, and is unlikely to return for more.

small molecules known as pentapeptides since each was made of five amino acids.

Hughes had been testing the different chemicals he obtained from the brains using several biological preparations which produced characteristic responses to morphine. These included the *vasa deferentia* of mice, in which morphine inhibited the release of norepinephrine, and the guinea-pig ileum in which morphine reduced the release of acetylcholine. Not only did the enkephalins have the same effects as morphine on these test systems, but the effects could be prevented by naloxone. Naloxone blocks the receptors for morphine and some related substances but does not affect, for example, receptors for other substances such as histamine, epinephrine, or insulin.

Soon after Hughes' discovery, it was realized that the enkephalin molecules were themselves part of larger molecules which were given the name endorphins. There appear to be several families of these 'opioid peptides'—molecules made up of amino acids but having actions related in some way to morphine and the other opiates. It seems that there are also several corresponding families of receptor, and the challenge facing pharmacologists is to identify which actions of the various morphine-related drugs are due to actions on which receptors.

Opiate receptors?

Just as there are alpha (α) and beta (β) receptors for epinephrine and M and N receptors for acetycholine (*see* Chapter 1), the opiate analgesics act on receptor molecules in the walls of nerve cells. The receptors for morphine and other opiate analgesics are of several types, known as the mu (Greek μ), kappa (κ), and delta (δ) receptors. Each of these has a different range of effects. The μ receptors produce analgesia but also euphoria and respiratory depression, and they seem to be largely responsible for the dependence on morphine. The κ and δ receptors also produce some pain relief, but the κ receptors can also cause some sedation. Activation of the κ receptors, however, does not usually induce addiction and may even reduce the ability of morphine to do so. One of the challenges facing pharmacologists is to create new opiates which act selectively on, say, the κ or δ receptors to produce analgesia without addiction or respiratory depression. One very promising drug is buprenorphine, which is not only an agonist at κ and δ receptors, but is also an antagonist at μ receptors.

Where are these receptors?

The receptors for morphine-like analgesics are in parts of the nervous system concerned with the feelings of pain. These include the spinal cord and the back of the brain.

The Spinal Cord

We have already seen that when any part of the body is stimulated, whether by touch, pressure, a warm or cold object, or movement of a hair, the stimulus initiates activity in a sensory cell which is specialized to respond to that stimulus. Each sensory cell is part of, or is connected to, a nerve fibre and it responds to a stimulus by producing a burst of electrical activity which travels along the nerve towards the spinal cord. Soon after the electrical impulse enters the cord, the nerve fibres release 'neurotransmitters' (*see* Chapter 1) which, in turn, stimulate or depress other cells in the area. Some of these cells send electrical 'messages' in the form of impulses travelling into the brain where they make us aware of the stimulus.

Pain is experienced in the same sort of way, except that the stimulus is usually the result of damage to part of the body—a cut, a knock, a burn. The damaging stimulus activates many sensory cells, some of which may be activated to a very abnormal, excessive degree. In addition, most tissues have free nerve endings, not associated with specialized sensory cells, which are activated by the various chemicals released by damaged cells—histamine, 5HT, prostaglandins, kinins, and other peptides. Together, this rather chaotic activation of nerve fibres sends signals to the spinal cord and brain that tissue damage has occurred or is likely to occur very soon. Our awareness of this is what we call pain.

The enkephalins and endorphins are produced by the brain and spinal cord during stress and they normally limit the amount of the chemical transmitters released by the incoming, sensory, nerve fibres. This is similar to the 'fight or flight' concept (*see* Chapter 1). When an animal is threatened or attacked it is vital that the brain ignores pain and protects itself from worse damage by fighting the adversary or fleeing the scene. The enkephalins are especially active in suppressing transmitter release from the nerves associated with free nerve endings. By acting upon the same receptors as the enkephalins and endorphins, morphine-like analgesics mimic this inhibition of transmitter release and suppress the transmission of 'painful' information from the tissues to the spinal cord and onwards to the brain.

The brain

Another part of the body which contains opiate receptors (receptors for enkephalins and endorphins) is in the back of the brain, an area known as the periaqueductal grey matter (PAG). This area sends nerve fibres to those parts of the spinal cord which receive sensory information from the skin and other tissues. These nerves trigger the local release of enkephalins and turn off the transmission of pain-related information. One fascinating aspect of this pathway is that it can be stimulated by nervous messages from higher parts of the brain: areas such as the cortex, which is responsible for our ability to think and reason, and from areas concerned with our moods and emotions. It is probably this pathway which is responsible for the fact that serious sportsmen and sportswomen and military personnel can continue playing or fighting even when they sustain serious injury. The enormous drive and committment of these people results in a suppression of pain sensitivity which dulls the pain produced by injury during a match or battle. Only when they are removed from the situation do they begin to feel pain.

Drugs of the future

Although many laboratories are trying to develop new drugs related to opiates but lacking their problems, there are several other ways in which drugs could be used to block pain. The most promising approach is to block the transfer of signals from the sensory nerve fibres in the skin into the spinal cord. The neurotransmitters involved in the transfer of information include the amino acid glutamate, peptides called tachykinins, and ATP. Several pharmaceutical companies and university laboratories are producing drugs which can block the effects of these transmitters. Since they have no effect on opiate receptors they should have none of the side-effects of morphine-like drugs and should not produce dependence.

Many animals and plants produce poisonous substances with which to kill or paralyse prey (see Chapter 25), and many of these have been studied by pharmacologists. A marine snail, Conus magus, produces a chemical which blocks the movement of calcium ions into nerve endings. As a result the nerves cannot release their transmitters. Since the release of transmitters is greatest from those nerves which are being activated strongly by painful stimuli or events, is it possible that the snail toxin could reduce the transfer of painful signals with much less effect on normal, sensory stimuli such as touch?

Vandana Mathur and colleagues at the American Neurex Corporation have shown that this is so. They have named the active chemical ziconotide and have shown that it blocks not only pain in animals but also in patients in whom pain could not be controlled fully by opiates. The drug is almost the only one we have which can control pain so intense that patients describe it as 'absolutely unbearable'. It is often pain which arises from a phantom limb—after amputation of a limb the damaged nerves may give rise to severe pain which is resistant to opiate drugs. Ziconotide is not associated with dependence or respiratory depression, and could represent the first in a line of new, safer drugs to treat very severe pain by an entirely new mechanism of action.

Another natural chemical is epibatidine, produced by the Ecuador tree frog and first isolated by John Daly at the National Institute of Health in Bethesda, USA. This substance is more than 200 times more effective than morphine as a painkiller, but because it is a totally different type of chemical it should not produce the problems of tolerance and addiction seen with opiates.

Table 6.1 Analgesic (painkiller) drugs

Mild analgesics	Opiate analgesics
acemetacin	alfentanil
acetaminophen (paracetamol)	anileridine (USA)
acetylsalicylic acid (aspirin)	buprenorphine
aspirin	butorphanol
benorylate*	codeine
benzydamine	dextromoramide
diclofenac	dextropopoxyphene
diflunisal	dezocine (USA)
etodolac	diamorphine (heroin)
fenbufen	dihydrocodeine
fenoprofen	dipipanone
ibuprofen	ethoheptazine
indomethacin	ethylmorphine
ketoprofen	fentanyl
meclofenamate (USA)	heroin (diamorphine)
mefenamic acid	hydrocodone (USA)
naproxen	hydromorphone (USA)
nefopam	levomethadyl (USA)
paracetamol (acetaminophen)	levorphanol (USA)
salicylate	meperidine (pethidine)
	meptazinol
Opiate antagonists	methadone
nalmefene	morphine
naloxone	nabumetone
	nalbuphine
Other analgesic agents	oxycodone (USA)
capsaicin	oxymorphone (USA)
phenazone (USA)	pentazocine
	pethidine (meperidine)
	phenazocine
	phenoperidine
	sufentanil (USA)
	tramadol

* Benorylate is converted in the body to aspirin and paracetamol. Like aspirin, it should not be given to children under 12 years of age.

Summary

- *Pain is produced when cells and tissues are damaged. The damage releases substances such as histamine, bradykinin, and prostaglandins which increase the sensitivity of nerve endings and cause the sensations of aching and pain.*
- *Aspirin and other mild analgesics (painkillers) stop the formation of prostaglandins and this reduces pain. They are known as non-steroidal anti-inflammatory drugs (NSAIDs). They also reduce high body temperature (anti-pyretic effect).*
- *By stopping the formation of prostaglandins, aspirin and similar drugs also reduce blood clotting and are now recommended for people who have had one heart attack, to reduce the chance of another.*
- *Paracetamol (acetaminophen) and ibuprofen are safer than aspirin, but paracetamol does not reduce inflammation.*
- *The long-term consumption of mild analgesics can cause stomach and kidney damage.*
- *New NSAIDs being developed are selective inhibitors or the enzyme COX-2. They should produce pain relief and reduce inflammation without dangerous side-effects on the stomach and kidney.*
- *Morphine and related chemicals from opium are much stronger analgesics. They act on the brain, interacting with receptors for enkephalins and endorphins—hormones produced in the brain.*
- *Some of these drugs can produce dependence (addiction) and can depress breathing. There is a continuing search for better and safer strong analgesics, of which meptazinol and tramadol show some promise.*

CHAPTER 7

Headaches and migraine

The first time I thought I was going blind. I was at work, just talking to a colleague, and I looked at her and saw lights and she was disappearing. I could see only half of her. I went home terrified. [The doctor] diagnosed it as migraine immediately. That was thirty-two years ago. I started by getting the classical ones. Things would change colour. I would get the flashing lights and the headache would come on within half an hour once they had stopped. ... I would get pins and needles in my face. I went through one point when I couldn't speak properly. It was as if the migraine was in my mouth and I was talking rubbish.*

Headaches

Headaches can be a real nuisance—disrupting work, and social and domestic relationships. Fortunately most people suffer from headaches only occasionally, such as after a long, dehydrating airline flight, overindulgence in alcohol, or as an accompaniment to a cold or influenza. They can also be brought on by drinking something cold or by abstaining from caffeine for a day or two.

We do not really understand what causes headaches in most of these situations. The view most popular amongst clinicians and scientists is that headaches are usually due to tension in the muscles of the head and neck. If we are worried, for example, we tend to frown and unconsciously contract muscles around the head, which stretch nerve endings in the muscles and surrounding tissues. This in turn causes the pain we call headache (Fig. 7.2). Very often people start to worry about a headache and so enter a vicious circle. This is the most common type of headache and is known as a 'tension headache'. The best way to treat such headaches is to break this cycle by taking a weak pain-killing drug such as paracetamol (see Chapter 6). Tension headaches usually involve a constant level of pain, rather than the throbbing headache of migraine.

Headaches can also be caused by many other factors, such as osteoarthritis in the neck in older people, causing pain which feels as if it comes from the

* Related by the patient Susan and reproduced from *The migraine handbook* by J. Lewis, British Migraine Association, Vermilion Publishers, London, 1993.

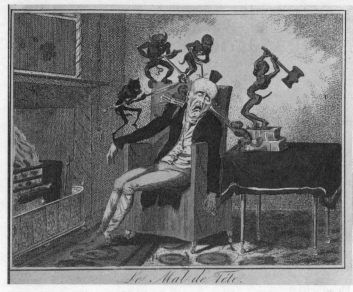

Fig. 7.1 'Headache'—an etching by W. Hogarth, summing up the distress which a severe headache can cause. (Science Photo Library)

head. Some people suffer from severe headaches several times over a period of a few days or weeks, and then will be trouble-free for months or years before experiencing another period of repeated headaches. Because of their arrival in closely-spaced groups, these are known as 'cluster headaches'.

Treatment

The usual treatment for these forms of headache is to use painkillers such as paracetamol or ibuprofen (*see* Chapter 6) which prevent the formation of the prostaglandin hormones. Ibuprofen acts in the skin and muscles so that prostaglandins are unable to increase the sensitivity of nerve endings in these tissues. Paracetamol acts mainly in the brain, where prostaglandins affect our awareness of pain.

Migraine

Migraines, which affect around 5 per cent of men and 15 per cent of women, are in a different league from a routine tension headache. A migraine attack sometimes begins hours or days before the actual headache, with what is called the 'prodromal phase'. The patient may yawn excessively or crave some foods, with unusual tiredness or euphoria. This may lead to an 'aura'—an abnormal sensory phenomenon which may include flashing zig-zag lights, smells, or visual hallucination-like images and which can itself occur several hours before the onset of the headache.* When it occurs, the migraine headache is usually an extremely severe, intense, throbbing headache that may last for hours or days. It is so severe that sufferers cannot think clearly and are often unable to work. Migraines are sometimes associated with nausea and vomiting.

The cause of migraines is believed to lie partly in the state of the blood vessels in the head. The aura phase seems to be due to a loss of activity in groups of nerve cells in the brain. This loss of function spreads across the brain at a rate of about 3 mm per minute and is called 'spreading depression'. Spreading depression is accompanied by a reduced blood flow through blood vessels in the brain and together these two phenomena cause the aural images. The spread across the brain explains why many of the flashing lights and other visual phenomena of the aura usually begin very small and gradually expand in size over several minutes.

This phase is followed by relaxation of the blood vessels (Fig. 7.2). As vessels relax, the nerve endings in their walls become stretched. Imagine a length of flexible rubber tube around which you have tightly wrapped a piece of tissue paper. If you then force something through the tube which stretches the walls (increasing the diameter of the tube), that stretch will tear the surrounding paper. In the same way if the walls of blood vessels relax, increasing the diameter of the vessel too much, this will stretch and damage the delicate nerve endings which run along them. The stretch will stimulate the nerve endings, which will cause pain.

The stretch of nerve endings also causes the formation and release of several chemicals, such as prostaglandins and peptide hormones† similar to those discussed in Chapter 6 and which are associated with tissue damage and inflammation. These are chemicals which further increase the sensitivity of the nerve endings to stretch. They also increase the leakiness of blood vessels, so that more substances gain access to the nerve endings and increase the pain, and cause mast cells‡ to release their load of chemicals including histamine and yet more pain-producing peptides.

People who develop migraines regularly (migraineurs) have lower than

---

* In older people the aura may occur without being followed by a headache. Migraine is often classified as 'classic migraine' (migraine with a preceding aura) or 'common migraine' (migraine without an aura).

† These include substance P, kinins, calcitonin gene related peptide (CGRP), and others.

‡ Mast cells are similar to white blood cells, but are found in and around tissues such as blood vessels.

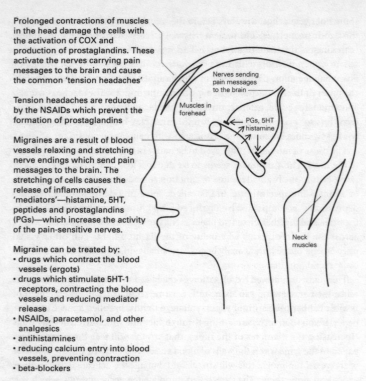

Prolonged contractions of muscles in the head damage the cells with the activation of COX and production of prostaglandins. These activate the nerves carrying pain messages to the brain and cause the common 'tension headaches'

Tension headaches are reduced by the NSAIDs which prevent the formation of prostaglandins

Migraines are a result of blood vessels relaxing and stretching nerve endings which send pain messages to the brain. The stretching of cells causes the release of inflammatory 'mediators'—histamine, 5HT, peptides and prostaglandins (PGs)—which increase the activity of the pain-sensitive nerves.

Migraine can be treated by:
• drugs which contract the blood vessels (ergots)
• drugs which stimulate 5HT-1 receptors, contracting the blood vessels and reducing mediator release
• NSAIDs, paracetamol, and other analgesics
• antihistamines
• reducing calcium entry into blood vessels, preventing contraction
• beta-blockers

Nerves sending pain messages to the brain

Muscles in forehead

PGs, 5HT, histamine

Neck muscles

Fig. 7.2 The actions of drugs used to treat headaches and migraine.

normal amounts of beta-endorphin in their blood. This is one of the body's own chemicals which helps to control pain sensitivity (*see* Chapter 6), so these patients may be more sensitive than normal people to some types of pain, such as that of the migraine headache.

Treatment

In some people migraines are triggered by chemicals in the food, such as amines in wine or cheese, and caffeine in coffee or chocolate. If a trigger can be identified, the best treatment, obviously, is to avoid it.

Mild migraines can be treated like most other headaches by taking painkillers such as paracetamol (*see* Chapter 6) which suppress the formation of prostaglandins by inhibiting the activity of the enzyme, COX, which produces them.

Some of these drugs, the NSAIDS, have anti-inflammatory activity as well as analgesic properties, and some of them, such as tolfenamic acid, seem to be especially effective in migraine. These drugs must be taken early in the course of an attack if they are to have much effect. They are not very effective in reducing the pain of a more severe migraine and in any case it is not desirable to take relatively large doses of aspirin-like drugs for days or weeks with the potential danger of ulcers and bleeding which accompany their use. A better strategy is to *prevent* a migraine attack, or at least to abort it, at the first signs of an impending attack.

Ergot

One group of drugs, the ergot alkaloids, has been used in the treatment of migraines for several years (Table 7.1, p. 115). Ergot is a fungus, *Claviceps purpurea*, which can attack rye plants. In a dry year there may be little infection, but this is much greater in a wet season. Rye grown today is inspected carefully for *Claviceps* infection. The amount of rye rejected by the inspectors varies, depending mainly on the recent climate, but it ranges between about 1 and 30%. *Claviceps* caused several serious infections in the Middle Ages, but its effects were not recognized by medical people at the time. Infected plants were simply harvested and processed with normal plants so that large numbers of people ate the fungus in the rye-based bread that was popular then. Those who ate infected products developed what became known as 'St Anthony's Fire', in which the blood vessels of the body, especially those of the exposed skin on hands and feet, contracted very tightly, shutting off the blood supply to those parts of the body. As a result the tissues of the hands and feet became blackened and dead, partly due to gangrene and partly due to infection of the skin with bacteria, which cause a condition known as 'erysipelas'. In the Middle Ages, however, people believed that sufferers had been burned by the fire of St Anthony, hence the name. The condition produced great pain and in many cases was fatal.

Some cases of 'witchcraft' in the Middle Ages may well have been due to poisoning by ergot, as those affected usually experience hallucinations and crawling sensations in the skin, both of which were said to be symptoms of some of those accused of being witches.

There are references to the effects of *Claviceps* in more ancient writings. There is an Assyrian reference dated about 600 BC to the 'noxious pustule in the ear of grain', and slightly later references to 'noxious grasses that cause pregnant women to drop the womb'. We now know that this last effect, premature labour, occurs because the ergot chemicals cause contractions of the womb or uterus, inducing early childbirth. These effects were first reported in detail by Adam Lonitzer at the University of Frankfurt in 1582 and ergometrine has been used ever since both to facilitate birth and to reduce blood loss after birth by contracting the blood vessels in the wall of the womb after delivery.

The reason for the contraction of the blood vessels and uterus is that ergot produces a group of chemicals known collectively as the ergot alkaloids. Beginning with Charles Tanret, a French pharmacist, in 1875, these have been extracted from the fungus and given names such as ergotamine, ergometrine, ergocornine, and ergocryptine. Several, especially ergotamine, ergometrine, and dihydroergotamine, act directly on the alpha receptors which normally respond to epinephrine and norepinephrine, the transmitters released by nerves which control the size of the blood-vessels (*see* Chapter 1). By activating alpha-receptors the ergot alkaloids mimic the effects of nerve activity and contract the blood vessels.

As in so many instances in medicine, what was a tragedy for some families in the Middle Ages led to a valuable treatment for millions of migraine sufferers in the twentieth century. If ergotamine or ergometrine are taken, ideally at the first sign of the aura which precedes a migraine, the blood vessels in the head can be made to contract partially, thus reversing the relaxation and stretching which causes the headache and nausea. Patients normally take these drugs only for a few days or in very low doses so there is little danger of the long-term effects such as tissue damage and gangrene which resulted from consuming infected bread for a year or so after each harvest five hundred years ago.

There are now many different ways of administering ergot drugs, most of them designed to increase the speed with which the drugs are absorbed by the body. The most recent preparation of dihydroergotamine is applied into the nose. This not only produces a rapid absorption into the bloodstream, but also removes some of the side-effects which result from taking the drug orally, in tablet form.

Unfortunately, ergot compounds must be taken within the first one or two hours of the first sign of a migraine, or they may be ineffective. This is because their ability to stop the release of the pain- and inflammation-producing chemicals is rather poor. Once the blood vessels have started to relax, the tissue damage and local inflammation will soon develop to the extent that the ergot-induced contraction of the vessels cannot stop their further development.

Problems

The main problems with ergot compounds are that the contraction of blood vessels reduces the blood supply to organs and this can lead to cramps in the abdomen and voluntary muscles. Ergotamine and dihydroergotamine cannot be used during pregnancy as they cause contractions of the uterus with a danger of abortion or premature labour.

The greatest problem is the production of ergotamine headaches. Ergotamine has little effect once the dilatation of vessels has started and local tissue damage and inflammation have begun. If sufferers continue to take ergotamine, they may keep blood vessels in the head contracted for so long that parts of the head will be deprived of blood and will start to show their own damage and inflammation. By this stage the patient is trapped. If she continues to take ergotamine she will shut off the blood supply to tissue in the head and prolong her headache; if she stops taking the ergotamine, the blood vessels in the head will all dilate and cause yet more headache. The patient is in a vicious circle.

The only way out of this is to reduce the dose of ergotamine gradually over several weeks. The patient will almost certainly have a continuous headache over that period, but at the end of it she will be free from ergotamine. She must then remember to take the drug only during the first 2 hours of an imminent attack, and no more for at least 24 hours.

Sumatriptan

Some of the ergot alkaloids can, in addition to activating alpha receptors, interact with receptors for another neurotransmitter 5HT.* 5HT is sometimes known as serotonin because it can increase the tone of involuntary muscle. It can, therefore, contract blood vessels. In fact 5HT activates at least a dozen different types of receptor with different effects, but one group of these seems to be important to our discussion of migraine. This is the 5HT-1 receptor group.

There are 5HT-1 receptors on blood vessels in the head and activation of these causes contraction just as does activation of alpha receptors for norepinephrine. The important difference between 5HT-1 receptors and alpha receptors for norepinephrine is that the 5HT-1 receptors do not cause contraction of other vessels in the body. Alpha receptors, when activated by norepinephrine cause widespread contraction with the possibility of side-effects (such as gangrene) as we have just described. 5HT-1 receptors only cause contraction of the blood vessels in the head. The pharmaceutical industry, therefore, became involved in a hunt for chemicals which would activate 5HT-1 receptors so that they could be used to prevent migraine without causing all the potential problems of ergot alkaloids.

A research team at Glaxo Pharmaceuticals led by the pharmacologist Pat Humphrey undertook several years of research which resulted in the discovery of a drug with this profile. This was sumatriptan, which was introduced into medicine by Glaxo (now GlaxoWellcome) in 1992. This is now one of the most valuable drugs for migraine, and has few side-effects, although it can cause feelings of tightness and pain in the chest which resemble angina. It has the advantage over ergotamine that it can abort a migraine at any stage of an attack,

* 5-hydroxytryptamine.

whereas ergotamine works best only if taken within the first one or two hours of the first signs of an attack. Why is this?

Inflammation

If migraine often lasts for several days or longer, why does a brief course of treatment at the onset of symptoms prevent or abort the development of a full-blown attack? The answer to this question seems to have many parallels with asthma (*see* Chapter 2) where the initial asthmatic attack can provoke the release of a series of chemicals, known as inflammatory mediators, which cause a delayed but relatively long-lasting (days or weeks) inflammation of the airways. In the same way, it looks as though the initial stretching of blood vessels and the damage caused to the nerve endings causes the release of prostaglandins, peptides, and enzymes which set up a local inflammatory response around the vessels. This leads to the local accumulation of fluid, increased chemical sensitivity of the nerve endings, and an accumulation of white blood cells.

Some of these changes interact with each other. Some of the peptides and proteins, such as tachykinins and cytokines, can trigger the release of prostaglandins from white blood cells. The prostaglandins and cytokines then attract more cells into the area and further increase nerve sensitivity. When the additional white blood cells arrive, they release more cytokines. In other words, a series of vicious circles is established which may prolong the inflammation for days. This inflammation is believed to account for the long duration of many migraine attacks. By preventing the initial relaxation of vessels using ergotamine or sumatriptan, the whole sequence can be prevented.

But does this mean that once relaxation has occurred there is little we can do to abort a migraine attack in progress except to take large doses of painkillers? Ergotamine affects only blood vessel diameter, not the inflammation, so it has relatively little effect once a migraine headache has started. However, activation of the 5HT-1 receptors by sumatriptan not only prevents relaxation of the vessels but also inhibits secretion of the inflammatory mediators. Apparently there are some 5HT-1 receptors on the tissues around the blood vessels and on the nerve endings. When these are activated by sumatriptan, they reduce mediator release and suppress the inflammation.

Several drugs similar to sumatriptan have now become available, including naratriptan and zolmitriptan, but these seem to have no real advantages or disadvantages over sumatriptan. Another related drug, eletriptan, is being tested clinically by Pfizer.

Isometheptene

Isometheptene is not related to the ergot compounds, but has a similar action, acting on alpha receptors on the blood vessels and causing them to contract.

Clonidine

Clonidine is an agonist at alpha-receptors for norepinephrine and thereby causes contraction of blood vessels. It is available for use in migraine, on the principle that this effect is similar to that of ergotamine.

Metoclopramide

In many people suffering from a migraine, movements of the stomach and intestine are reduced. This means that some drugs, including those being taken to treat the migraine, will not be absorbed well and will take much longer to act. Substances such as aspirin may stay in the stomach long enough to cause marked irritation and bleeding. The drug metoclopramide (*see* Chapter 4) can be used in this situation. It can be given by injection and increases movements of the stomach and intestine, so improving the absorption of drugs.

Prevention of frequent attacks

β-blockers

Many patients experience a migraine only occasionally, but some have two or more attacks each month. These are considered to be frequent, and they can seriously disrupt a person's life. Fortunately, there are some drugs which seem to prevent the occurrence of frequent migraines, or at least to reduce their frequency. These include propranolol, one of the first beta-blockers introduced in 1962, timolol, nadolol, and metoprolol. All these drugs are beta-blockers, but their antimigraine activity may not be due to blocking beta-receptors (*see* Chapter 1) because several other beta-blockers are not effective. How propranolol and these other beta-blockers work in migraine is not yet understood. Most of these drugs, however, can precipitate asthma in susceptible people because the activation of beta-receptors normally helps to keep the airways open (*see* Chapter 2).

Antidepressant drugs

The antidepressant drugs (*see* Chapter 11), such as amitriptyline, are also effective in preventing recurrent migraines, probably because they can block alpha receptors on the blood vessels.

5HT antagonists

Although activating 5HT-1 receptors helps to stop a migraine, activation of 5HT-2 receptors makes it worse, probably because they oppose some effects of the 5HT-1 receptors. Pizotifen and cyproheptadine are drugs which block 5HT-2 receptors as well as receptors for histamine and they may be useful in patients in whom propranolol does not prevent migraines. By blocking 5HT receptors in the brain, both these drugs can increase the appetite and lead to weight gain.

Methysergide is another of the ergot alkaloids, but it has complex actions which include the ability both to activate and block 5HT receptors as well as alpha-receptors for norepinephrine. It may be worth trying when other drugs fail although it has a worrying tendency to cause scar tissue formation after prolonged use, especially at the back of the abdomen. This tissue may trap and damage other organs and if it occurs the drug must be withdrawn at once.

Antihistamines

Histamine is one of the substances released by the mast cells as a result of local damage and, as it dilates many blood vessels, it may play a small role in producing the migraine headache. Pizotifen has just been mentioned as having some antihistamine activity and oxeterone is also used as an antihistamine in the treatment of migraine.

Calcium antagonists

A final group of compounds may also be tried. These are the calcium blockers, drugs such as verapamil, nifedipine, and flunarizine, which prevent calcium from entering the muscle cells of the blood vessels and prevent their contracting. As this effect occurs on all blood vessels in the body, there is a greater possibility of side-effects, such as a fall in blood pressure and slowing of the heart.

Drug combinations

Many preparations for migraine consist of combinations of drugs. They may include a mixture of painkillers with a drug to reduce the feelings of nausea and the vomiting that often accompany more severe migraines. These anti-sickness, (or anti-emetic drugs, *see* Chapter 4) include buclizine, prochlorperazine, and cyclizine, but it must be remembered that these are antihistamine drugs and can cause drowsiness.

Another popular drug combination is ergotamine and caffeine, best known under the trade name Cafergot. Caffeine acts on receptors for a natural substance called adenosine which dilates blood vessels. By blocking these receptors, caffeine induces some contraction of the vessels. When these drugs are present in the same tablets, the similar effects of caffeine and ergotamine combine to constrict the blood vessels more effectively and suppress an impending migraine attack more completely.

Table 7.1 Drugs used in migraine

Ergot derivatives	Beta-blockers (see Chapter 2)
dihydroergotamine	metoprolol
ergotamine	nadolol
methysergide	propranolol
	timolol
5HT-1 agonists	
naratriptan	**Antihistamine**
rizatriptan	oxeterone
sumatriptan	pizotifen
zolmitriptan	
	Calcium blockers
5HT-2 antagonists	verapamil
cyproheptadine	nifedipine
methysergide	flunarizine
pizotifen	
	Other drugs
Analgesics (*see* Chapter 17)	clonidine
aspirin	isometheptene
paracetamol	
tolfenamic acid	

Summary

- *The most common headaches are caused by stress and tension in the muscles around the head and neck. They are most safely treated with mild painkillers such as paracetamol and ibuprofen.*
- *Migraines are severe headaches, often associated with dizziness, nausea, and vomiting. They are caused by relaxation of blood vessels in the head, stretching nerve endings and setting up an inflammatory reaction.*
- *Drugs to treat migraines contract the blood vessels by acting on norepinephrine receptors or 5-hydroxytryptamine (5HT) receptors. They include ergot chemicals such as ergotamine, and sumatriptan.*
- *The frequency of attacks can be reduced by drugs which prevent blood vessel contraction.*

CHAPTER 8

Parkinson's disease

Judith first noticed a slight trembling of her left hand at the age of 69. She thought little of it at first, but cut down on her drinking of tea and coffee, as she was told that the consumption of six or more strong cups a day over several years could produce a mild tremor of the hands. At first that seemed to work, but within a few weeks the tremor was back. It became progressively worse over the next year or so, spreading to the other hand. The tremor was a coarse shaking of the hands, turning back and forth at the wrist at a rate of 4 or 5 shakes a second. It was worse when she was sitting quietly. It stopped when she fell asleep, and was much less obvious when she tried to do something with her hand, such as lifting a heavy cup.

The tremor seemed to concern her husband more than Judith. When they were out shopping together, Judith would usually insist on fumbling in her purse to find money, waving away her husband's pleas to allow him to help. While Judith's husband avoided arguing too much in public, he always felt acutely embarrassed at standing by helplessly.

Soon, Judith noticed other changes too. She was finding it difficult to write: her handwriting would begin adequately, but would get smaller and smaller so that after a few sentences it was totally illegible. Her husband noticed that she was walking more slowly and not lifting her feet—more like shuffling than walking—and she was starting to stoop as she walked, as if afraid of falling over. She was even having difficulty starting to make movements. If she was standing still and then decided to go into the kitchen, it could take many seconds of concentrated effort to start her legs moving. And once she had started, she seemed to have difficulty stopping again, so she would often walk up to a cupboard or the table which would act as a brake for her. If she were sitting down, it could take a minute or two for her to shuffle her body into a position from which she could raise herself into a standing position.

The difficulty in moving eventually seemed to involve Judith's ability to talk. Her speech became rather slurred and at times she would stop in the middle of a sentence, look totally lost, and say that she had forgotten what she was saying.

Parkinson's disease

The description above is of a patient suffering from a disorder of the brain known as 'Parkinson's disease'. The disorder is named after James Parkinson, who first published a description of the disease in 1817. At the time, he called it *paralysis agitans* in view of the tremor, or agitation, of the hands, and the apparent paralysis, or difficulty in making movements. Parkinson was astute enough even in 1817 to describe the disease as distinct from 'the trembling consequences of indulgence in the drinking of spiritous liquors, that which proceeds from the immoderate employment of tea and coffee ... and that which appears to be dependent upon advanced age'.

Parkinson's disease is usually a disorder of the elderly, occurring after the age of 65. It is caused by the death of a group of nerve cells in the brain called the *substantia nigra* or 'black substance' because they look dark in appearance. The nerve processes from these cells normally extend up to another area of brain called the striatum, where they make connections (synapses) and release a chemical called dopamine as their neurotransmitter. The pathway from the *substantia nigra* to the striatum is known as the 'nigrostriatal pathway'. It was Oleh Hornykiewicz and his team at the University of Vienna who, in 1960, first examined the brains of patients with Parkinson's disease after death and showed that this pathway had degenerated and the amounts of dopamine in the diseased brains were less than one tenth of those in normal people.

The *substantia nigra* and the striatum help to control movement, including our ability to initiate movement. This is a feature of life which most of us take for granted. We move almost without thinking. We can easily perform two or more actions at the same time. Moving our limbs or our body is as natural, unconscious, and effortless as breathing.

But for the patient with Parkinson's disease this luxury has gone. With the loss of the nigrostriatal pathway, the patient has to bring all his or her attention to bear on a simple act like getting out of a chair, or starting to walk. Nor is that all. Most patients also have to contend with the marked tremor described in Judith, and with muscles which become more rigid due to their being partially contracted. Both these symptoms make the problems of moving even more difficult. The tension, or rigidity of the muscles can lead to a generalized aching, especially in the neck and arms. Fine movements such as fastening a button or cutting food are difficult, as are repetitive movements such as stirring, brushing, or writing. The loss of movement in the face can sometimes make patients appear to be intellectually vacant when in truth their mental faculties are unimpaired, but are trapped in a body which refuses to express their feelings facially or verbally.

Movements are often slow, partly due to a feeling of being about to fall over.

Patients often have the greatest difficulty walking downhill and may lose balance easily, especially when turning round. The effort of moving at all results in profound tiredness and the need for sound sleep. The lack of mouth movements and swallowing may result in saliva dribbling out of the mouth, while the lack of body movements may lead to constipation and swelling of the legs and ankles.

Patients, not unreasonably, may become depressed, and some develop a degree of intellectual impairment including loss of memory, confusion, and 'thought block' in which a thought sequence may suddenly be lost—patients may stop in mid-sentence as they forget what they were saying.

In some patients with Parkinson's disease the symptoms develop very slowly, over many years, and the patient may die before being affected too severely. In others, in whom the disease progresses more rapidly or who live to be very old, the inability to move may eventually result in their being bedridden, and requiring help for all their daily activities.

Causes of Parkinson's disease

We still do not know what causes Parkinson's disease. There is evidence for a weak hereditary link in a few cases, but this appears to determine only a predisposing factor. A theory being considered carefully is that it is caused by an environmental toxin (poison). This idea arose from the unfortunate experience of a group of young drug addicts.

James Langston, a neurologist in California, found himself one morning faced with a series of patients who seemed to have developed Parkinson's disease literally overnight. Langston soon established that these young sufferers had consumed an adulterated drug. They had consumed what they believed to be the morphine-like drug pethidine which they had bought from someone in the street. In fact the powder had been made by an amateur chemist and was a chemical called MPTP.* This can destroy the nerve cells containing dopamine within a few hours, causing the symptoms of a disease which usually takes decades to develop.

Although tragic for the young people concerned, the discovery of MPTP has had two important results for sufferers of Parkinson's disease. Firstly, by giving MPTP to animals it is now possible to produce Parkinson's disease artificially. This is a breakthrough for research as it provides a means of testing new drugs which may be of value in human patients.

Secondly, the incident has raised the possibility that Parkinson's disease in humans may be due to people being exposed to a substance like MPTP. One of the most striking possibilities is based on the similarity in the molecular

* MPTP is an abbreviation for 1-Methyl-4-phenyl-tetrahydropyridine.

structure between MPTP and herbicides such as paraquat and rotenone, used in agriculture and garden weedkillers. People living in third world countries where vast quantities of paraquat are used appear more likely to develop Parkinson's disease.

Drug treatment of Parkinson's disease

L-dopa[2]

Since the cause of Parkinson's disease is a loss of dopamine-releasing nerve cells, one approach to treating the disorder is to restore the levels of dopamine in the brain. Dopamine itself cannot be used because it will not pass readily from the blood into the brain. Within nerve cells, dopamine is produced by a series of chemical reactions catalysed by enzymes. The last stage in the sequence is the formation of dopamine from the amino acid L-dopa,* which does cross easily into the brain (Fig. 8.1). The most popular and effective treatment for Parkinson's disease in most patients, therefore, is the administration of L-dopa in tablets. The L-dopa passes into the brain, where local enzymes convert it into dopamine.

To many people, L-dopa has been a miracle drug. Oliver Sacks wrote a moving and dramatic account of the use of L-dopa in Parkinson's disease in his best-selling book *Awakenings*, of which a film was later made with the same title. Patients who may have been virtually immobile with Parkinson's disease, even for several years, suddenly come alive within an hour or so of taking L-dopa. They are able to walk easily and at will, to speak freely, and to use their hands again. In the case of Judith, she could move around her house normally, her face showed emotion and laughter where previously it had been expressionless, and she was able to communicate better than she had for months. Initial side-effects such as a feeling of nausea passed after a few days, and her life was vastly improved.

Certainly, L-dopa produces in most patients a very marked improvement in general movement, facial expression, and body posture. There is usually less effect on the tremor, swallowing, balance, and the slow initiation of movements.

Combining other drugs with L-dopa: carbidopa and benserazide

There are a few problems with this deceptively simple approach. The conversion of L-dopa into dopamine in the brain is achieved by an enzyme—dopa decarboxylase (DDC), but the same enzyme exists in the blood and body tissues. After being absorbed from the intestine, some L-dopa will be changed into dopamine before it can reach the brain. A large fraction (90 per cent or more) of a dose of L-dopa will be lost in this way. Fortunately, there are drugs

---

* Dopa, which is also known as L-dopa or Levodopa, is actually an abbreviation for the chemical 3,4-DihydrOxyPhenylAlanine.

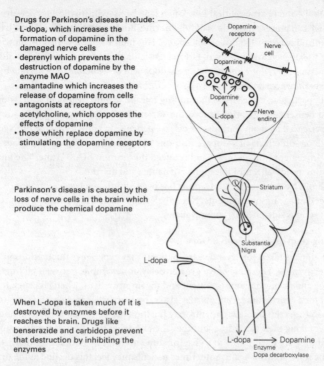

Drugs for Parkinson's disease include:
• L-dopa, which increases the
  formation of dopamine in the
  damaged nerve cells
• deprenyl which prevents the
  destruction of dopamine by the
  enzyme MAO
• amantadine which increases the
  release of dopamine from cells
• antagonists at receptors for
  acetylcholine, which opposes the
  effects of dopamine
• those which replace dopamine by
  stimulating the dopamine receptors

Parkinson's disease is caused by the
loss of nerve cells in the brain which
produce the chemical dopamine

When L-dopa is taken much of it is
destroyed by enzymes before it
reaches the brain. Drugs like
benserazide and carbidopa prevent
that destruction by inhibiting the
enzymes

Dopamine
receptors

Nerve
cell

Dopamine

Dopamine

L-dopa

Nerve
ending

Striatum

Substantia
Nigra

L-dopa

L-dopa ⟶ Dopamine
Enzyme
Dopa decarboxylase

Fig. 8.1 The actions of drugs used to treat Parkinson's disease.

which block the activity of this enzyme outside the brain. These include
carbidopa and benserazide. These are combined with L-dopa in preparations
such as Sinemet® and Madopar®, so that less dopa is lost in the gut and other
tissues and more is available to the brain. Carbidopa and benserazide themselves do not pass into the brain, so the conversion of L-dopa into dopamine in
the brain is not affected.

Most patients are nowadays given tablets which contain both L-dopa and one
of these enzyme inhibitors in the same tablet. The combination not only means
that far more L-dopa passes into the brain, but also that a lower dose can be
given and the patient has fewer side-effects.

Tolcapone and entacapone

Unfortunately for Parkinson's disease patients dopa decarboxylase is not
the only enzyme able to destroy L-dopa. Some is removed by the enzyme

COMT,* and pharmaceutical companies have been trying to produce new drugs which can prevent the actions of this enzyme. Roche pharmaceuticals have tried to introduce one such drug—tolcapone. This inhibits COMT, thereby allowing the use of even lower doses of L-dopa. Patients should experience fewer side-effects of the L-dopa and also more L-dopa will be available to penetrate into the brain where it is needed.

In particular, it is claimed that adding tolcapone onto treatment with L-dopa and benserazide greatly reduced the variations in responsiveness to L-dopa experienced by many Parkinson's disease patients. In patients having problems with on–off effects of L-dopa, tolcapone increased the duration of periods of improvement ('on' periods) and reduced the amount of 'off' time. The most common side-effects of tolcapone are nausea and diarrhoea.

From November 1998, tolcapone has been withdrawn because of reports of liver damage in some patients. Nevertheless, a similar drug, entacapone, without serious side-effects, is now available.

Long-term problems with L-Dopa

If L-dopa is taken for several years, patients may experience fluctuations in its effectiveness. There may be a greater delay, for example, between taking the drug and feeling any improvement and the improvement, when it occurs, may last for a shorter time. Patients may also experience what are known as 'on–off' periods. As this implies, patients may function perfectly well for several hours after taking their usual dose, but they then find that the effect of the drug stops and they are hardly able to move for some minutes or hours. Eventually the drug starts to work again. Sometimes patients may feel this decline in the drug effect as it starts to happen, so they can make sure that they get themselves to a safe and comfortable place. They would want to get out of a bath, for example, otherwise they could find themselves sitting in a very uncomfortable, cold bath of water. They may also turn off any food cooking in the kitchen. Some of the receptor agonist drugs described below help to smooth out these on–off periods, giving the patient a more continuous benefit from L-dopa.

Very often, however, patients may have little warning of an impending 'off' period until it is too late. This is why advanced sufferers of Parkinson's disease require watchful care and attention.

Side-effects of L-dopa

Most patients feel some nausea when they start taking L-dopa, although it usually disappears after a few days.

Unfortunately, L-dopa increases the amount of dopamine throughout the

* COMT is an abbreviation for Catechol O-Methyl Transferase.

brain: it is not confined to the nigrostriatal pathway. The areas in which dopamine levels are increased include the limbic system, which is discussed in Chapter 9. There, overactivity of dopamine neurons or receptors can cause schizophrenia. One of the major problems with L-dopa, therefore, is that after prolonged use it may induce some of the symptoms of schizophrenia, especially hallucinations, which may be vivid enough to appear as nightmares and to give the patient some very disturbed nights' sleep.

Lastly, the effect of L-dopa on the striatum may be to cause overstimulation. After some months of treatment patients may develop slow, involuntary movements in which the limbs or the trunk move almost of their own accord. The patient has the appearance of continual fidgeting, of not being able to sit or stand still. But these movements are out of the patient's control. In many cases they may be reduced by lowering the dose of L-dopa, but it may be difficult to find a dose of L-dopa which provides adequate overall improvement while not inducing these movements.

Other drugs

MAO inhibitors

An alternative to increasing the formation of dopamine in the brain by administering L-dopa, is to decrease the breakdown (metabolism) of dopamine. Dopamine is broken down by the enzyme monoamine oxidase (MAO) (*see* Chapter 11). MAO exists in two forms, A and B, one of which—MAO-B—is responsible for the breakdown of dopamine. One of the drugs which can be used in conjunction with L-dopa is deprenyl which inhibits MAO-B and thereby prevents it from destroying dopamine. This increases the amount of dopamine in the striatum. Deprenyl is not usually used alone, but in combination with L-dopa to help preserve the dopamine formed from the amino acid in the brain. The combination is especially useful in reducing the 'end-of-dose' deterioration—the decline in function which appears as the effect of each dose of dopa wears off.

Receptor agonists

In addition to restoring dopamine levels with L-dopa, it is also possible to compensate for its loss by using drugs which act directly on dopamine receptors. These drugs, which include bromocriptine, lisuride, and apomorphine, are agonists. They stimulate the receptors which would respond to dopamine and act as replacements for the dopamine normally released by the nigrostriatal neurons. The main problem with this group of drugs is that, like dopa itself, they induce a range of involuntary movements. They also act on dopamine receptors in the pituitary gland, a part of the brain which controls hormone secretion. The activation of dopamine receptors here suppresses the release of the hormone prolactin, which can lead to infertility and menstrual disorders.

These drugs are used primarily in two situations. Firstly, if they are taken early after the diagnosis of Parkinson's disease, they can suppress the symptoms enough to delay the initiation of therapy with L-dopa. This may be valuable because L-dopa, despite its excellent effectiveness when first used, becomes less effective with time. The longer its use can be delayed, therefore, the longer the overall time for which the patient can be treated.

The second use of drugs acting directly on dopamine receptors is to reduce the variability in responsiveness which often occurs in patients taking L-dopa for several years (such as the on–off effects described above). It is not understood exactly why these drugs should smooth out the effects of L-dopa, but the effect is clear and is of major help to advanced patients.

Amantadine

Introduced into medicine as an antiviral drug, amantadine prevents viruses from entering cells and starting an infection. It was noticed that when patients with both Parkinson's disease and viral disorders were treated with this drug, their parkinsonism improved. This is another example of a drug being found accidentally. Research showed that amantadine stops the removal of dopamine by nerve cells in the brain, and also increases the quantity released by nerve cells as a neurotransmitter. It is not a very strong drug, and seems to work only in a few patients, but it is useful in treating the early stages of Parkinson's disease. Because of the development of the long-term side-effects of L-dopa treatment, any drug which can reduce the early symptoms of Parkinson's disease and delay the patient's taking dopa is considered to be useful.

Anticholinergic drugs

Within the striatum of the brain, both dopamine and acetylcholine are neurotransmitters. The effects of dopamine and acetylcholine are opposite, dopamine causing inhibition of nerve cells, acetylcholine causing excitation. When the brain loses the dopamine cells, the activity of acetylcholine is left unrestrained. Another method of treating Parkinson's disease, therefore, is to reduce that activity by giving drugs which block the effect of acetylcholine on the muscarinic receptors (*see* Chapter 1). The anticholinergic drugs are more effective than L-dopa at reducing the tremor of Parkinson's disease, although they have little effect on the muscular rigidity and difficulty of movement.

These drugs, listed in Table 8.1 (p. 126), produce a range of side-effects due to their blocking acetylcholine receptors outside the brain. These include reduced salivation (dry mouth), poor visual accommodation (blurred vision), and decreased intestinal movements (constipation). They may also make urination more difficult as acetylcholine receptors are involved in contracting the bladder. Since there are acetylcholine receptors in many parts of the brain in addition to those involved in Parkinson's disease, the anticholinergic drugs can worsen the confusion and memory loss sometimes seen in patients.

Remaining problems

In addition to the motor difficulties, elderly Parkinson's disease patients often show signs of dementia—confusion, memory loss, sudden interruptions of thoughts or speech. These may partly be a result of the ever-decreasing number of nerve cells in the brain and at present there are no drugs which will treat these problems. Given the huge amount of research into the mechanisms of memory and cognition in order to treat related disorders such as Alzheimer's disease, it cannot be long before drugs are available to help with mental deterioration in Parkinson's disease.

Drugs of the future

The pharmaceutical industry is trying to develop several new types of drug for use in Parkinson's disease. One approach is to obtain drugs which act directly on the dopamine receptors, like bromocriptine, but with fewer side-effects. Several such drugs, including pramipexole and ropinirole, have been found to be effective in clinical studies, with very few side-effects, and are likely to be available in the near future. Both can be used to treat patients for several years before starting treatment with L-dopa, or can be used together with L-dopa to reduce the dose of this drug needed.

Another approach is to increase the activation of receptors by any dopamine remaining in the brain of Parkinson's disease patients. Adenosine is a substance produced by cells which inhibits the activation of dopamine receptors. Drugs which block adenosine receptors allow dopamine to have a greater effect than usual and are being tested as possible new drugs for Parkinson's disease.

Many of the cells in the brain use the amino acid glutamate as their neurotransmitter, and research in rats has shown that drugs which block the effects of glutamate can restore the balance between cells caused by the loss of dopamine. Several drug companies are developing glutamate antagonists which might be useful in Parkinson's disease as well as other disorders. One drug, riluzole, does not block glutamate receptors but reduces the release of glutamate from nerve cells, producing the same overall effect as glutamate antagonists. Riluzole has been tested in humans for the treatment of multiple sclerosis (amyotrophic lateral sclerosis) and has been found to be quite safe. It is now also being tested in patients with Parkinson's disease.

Table 8.1 Drugs used in the treatment of Parkinson's disease

Anticholinergic drugs	Dopamine receptor agonists
benzhexol*	apomorphine
benztropine	bromocriptine
biperiden	cabergoline
orphenadrine	lysuride
procyclidine	pergolide
trihexyphenidyl*	quinagolide
	ropinirole

L-dopa and combinations	Other drugs
L-dopa (Levodopa)	amantadine
Mixtures containing L-dopa	
Co-beneldopa (contains levodopa and	**MAO inhibitor**
benserazide in a ratio of 4: 1 [Madopar®])	deprenyl (selegiline)
Co-careldopa (contains levodopa and	
carbidopa in a ratio of 10: 1 [Sinemet®]	**COMT inhibitors**
or 4: 1 [Sinemet-Plus])	entacapone
	tolcapone†

* These are different names for the same drug.
† Introduced in November 1997; withdrawn from November 1998.

Summary

- Parkinson's disease is a disorder of movement caused by the degeneration of nerve cells in the brain which secrete the transmitter dopamine. The main symptoms are tremor, rigid muscles, and slowness in moving.

- The main treatment is to replace the missing dopamine by giving L-dopa, an amino acid which the brain converts into dopamine.

- L-dopa is normally given with other drugs like benserazide and carbidopa which stop L-dopa from being destroyed in the blood and tissues.

- Long-term use of L-dopa brings side-effects to many patients, including difficulty in thinking, hallucinations, and swaying movements of the body which the patient cannot control.

- Amantadine increases the release of dopamine from nerve cells and reduces its destruction.

- Deprenyl (selegiline) prevents the destruction of dopamine in the brain and improves the efficacy of L-dopa.

- Agonist drugs which activate dopamine receptors, such as bromocriptine, can be used even when all the dopamine cells have died.

- Anticholinergic drugs such as benxhexol, which block the receptors for acetylcholine, restore the balance between dopamine and acetylcholine in the brain and reduce the signs of Parkinson's disease.

CHAPTER 9

Schizophrenia

We apply a variety of names to people who differ mentally from the majority. They have been called 'deranged', 'insane', or just 'mad'. Many of them suffer from a mental disorder called schizophrenia, a disorder of the brain about which we are beginning to understand more. One sociological breakthrough this century has been the acceptance that people once locked away because of uncontrollable and sometimes dangerous insanity, are now recognized as suffering from this disease of the brain. It remains a disease from which the

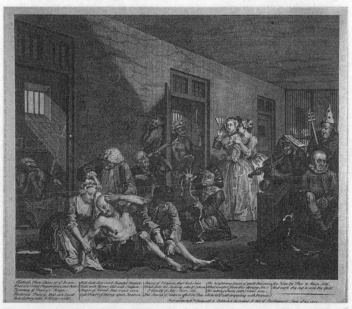

Fig. 9.1 An engraving by W. Hogarth in 1735, showing 'an insane man clutching his head, while his lover cries and two attendants chain his legs'. They are surrounded by other mentally ill patients at Bethlem Hospital, London.

general public may need to be protected by restraining the patient, but it is a disease which, in principle, is no different to treat than high blood pressure or asthma.

Schizophrenia affects about 5 people in every 1000. Despite its popular description as 'split personality', it does not involve a division of personality into two different characters of the 'Jekyll and Hyde' type, but a separation of the emotions and the intellect. Its key feature is a disordered perception of reality and it is usually quite distinct from disorders of mood, such as depression and mania, in which the patient experiences extremes of these moods, sometimes for periods of weeks or months, but with relatively well-organized thoughts, modified only by their mood at the time. Schizophrenia is also quite different from Alzheimer's disease in which the patient is very forgetful and mentally confused, but their overall perception of the world remains within normal bounds.

A schizophrenic patient, on the other hand, sees the world very differently from normal people. Patients may, for example, see colourful patterns dancing around in the air or on walls. The walls themselves may appear to be curved, perhaps even shaking or moving aggressively towards the patient. One patient* has written:

> Objects would sometimes pop out of their backgrounds ... Perspective was often disordered and confusing. Sometimes I would look down at my feet and they would seem to be very far away from me ... Or my knees might appear too big and perhaps shrink again. There were times when I could see the room breathing, the walls contracting and expanding. A lamp was not just a lamp: it had a personality and it was trying to communicate with me. A chair was not just a chair: it seemed more real than reality itself. It scared me.*

These are examples of visual hallucinations, but perhaps the most frightening and characteristic example of disordered perception in schizophrenia is that of auditory hallucinations—hearing voices. Patients may hear a voice talking to them almost all the time. These may be the voices of persons from history, or religious characters, or an indeterminate voice commenting on the patient's every action, often very critically, sometimes abusively. Inanimate objects may appear to be speaking—windows, buildings, books, rocks. Elizabeth Farr* wrote that:

> I remember once asking my next-door neighbour to come over and listen to my house-plants. I thought they were talking.
> ... the voices might be having a war with each other, yelling and screaming at me ...

* From the report by Elizabeth L. Farr in *Schizophrenia: the facts* by M. T. Tsuang, Oxford University Press, Oxford, 1982.

Patients are often convinced that their own thoughts, even the most private and intimate, are audible, being broadcast and heard by everyone around them. There are also motor disabilities in some patients. Elizabeth Farr* again:

> In conversation I sometimes noticed that after I gestured my hand would stay suspended in the air, forgotten, and it would not occur to me to move it for a long time. I used to sit in the corner of my apartment for days at a time, motionless, petrified.

This last feature is characteristic of 'catatonic' schizophrenia. Catatonia is a state in which the body, or parts of it, may be placed in unusual positions and will remain there for several hours, apparently 'forgotten' by the rest of the body.

Perhaps the most difficult aspect of schizophrenia for normal people to appreciate is that it is a *psychosis,* which means that the patient is not aware, at the time, that they are ill. The colourful fantasies, the moving walls, the voices, the talking plants—these are all as real to the schizophrenic patient as people seen on the television or heard on the radio are to you or me. Only when a patient enters a period of remission, or is treated successfully by drugs, can he or she look back and see how irrational and abnormal were their earlier thoughts and experiences.

Schizophrenia often appears during the teens and continues through the twenties. The hallucinations and other symptoms are prominent during these years, and are known by doctors as the 'positive' symptoms. The ability to think and reason, to learn and understand, is not greatly impaired, so that some schizophrenic patients may continue to hold a job and to have friends. The positive symptoms can usually be treated by drugs, so that the patient can conduct a reasonably normal life provided he or she continues to take the drugs.

In contrast, older patients may become increasingly withdrawn from society, friends, and family, showing very little emotion (or even showing inappropriate emotions such as laughing at very bad news) and losing the ability to think clearly and rationally. Patients may show bizarre behaviours such as repeated, purposeless movements, prolonged rocking, or the maintenance of abnormal positions. These are the 'negative' symptoms. Dr Tim Crow, working mainly at the Medical Research Council Clinical Research Centre at Harrow in England, and others, have found that these are associated with a general deterioration of the brain, which shrinks and loses many nerve cells. These changes are much more resistant to drug treatment.

Clearly schizophrenia represents a very frightening state of mind. Abusive voices, the belief that everyone can hear your thoughts, and in some cases paranoid delusions that people around are victimising you, telling lies about

---

* From the report by Elizabeth L. Farr in *Schizophrenia: the facts* by M. T. Tsuang, Oxford University Press, Oxford, 1982.

you, or even trying to kill you, may cause some patients to become very aggressive, suicidal, or homicidal. Schizophrenia is a disorder which requires treatment at the earliest possible stage. Trying to explain it scientifically, in terms of chemical events in the brain, so that new and better drugs can be developed, remains one of the most sought-after targets in neuroscience research.

Causes of schizophrenia

There is no question that schizophrenia is a disorder of the brain and needs to be treated as a disease in just the same way that we treat other people with disorders of the brain such as epilepsy or Parkinson's disease. As to what causes schizophrenia, we have made little progress in a hundred years. Studies of identical twins suggest that the cause is not a simple hereditary transmission, since they do not always both develop the disorder. On the other hand, there is a definite hereditary link, since the chances of developing schizophrenia are increased with a schizophrenic relative. If both parents have schizophrenia, there is a fifty–fifty chance that a child will also be affected.

It is possible that there is a genetic tendency making some individuals more susceptible to other precipitating factors. Scientists have considered bacteria, viruses, diet, and toxins in the environment, but with, as yet, no conclusive evidence for any one particular cause being responsible for initiating the changes within the brain. However, some kind of chemical abnormality in the brain is certainly responsible for schizophrenia, an idea which dates back to the discovery that some substances could produce schizophrenic-like symptoms.

This concept arose partly from the experience of a Swiss chemist, Albert Hofmann. In 1943, Hofmann was working for the pharmaceutical company Roche, and was investigating chemicals obtained from the fungus, ergot (*see* Chapter 7). One afternoon, Hofmann began to feel unwell and dizzy, so he went home. Over the next couple of hours, Hofmann experienced vivid visual hallucinations and distortions in his perception of objects—solid objects moved or changed their shape, for example. The chemical he had been working on was lysergic acid diethylamide—which we now abbreviate to LSD—and he had probably inhaled minute quantities of the powder during the day. In order to confirm that the powder was responsible for the hallucinations, Hofmann deliberately swallowed 250 micrograms the next day. This is still a very tiny amount of powder, but is about 10 times the dose used by 'hippies' in the 1960s. Hofmann's visual and psychological disturbances were much more intense this time and lasted for about 24 hours. His experiences led to the idea that the body may produce a chemical similar to LSD, and that too much of it may cause the disturbed behaviours and hallucinations characteristic of schizophrenia.

Localizing the abnormalities in schizophrenia

Which parts of the brain are affected in schizophrenia? We know that many functions of the brain are carried out partly on the left side, and partly on the right side, and that normal behaviour depends on the two halves communicating with each other. In patients in whom the connections between the two halves have been cut (usually to control epilepsy which is resistant to drugs) there are some strange consequences. Since the left side of the brain contains the areas for speech (in most people), it is possible for a researcher to show an object to the right side of the brain and find that the patient cannot say what the object was. But if the patient is asked to pick the object out of a group, they will do so. In other words, the 'speaking brain' (left side) has been cut off from the 'recognition brain' (right side in this case).

What has this to do with schizophrenia? One idea, proposed by Tim Crow, is that the connections between the speech areas and thinking areas of the brain are disturbed in schizophrenia, so that patients do not realise that the voices they hear are their own thoughts. However, some patients are well aware that the voices are coming from inside their heads and not from an external source.

The limbic brain

Those parts of the brain which have been the focus of most attention in the study of schizophrenia for around thirty years, are known as the limbic system.* This is a group of areas which have important functions in regulating the flow of information from sensory and motor pathways into consciousness, and in controlling the interplay between these different types of information. One of the most important pathways of nerve cells in the limbic system releases dopamine as its neurotransmitter. When the brains of schizophrenic patients are examined after death, this pathway† can be shown to contain more receptors for dopamine than do brains taken from patients who had been psychiatrically normal.

If normal people take amphetamines repeatedly for several weeks, they often develop symptoms which psychiatrists may find difficult to distinguish from schizophrenia. This condition, called 'amphetamine psychosis', probably occurs because amphetamines induce the release of dopamine in large quantities from nerve cells.

These and related pieces of evidence have led to the belief that the major chemical disorder in schizophrenia is overactivity in the nerve cells using dopamine as a neurotransmitter in the brain (Fig. 9.2). This may involve an

---

* The limbic system includes areas of the brain such as the hippocampus, amygdala, and the ventral striatum.
† This is the 'mesolimbic' pathway from the ventral tegmental area (VTA) to the ventral striatum (*nucleus accumbens*).

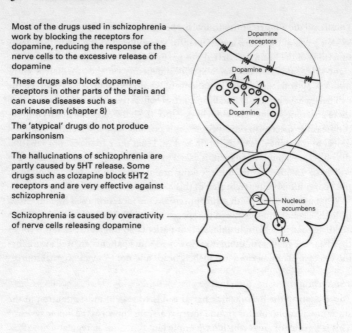

Most of the drugs used in schizophrenia work by blocking the receptors for dopamine, reducing the response of the nerve cells to the excessive release of dopamine

These drugs also block dopamine receptors in other parts of the brain and can cause diseases such as parkinsonism (chapter 8)

The 'atypical' drugs do not produce parkinsonism

The hallucinations of schizophrenia are partly caused by 5HT release. Some drugs such as clozapine block 5HT2 receptors and are very effective against schizophrenia

Schizophrenia is caused by overactivity of nerve cells releasing dopamine

Dopamine receptors

Dopamine

Dopamine

Nucleus accumbens

VTA

Fig. 9.2 How drugs work in schizophrenia.

abnormally high release of dopamine at the synapses, or an increase in the sensitivity of cells to dopamine. As first pointed out by the pharmacologist Philip Seeman in 1976 at the University of Toronto, most of the drugs now used to treat schizophrenia act on this pathway to block the receptors for dopamine. They are known as antipsychotic, antischizophrenic, or neuroleptic drugs.

Drug treatment

Reserpine

An Indian plant known as snakeroot,* because of the appearance of its roots, had been in use in India for treating snakebites and other disorders for at least a thousand years before it was first studied scientifically. In 1931 two physicians based in Calcutta, Gananath Sen and Kartick Bose, published a report which confirmed and drew attention to the fact that the plant produced a fall of blood pressure, induced sedation, and calmed violently insane patients. Its proper

---

* The proper name of the plant is *Rauwolfia serpentina*, named by Charles Plumier in 1703 after the explorer Leonard Rauwolf who described the plant in 1582.

name is *Rauwolfia serpentina*, after the German botanist Leonard Rauwolf who first studied it botanically, and the powdered roots of *Rauwolfia* soon became a standard treatment for hypertension in India.

Another report of the sedative activity of *Rauwolfia* was published in 1933 by the Indian doctor Ram Nath Chopra working in the Department of Pharmacology, at the University of Calcutta and this came to the notice of two chemists, Emil Schlittler and Hugo Bein, working for the drug company Ciba in Switzerland. They decided to try to isolate the chemical responsible for the effects of *Rauwolfia* and eventually succeeded in 1951. They called the chemical reserpine and this was soon being marketed by Ciba under the trade name 'Serpasil'. Despite an early period of popularity, its use began to decline when it was realized that it produced not only sedation, but also depression in some patients, leading them to suicide. At the same time, several new and more effective drugs became available to treat high blood pressure. Nevertheless, two American psychiatrists, Meltzer and Stahl noticed in the 1960s that when schizophrenic patients were being treated with reserpine for high blood pressure, their schizophrenia improved. They also noticed that amphetamine made the schizophrenia worse.

At about the same time that *Rauwolfia* was being studied, a parallel series of developments was taking place which would have far-reaching consequences.

The discovery of anti-schizophrenic drugs

In the late nineteenth century, following the Industrial Revolution, many chemical companies sought to manufacture new dyes which would provide a wider range of colours, or which could dye different types of material such as fabrics for clothes, paper for books and decorations, solutions for paints and inks, and so on. Many thousands of new chemicals were produced. It was from these early chemical companies that many of the major pharmaceutical companies developed in the twentieth century and one of the first tasks of scientists in the new pharmaceutical industry was to test the range of chemicals on the shelves to determine their biological properties. One group of chemicals, the phenothiazines, were antagonists of several neurotransmitters and hormones including histamine.

In 1949, a French anaesthetist, Henri Laborit, began seeking a drug which would reduce the shock and trauma of major surgery, perhaps by antagonizing the effects of histamine. He began a collaboration with the pharmaceutical company Rhone-Poulenc in Paris and in 1950 he tested one of their anti-histamine compounds on several patients due to have surgery. He noticed that the drug did indeed reduce the traumatic effects of surgery, but it also made the patients seem quite unworried during the stressful pre- and post-operative periods. Pursuing this observation, Laborit tested the drug on an aggressive psychiatric patient and found it rapidly calmed him. Two other doctors, Jean Delay and Pierre Deniker, working at the Hopital St Anne in Paris, were involved in this work and subsequently introduced the drug as a standard treatment for their psychotic patients. It was called chlorpromazine and proved to be the first of dozens of effective drugs that would be developed over the next few years.

How do these drugs work?

The first clues to the chemical abnormality responsible for schizophrenia came from studies of LSD and reserpine—the drug isolated from *Rauwolfia* roots. Reserpine destroys the ability of nerve cells to store and release amine neuro-transmitters such as norepinephrine, 5HT* and dopamine. LSD, on the other hand, activates the receptors for 5HT. Since reserpine improves schizophrenic symptoms, these results suggested that schizophrenia might be due to an excess of amine transmitters, especially 5HT, in the brain. That clue prompted research to find out whether other drugs also affected these amines. Eventually it was realized that, except for reserpine, drugs which were effective in treating schizophrenia had one biological property in common—they were all able to block receptors for the neurotransmitter dopamine in the brain, i.e. they were dopamine antagonists.

Paradoxically, science has now come almost full circle back to Hofmann and LSD. We now know that the hallucinogenic effects of LSD and similar drugs are produced by stimulating a type of 5HT receptor known as 5HT-2. Many of the newer antischizophrenic drugs, which are better than the older drugs at treating schizophrenia, and also have fewer side-effects, act on 5HT receptors as well as dopamine receptors. The best antipsychotic drugs may, therefore, work as dopamine antagonists to reduce the agitation of psychotic patients, and as 5HT-2 antagonists to reduce the hallucinations and delusions.

Side-effects

There is a large range of drugs which act in this way (Table 9.1, p. 138), although they belong to different chemical classes. Most of these differ mainly in the side-effects which they can produce. For example, drugs such as chlorpromazine and thioridazine are strongly sedative and are often the preferred drugs to treat schizophrenic patients who are aggressive. These same drugs also block receptors for acetylcholine and norepinephrine, so that patients experience the effects of blocking the parasympathetic nerves (*see* Chapter 9)—dry mouth, blurred vision, and some constipation, and blockade of the sympathetic nerves leading to low blood pressure. There are also several drugs which are less likely to produce these side-effects.

* 5HT is an abbreviation for 5-hydroxytryptamine.

In the 1950s Paul Janssen in Belgium was trying to synthesize a new type of chemical with the properties of morphine. One of these did produce analgesia in animals but it also produced a marked calming, sedating effect. From this accidental beginning, Janssen developed the drug haloperidol, which was much more selective for brain dopamine receptors than other drugs available at the time and which was marketed for the treatment of schizophrenia in 1958. It is around one hundred times more effective as a dopamine receptor blocker and has little effect on acetylcholine and norepinephrine receptors. Unfortunately, haloperidol brings with it a different kind of problem—parkinsonism.

Parkinsonism

As discussed in Chapter 8, another dopamine-releasing pathway—the nigro-striatal pathway—is involved in the control of movement. Its gradual degeneration causes Parkinson's disease, but the symptoms of Parkinson's disease can also be produced by any procedure or drug which suppresses the effects of dopamine. Almost any drug which blocks dopamine receptors in the limbic system and reduces the symptoms of schizophrenia will also block some dopamine receptors in the nigrostriatal pathway and may, therefore, produce symptoms of Parkinson's disease. Haloperidol is one of the drugs most likely to produce this problem.

Why some drugs effective in schizophrenia should induce parkinsonism while others do not is only partly understood. Chapter 8 indicates that drugs which block acetylcholine receptors in the brain could reduce the symptoms of Parkinson's disease. Drugs such as chlorpromazine which can block acetyl-choline receptors as well as dopamine receptors are less likely to produce parkinsonism than drugs such as haloperidol which do not block acetylcholine.

Another possibility is based on the fact that there is a family of several types of receptor for dopamine. The receptors most important for parkinsonism are the D1 and D2 types, whereas those that are important in schizophrenia are D2, D3, and D4 receptors. Drugs which reduce schizophrenia and cause parkinsonism do so by blocking D2 receptors. One of the major targets for developing new drugs against schizophrenia may be to find compounds which will block D3 and D4 receptors and not D2 receptors.

Endocrine effects

The pituitary gland is a part of the brain which controls the secretion of several hormones. One of these is the hormone prolactin, which helps to maintain activity in the sex organs of women. The secretion of prolactin is inhibited by neurons releasing dopamine as their transmitter. Since the antipsychotic drugs block dopamine receptors, they remove this inhibition and the secretion of prolactin increases. The result can be enlargement of the breasts and menstrual irregularities in women, and enlargement of the breasts and impotence in men.

Other side-effects

Most of the antischizophrenic drugs have some side-effects because they interfere with the effects of norepinephrine or 5HT in the brain. For example, they tend to cause patients to put on weight and reduce their sexual activity.

Effects of long-term treatment

One of the effects of stimulating dopamine receptors in the brain is to produce repeated movements of the face, tongue, and mouth. If a dose of amphetamine is given to a rat, for example, the animal will stand in one corner of its cage for a couple of hours, sniffing the same small area of cage, and often gnawing at the bars of the cage. These movements are called 'stereotyped movements'. Exactly the same phenomenon appears in some schizophrenic patients who have been treated with antipsychotic drugs, usually for several years. The patients cannot stop themselves from smacking and moving their lips, or sticking out or moving their tongue. Sometimes the whole face is involved, with continuous, grimacing movements of the cheeks and mouth.

In both the rats and the patients the cause of these movements* may be activation of dopamine receptors. For the rats, this is due to the experimental administration of amphetamine. But why do symptoms of dopamine receptor stimulation occur in schizophrenic patients being treated with drugs which block dopamine receptors?

There is still no certain explanation, but it may result from the phenomenon called 'denervation supersensitivity'. When any receptor is blocked for a long time, the cells bearing those receptors try to compensate by producing more receptors. In the case of the dopamine receptors blocked by antischizophrenic drugs, it is believed that some cells in the brain overcompensate, producing so many dopamine receptors that they become supersensitive to dopamine and we see the facial symptoms of *tardive dyskinesia* just described. Presumably this supersensitivity is limited to brain cells involved in facial movements, because in most of these patients their schizophrenia remains under control despite the emergence of these involuntary movements.

Another explanation is that some of the nerve cells which normally release the transmitter GABA† die during prolonged treatment with antipsychotic drugs. GABA restrains the activity of dopamine nerve cells, so as the levels of GABA fall, the dopamine nerve cells become more active, causing the facial movements.

Elderly patients seem more likely to develop these *dyskinesias*, but recent

---

* The phenomenon is called *tardive dyskinesia*. The word 'tardive' refers to the tardy or slow development of the movements, while 'dyskinesia' means abnormal movement.
† GABA is Gamma-amino-butyric acid.

research suggests that changing the anti-schizophrenic drug used to one of the newer ones such as olanzapine can reduce them. Trials with vitamin E also indicate that this antioxidant may greatly reduce the symptoms.

Atypical antipsychotic drugs

Clozapine

At least one drug already available does act at dopamine D4 receptors and also has strong antagonist activity at acetylcholine receptors. This is clozapine, which hardly ever produces symptoms of parkinsonism. For this reason it is called an 'atypical' antischizophrenic drug, to distinguish it from most other drugs used in this disorder which can induce parkinsonism.

Clozapine has other actions too which may help its antischizophrenic action, such as blocking receptors for 5-hydroxytryptamine. Sadly, few drugs are perfect, and clozapine was withdrawn from general medical use in 1980, only a few years after its introduction, because it produced serious and potentially fatal blood disorders in about 2 per cent of patients. However, this is a small risk for such a powerful and useful drug and clozapine was eventually reintroduced into clinical practice in 1990, under carefully controlled conditions. Firstly, other drugs must have proved to be ineffective, or to produce serious side-effects in the patients concerned. Secondly, the patient must undergo a blood test every few weeks to check for the development of blood disorders, and thirdly, patients must be registered with an official monitoring service. With these safeguards, clozapine is once again being used for seriously ill schizophrenic patients who cannot use, or do not respond to, other drugs.

Other 'atypical' drugs

The main objective of research is to produce more and safer 'atypical' antipsychotic drugs. In addition to clozapine, the drugs already available are sertindole, risperidone, olanzapine, quetiapine, and amisulpride, but all of these should be used with caution in patients with heart disease or a history of epilepsy.

Amisulpride seems to have a more selective action on dopamine receptors in the limbic system, so that involuntary movements are less likely to arise. This is because it acts at D3 receptors which are found almost exclusively in the limbic brain, as well as D2 receptors in the limbic and motor areas.

Treating negative symptoms

While most of the drugs currently available can control the early, or positive, symptoms of schizophrenia, there are few which modify the more advanced, negative symptoms. Those which do include the newer drugs, such as olanzapine, ziprasidone, sertindole, zotepine, and ritanserin as well as clozapine and some of the antidepressants (*see* Chapter 11). These drugs represent, after years of research in universities and the pharmaceutical industry, real promise for the treatment of schizophrenic patients. They are regarded by many people as such an important medical advance that olanzapine, launched by Eli Lilly and Company in 1996, was awarded the 'Prix Galien' by the pharmaceutical industry in 1998. This is the industry's equivalent of a Nobel Prize. How do these new drugs work to reduce the negative symptoms?

In advanced schizophrenic patients there is a decline in the number of D1 dopamine receptors in the frontal cortex of the brain. This area is associated with the ability to think and control one's emotions, and the loss of cells and receptors in this region probably accounts for the loss of emotional responses of patients in the more advanced stages of schizophrenia, and who are showing this and other 'negative' symptoms. At low doses, amisulpride and some of the other new drugs increase the release of dopamine by nerve cells in the frontal cortex, an action which would help to compensate for the loss of dopamine receptors and which would explain the activity of these drugs in patients who exhibit the 'negative' symptoms.

Drugs of the future

Research to find new drugs to treat schizophrenia is one of the most active areas in pharmacology. New drugs are being developed, such as zotepine which act on a range of receptors including dopamine receptors and 5HT receptors, and which seem to show great promise in treating schizophrenia without the production of abnormal parkinsonian movements or *tardive dyskinesias*.

Table 9.1 Drugs used in schizophrenia

acetophenazine (USA)	pericyazine
amisulpride	perphenazine
benperidol	pimozide
chlorpromazine	pipothiazine
chlorprothixene (USA)	prochlorperazine
clozapine	promazine
droperidol	quetiapine
fluopromazine (USA)	risperidone
flupenthixol	sertindole
fluphenazine	sulpiride
haloperidol	thioridazine
loxapine	thiothixene (USA)
mesoridazine (USA)	trifluoperazine
methotrimeprazine	ziprasidone
molindone (USA)	zotepine
olanzapine	zuclopenthixol
oxypertine	

Summary

- Schizophrenia is a disorder of the brain in which nerve cells secreting or responding to the transmitter dopamine are overactive.
- The main symptoms are hallucinations, usually auditory (hearing voices), confused thinking, and abnormal emotional responses. These are the 'positive' symptoms.
- As patients get older they may develop 'negative' symptoms of withdrawal from society, lack of emotion, an inability to think rationally and logically, and bizarre movements or the adoption of strange positions.
- Most of the anti-schizophrenic drugs (also called antipsychotic or neuroleptic drugs) block the receptors for dopamine in the brain.
- Because they block dopamine receptors in all parts of the brain, some patients develop signs similar to Parkinson's disease.
- The 5HT2 receptors are also involved in hallucinations and may cause some of the symptoms of schizophrenia. The most effective drugs at present, such as clozapine, block these receptors in addition to dopamine.
- Clozapine and a few other drugs also block acetylcholine receptors, an action which reduces parkinsonian symptoms.

CHAPTER 10

Alzheimer's disease and other dementias

George startled his wife by dragging the lawnmower up to the bathroom. She had asked him for a ladder. Formerly the manager of a large engineering works, George was finding that his knowledge of everyday objects and what they were used for was beginning to fragment, leaving him increasingly at a loss to make sense of the world around him. Yet he knew perfectly well who he was and where he was, and could competently recall events that had taken place in recent days or weeks.*

Dementia

Dementia refers to a range of disorders characterized by different degrees and types of mental confusion and memory loss. It can occur as a result of chronic and excessive alcohol intake, chronic vitamin B12 deficiency, infection with syphilis, a stroke, or a brain tumour. Most often, it is the result of small clots forming in the blood vessels of the brain and cutting off the blood supply to small areas when it is called 'multi-infarct dementia', or to the condition known as Alzheimer's disease. George was suffering from one form of dementia in which the names and functions of objects become forgotten or totally confused. This type of dementia is called 'semantic dementia' and is often seen in patients with Alzheimer's disease.

Brain cells

Most of the many billions of cells in the body continue to divide throughout life, providing two new cells from each parent cell. In this way cells that die or are damaged are continually replaced. The brain is different: the nerve cells stop dividing around the time of birth. From then, about 10 000 nerve cells die every day of our lives, never to be replaced. Fortunately, this is not quite as depressing a thought as it sounds because, as we start with about 10 million million cells at birth, we normally have enough to last each of us for around 30 000 years.

The inability of brain cells to divide means that, if part of the brain is

* Related by J. Hodges in *Wellcome News*, supplement 2, page 24, 1998.

damaged, the nerve cells cannot be replaced. We become dependent on the remaining cells to take over the functions previously carried out by the dead cells, a process which can take many months or years. This is the reason why recovery from a stroke, for example, can be a slow process, even though many patients do eventually regain some of the abilities they lost immediately afterwards. It also means that as cells in the brain concerned with learning and understanding die, they cannot be replaced to retain those faculties; in those people in who cells die at a relatively high rate this can result in dementia.

Alzheimer's disease

Alzheimer's disease is the fourth leading cause of death in industrialized countries, after heart disease, cancer, and stroke. There are about four million Alzheimer's patients in the USA and nearly half a million in the UK. As life expectancy increases, the proportion of people with Alzheimer's disease will also increase.

Alzheimer's disease develops very slowly, starting with forgetfulness, tiredness, and difficulty learning new things and recalling familiar words. It may progress over twenty or more years with patients becoming more and more forgetful, confused, and disoriented, unable to understand simple statements or carry out simple tasks. They may forget the names of familiar objects, of people they see every day, or even where they live. They may forget common words in sentences, put clothes on inside out, and lose things by putting them in completely inappropriate places (such as leaving shoes in the fridge). Patients lose the ability to think clearly and rationally, and eventually lose motor coordination and the ability to wash, dress, and look after themselves, becoming dependent on carers for most aspects of their daily lives.

The early diagnosis of Alzheimer's disease is often made on whether a patient can complete the set of tasks known as the 'Mini-Mental State Examination'. The number of people affected increases from about 1 in 100 at ages between 60 and 69 years, up to 1 in 5 for those over 85. It is, therefore, a disease which creates enormous social and economic problems as well as a strain on welfare services, family, and friends of those affected.

Who was Alzheimer?

Alzheimer's disease is named after a German neurologist, Alois Alzheimer, who described the symptoms of a 56-year-old female patient, Auguste, from Frankfurt. Auguste had shown progressive mental deterioration for several years, with confusion and serious losses of memory. After her death in 1906 Alzheimer examined her brain, taking thin slices and viewing them under a microscope. He observed, firstly that the brain was smaller than in normal people and that many of the nerve cells had died, especially in areas such as the cerebral cortex which is responsible for reasoning and some aspects of memory. He also saw dark, dense deposits, mainly in those areas showing the most cell death. These dense deposits of material are known as 'plaques' and 'tangles' and much research has been directed at establishing their composition and origin and why they seem to be associated with cell death.

Plaques consist of a starch-like substance known as beta-amyloid. We still do not understand for certain why the brain produces beta-amyloid at all. One theory is that it is important for the movement of fatty substances, including cholesterol, around cells and into membranes. Normally nerve cells produce a form of amyloid which dissolves easily and washes out of the brain. In Alzheimer's disease, nerve cells produce an incorrect form of amyloid which does not dissolve and therefore accumulates to form the plaques.

The tangles consist of a twisted mass of proteins which normally exist only inside cells and help to maintain cell shape and structure. When the brains of Alzheimer's disease patients are examined after death, it is the number of tangles which relates most closely to the amount of mental deterioration of the patient.

The reason why plaques and tangles are associated with cell death remains unknown. The abnormal beta-amyloid may allow much more calcium to enter cells than usual, and large amounts of calcium kill nerve cells.

What causes Alzheimer's disease?

No-one knows for certain why some people develop Alzheimer's disease. There are many theories, such as the idea that a slowly acting virus is involved, or that the disorder is due to an accumulation of aluminium in the brain, but none of these theories is widely accepted. Relatives of people with the disorder are slightly more likely to develop it themselves, and people with a history of severe depression, epilepsy, or head injury are also slightly more likely to succumb.

One of the few sure facts is that patients with Down's syndrome often develop some features of Alzheimer's disease. The cause of Down's syndrome is the presence of an extra chromosome (chromosome 21) which happens to be the same one which causes the formation of beta-amyloid. An obvious explanation of this coincidence might be that chromosome 21 causes the overproduction of beta-amyloid or some related substance which leads to Alzheimer's disease. However, although most Down's patients do have high levels of beta-amyloid in their brains, not all of them develop Alzheimer's disease.

Which parts of the brain are affected in Alzheimer's disease?

The first real clue to the nature of the chemical defect in Alzheimer's disease came from David Bowen in Liverpool. In 1976 he found that the brains of

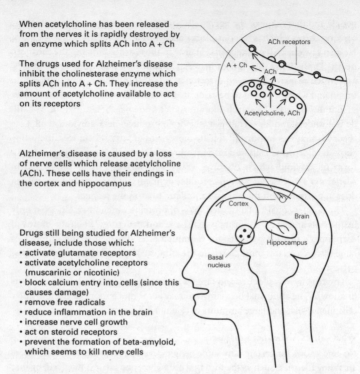

When acetylcholine has been released from the nerves it is rapidly destroyed by an enzyme which splits ACh into A + Ch

The drugs used for Alzheimer's disease inhibit the cholinesterase enzyme which splits ACh into A + Ch. They increase the amount of acetylcholine available to act on its receptors

Alzheimer's disease is caused by a loss of nerve cells which release acetylcholine (ACh). These cells have their endings in the cortex and hippocampus

Drugs still being studied for Alzheimer's disease, include those which:
• activate glutamate receptors
• activate acetylcholine receptors (muscarinic or nicotinic)
• block calcium entry into cells (since this causes damage)
• remove free radicals
• reduce inflammation in the brain
• increase nerve cell growth
• act on steroid receptors
• prevent the formation of beta-amyloid, which seems to kill nerve cells

Fig. 10.1 The actions of drugs used to treat Alzheimer's disease.

patients who had died with Alzheimer's disease contained far less acetylcholine than those of normal individuals.

Cells in some parts of the brain seem to be more susceptible than others to damage in Alzheimer's disease. These include cells in those areas involved in learning and memory,* especially cells in the basal nucleus, which secrete acetylcholine as their neurotransmitter (Fig. 10.1). Cells in this region also have branches which travel to the cerebral cortex, the area of brain which is important for the ability to think and reason clearly and logically.

Learning and memory

Whenever we learn something new, a change occurs in a nerve cell or group of cells which lasts for some time. Acetylcholine is involved in producing those changes. If animals or people are given drugs which block the effects of

---

* These areas include the basal forebrain, the amygdala, and hippocampus.

acetylcholine in the brain, they have difficulty in learning, and may forget recently-learned facts or tasks. These are often the earliest symptoms of Alzheimer's disease: people forget simple, everyday things and eventually, after several years of this progressive disease, may not even remember the names, or recognize the faces of their husband, wife, or children.

Drugs to treat Alzheimer's disease*

This chapter is unusual in that very few drugs are as yet available to treat Alzheimer's disease. Since this is one of the developed world's greatest killers and brings enormous distress and suffering for entire families, there is probably more research in the pharmaceutical industry to find drugs to treat this disease than for any other disorder of the brain. Most of the drugs being developed are intended to replace or restore the functions of specific groups of cells which appear to be damaged in Alzheimer's disease, most emphasis being placed on those cells releasing acetylcholine.

Until recently no drugs were approved officially for Alzheimer's disease. That changed on 9 September 1993, when the Federal Drugs Administration (FDA)† in America approved the use of tacrine for Alzheimer's disease.

Acetylcholinesterase inhibitors

Since one of the major changes in the brain is the loss of cells producing acetylcholine, which is important for learning, memory, and thinking, one approach to treatment is to increase the amounts of acetylcholine in the brain by inhibiting the enzyme which breaks it down. The enzyme is acetylcholinesterase and the substances which inhibit it are anti-cholinesterase drugs (*see* Chapter 1). By stopping the breakdown of acetylcholine, these compounds increase the amount of this transmitter in the brain, and can slow down the progressive development of Alzheimer's disease (Table 10.1).

Two of the drugs being used are tacrine and eserine (also called physostigmine) but they are far from ideal. Tacrine has many effects in addition to blocking cholinesterase, and can cause serious liver damage. Both tacrine and eserine inhibit cholinesterase throughout the body, not just in the brain, so that there are many side-effects. These include increases in the flow of saliva, sweating, activity of the intestine (leading to diarrhoea), and acid secretion in the stomach, together with difficulty focussing the eyes and muscle cramps. All of these make life unpleasant both for patients and carers.

---

* Drugs used to treat dementias are sometimes known as no-otropic drugs, from the Greek words *noos*, meaning 'mind', and *tropos*, meaning 'moving towards', or 'developing'. The word no-otropic, therefore, refers to drugs which develop or improve the mental state.
† The body which has to approve drugs for use in patients.

Newer anticholinesterase drugs

The pharmaceutical industry is trying hard to improve on these two drugs, with the result that several cholinesterase inhibitors are now available on prescription or are being tested in clinical trials. They include metrifonate, galanthamine, and eptastigmine. Metrifonate has the advantage that it has been used for an entirely different purpose—as an anthelmintic to kill intestinal parasites—for over 30 years, so that it is already established as a safe drug with no serious or long-term side-effects.

We also now know that the cholinesterase molecule in the brain is slightly different from that in the rest of the body, so that it should be possible to develop drugs which only act on the brain molecule. Several laboratories have had some success, and their drugs are now available. These include rivastigmine and donepezil, which improve the ability of Alzheimer's disease patients to think clearly, remember things, and perform simple motor tasks for themselves without producing many of the troublesome side-effects of eserine and tacrine.

Donepezil is particularly valuable as it lasts a long time in the body. A single dose each day lasts for more than 24 hours, so that patients or their carers need remember only to take a single tablet at the same time each day.

Keep taking the tablets!

One feature of clinical trials is that new drugs are given for a defined period of time. When patients were taken off treatment with donepezil or metrifonate, however, their condition rapidly deteriorated again. Patients may, therefore, need to continue taking these drugs for life.

Unfortunately, the side-effects may make this difficult. Since these drugs increase the amount of acetylcholine in the body (*see* Chapter 1), there will be a tendency to increased salivation, slowed heart rate, and diarrhoea, as well as the nausea often produced by drugs acting on the brain. Most patients tolerate these very mild effects to gain the improvements in memory and thinking produced by the drugs, but a few may find them too unpleasant.

Acetylcholine receptor agonists

Rather than increasing the amount of acetylcholine in the brain by inhibiting cholinesterase, an alternative strategy is to use drugs which act directly on the receptors for acetylcholine.

The earliest attempts to treat Alzheimer's disease involved increasing the amount of choline (an amine present in high quantities in fish) in the diet. Nerve cells use choline to make acetylcholine and the idea was that by increasing the amount of choline available, the synthesis of acetylcholine would be increased. The results, however, were not impressive and this strategy is no longer used.

There are two types of receptor for acetylcholine—nicotinic and muscarinic (*see* Chapter 1)—both of which exist in the brain as well as in the rest of the body. However, the receptors in the brain are slightly different from those found in other organs, so that it has been possible to develop drugs which can act mainly in the brain without producing many side-effects. These include xanomeline, an agonist at muscarinic receptors which improves attention, cognition (thinking), and memory. A major advantage of this drug is that it also reduces the activity of cells which release dopamine as their transmitter. This means that xanomeline reduces the aggression, agitation and hallucinations which can sometimes occur in patients with Alzheimer's disease. However, because this drug activates acetylcholine receptors throughout the body, it can produce a marked drop in blood pressure, with fainting.

Drug companies are now assessing several similar drugs such as sabcomeline and milameline to see if they might be more effective and have fewer side-effects than xanomeline (Table 10.2, p. 151).

Nicotine

Several areas of the brain affected by Alzheimer's disease contain nicotinic receptors for acetylcholine, but the number of these receptors is greatly reduced in Alzheimer's disease patients.

If nicotinic receptors are blocked in normal people by drugs such as mecamylamine, the subjects perform less well in learning and reasoning tests. Conversely, the receptors can be activated by nicotine itself, and tests in animals and humans show that nicotine increases the ability of patients to pay attention to events and to remember new things. Smokers, of course, will not be surprised by this, as it has long been claimed that increased alertness, attention, memory, and thinking are enhanced by smoking.*

Nicotine patches are now being developed for use in Alzheimer's disease, as this should help the mental condition without the serious health problems which accompany smoking. However, nicotine activates receptors in the muscles, intestine, and nerves, leading to digestive and cardiovascular problems. Several companies are, therefore, developing drugs which only activate the nicotinic receptors in the brain. As yet, these are not available clinically.†

Metabolic enhancers

Since dementia can be caused by the blockage of small blood vessels in the brain (multi-infarct dementia), drugs which relax blood vessels and increase blood

---

* It has often been pointed out, however, that memory and reasoning may be relatively poor to begin with in some people who smoke, and smoking helps them to improve towards the standard of the majority of the population, just as giving nicotine as a drug improves patients with Alzheimer's disease much more than normal subjects. Furthermore, the long-term side-effects of smoking make it a completely unacceptable and dangerous way of trying to improve concentration.

† These drugs are known only by their code numbers such as GTS-21 and RJR1401.

flow to the brain have been tested in patients. Their effects vary greatly, probably because the importance of blocked vessels varies greatly between different patients. Nevertheless some of these drugs, such as nicergoline and hydergine, have been claimed to benefit some patients. They work by blocking alpha-receptors for norepinephrine (see Chapter 1) and receptors for 5-hydroxytryptamine (5HT) on blood vessels, dilating them and improving the blood flow to damaged areas of brain. Because they also block receptors on other blood vessels, patients may find that their blood pressure falls when they stand up quickly, causing fainting.

Drugs of the future

Drugs acting on 5HT receptors

The 5HT3 receptors reduce the release of acetylcholine from nerve cells, so drugs such as ondansetron, granisetron, and tropisetron which block 5HT3 receptors cause the opposite—an increase in the release of acetylcholine. These drugs are already being tested or used clinically for disorders such as migraine, nausea, and vomiting (see Chapters 4 and 7) and will soon be tested in Alzheimer's disease.

Glutamate receptor agonists

As the number of nerve cells declines in Alzheimer's disease, one strategy for treatment is to increase the activity of the cells that remain. One way of achieving this is to activate the receptors for the excitatory neurotransmitter glutamate. There are several types of glutamate receptors, including those known as NMDA* and AMPA† receptors. Drugs are in development which can act on both types of receptor: D-cycloserine and milacemide activate the NMDA receptors, and are being tested in humans. In animal tests both drugs increase the ability to learn and remember.

When glutamate acts on AMPA receptors, they stop responding after a short time, a process known as 'desensitisation'. There is a range of drugs able to prevent this loss of sensitivity, thereby increasing the activation of AMPA receptors by glutamate already in the brain. These include aniracetam, pramiracetam, and rolziracetam. Some have been available in some countries for several years without any knowledge of how they worked. Similar but more powerful drugs are being developed for testing in the future.

Glutamate receptor antagonists

Since glutamate can kill nerve cells, an alternative approach is to slow down the rate of cell death by using drugs which block the receptors for glutamate. There

* NMDA is an abbreviation for N-methyl-D-aspartate.
† AMPA is an abbreviation for α-amino-3-hydroxy-5-methyl-4-isoxazole-propionic acid.

are many of these drugs under development because they may also be valuable in epilepsy and other brain disorders.

Calcium blockers

The movement of calcium into nerve cells is often part of the sequence of events leading to cell death and is increased by substances such as glutamate and beta-amyloid. Several drugs, such as nimodipine, block this movement of calcium and should protect cells against damage.

Antioxidants

The damaging effects of 'free radicals' on cells is described in Chapter 22. Nerve cells in the brain are especially susceptible because their activity is so dependent on complex fatty molecules which are easily oxidized and disrupted by free radicals. Some research has shown that beta-amyloid can increase the formation of free radicals in the brain, so another approach to treating Alzheimer's disease may be to use antioxidant drugs. One being tested is idebenone, which can 'mop up', or scavenge, the free radicals, limiting their ability to injure the cells.

A series of steroid-like drugs called lazaroids* are also able to scavenge free radicals and protect nerve cells from death.

Anti-inflammatory agents

When nerve cells in the brain die, other nearby cells called 'glia' seem to react and produce localized inflammation. Glia can produce substances which can damage the brain further. One possibility, therefore, is to treat Alzheimer's disease with drugs known to reduce inflammation. These have been described in Chapters 6 and 20, and include aspirin and indomethacin. Aspirin is too dangerous a drug to take in large amounts for several years, because of its tendency to damage the stomach wall. At least one trial using indomethacin in humans has shown that it can slow the progression of Alzheimer's disease symptoms, although it carries the risk of causing bleeding from, or ulceration of, the stomach (see Chapter 6). It is likely that more drugs of this type will be developed with effects that are limited to the brain. However, it is still not clear whether these drugs work by inhibiting the COX enzyme (see Chapters 6 and 16) or by mopping up free radicals—molecular fragments which can wreak serious damage to cells (see Chapter 22). Aspirin is very efficient at removing free radicals, and is even used in some methods of detecting the rate at which free radicals are being produced.

Growth factors

Nerve cells need a 'soup' of hormones to survive. The acetylcholine-releasing cells of the nucleus basalis need, most of all, a hormone called Nerve Growth

* So-called after the biblical character Lazarus who was brought back from dead.

Factor (NGF). In Alzheimer's disease, cells may die because they are starved of this hormone, so one possible treatment being examined is to replace the NGF, either by delivering the hormone directly into the brain, or by using chemicals which act on the NGF receptors to increase the survival of the nerve cells—in other words, by replacing the natural NGF.

The drug propentofylline seems to increase the formation of NGF in the brain and is being tested in clinical trials for Alzheimer's disease.

ACE inhibitors

The Angiotensin converting enzyme (ACE) is responsible for making the hormone angiotensin II in the blood (see Chapter 15). It performs the same function in the brain and its product, angiotensin, inhibits the release of acetylcholine from nerve cells. In addition, the same enzyme helps to break down several other peptide hormones and neurotransmitters such as the enkephalins and endorphins (see Chapter 6) which also affect learning and thinking. Drugs which inhibit ACE prevent the formation of angiotensin and other peptides and increase the release of acetylcholine. As a result these drugs, such as captopril, increase the ability of animals to learn and remember and they are likely to be tested soon in humans.

Steroids

Experiments in animals have shown that steroid hormones can determine whether nerve cells live or die. The female steroids, oestrogens, seem to protect cells, so that drugs which activate the receptors of oestrogens in the brain may be of use in Alzheimer's disease.

Conversely, the steroids which are produced by the adrenal glands in response to stress (the glucocorticoids, Chapter 19) enhance the death of nerve cells. Long-term exposure to stressful situations may, therefore, turn out to be one of the factors which predisposes people to develop Alzheimer's disease. Equally, drugs which block the receptors for these steroids in the brain might reduce the development of the disease.

Drugs affecting beta-amyloid

Finally, a vast amount of research is underway to find substances which can stop the formation of beta-amyloid. We have seen that there is a close association between the existence of amyloid in the brain and the development of Alzheimer's disease. Animals which secrete abnormally large amounts of beta-amyloid show increased cell death in the brain, as well as a poor ability to learn. Drugs which either interfere with the production of beta-amyloid, or which speed its destruction and removal might, therefore, be of benefit in delaying or slowing the progression of Alzheimer's disease.

Other dementias

Alzheimer's disease is only one form of dementia. It arises because cells in the brain die at a rate far higher than can be compensated by other cells. Other forms of dementia, as mentioned at the beginning of this chapter, can be caused by a stroke, infections of the brain (as can happen in syphilis), or a long-term deficiency of vitamin B_{12} (which can occur in chronic alcoholics). Forms of dementia can also occur in Parkinson's disease and Huntington's disease. Unfortunately, the cellular changes which occur in these dementias are less clear even than in Alzheimer's disease, so that drugs to treat them are not yet becoming available. This is partly because they are far less common than Alzheimer's disease, so that the testing of drugs in patients is much more difficult. Perhaps, as we learn more about Alzheimer's disease and the ability of drugs to treat it, we may also learn more about these other forms of dementia. Perhaps some of the same drugs being developed for Alzheimer's disease may in time prove to have some beneficial effect in other dementias.

Table 10.1 Drugs used in Alzheimer's disease

Cholinesterase inhibitors
donepezil
eptastigmine
eserine (physostigmine)
galanthamine
metrifonate
physostigmine (eserine)
rivastigmine
tacrine

Table 10.2 Drugs being developed for Alzheimer's disease

Acetylcholine receptor agonists	Glutamate receptor modulators
muscarinic	Aniracetam
xanomeline	Oxiracetam
	Piracetam
nicotinic	Pramiracetam
nicotine	Rolziracetam
Glutamate receptor agonists	**Metabolic enhancers**
D-cycloserine	Hydergine
Milacemide	Nicergoline
	Free radical inhibitors
	idebenone

Summary

- *Dementias are disorders of the brain characterized by mental confusion and a loss of memory. Alzheimer's disease is one of these disorders.*
- *Alzheimer's disease involves a loss of nerve cells releasing acetylcholine as their transmitter.*
- *The drugs available to treat Alzheimer's disease increase the activation of acetylcholine receptors in the brain, either by inhibiting the breakdown of acetylcholine or by acting directly on the acetylcholine receptors.*
- *Many other types of drug are being studied in the hope of alleviating the enormous social and financial costs of Alzheimer's disease.*

CHAPTER 11

Depression

There were rows of beds and near them immobile people, seemingly petrified, with gloomy, hostile faces. A few smiled falsely and were over-pleasing, whereas others were strange and incomprehensible. Silence and immobility dominated the ward. Where was the unrest, the excitement, the agitation, the chaos, the turbulence, the out-of-control actions, the characteristics of insanity anticipated in my student eyes and in the eyes of the average person? Was this madness I was seeing? Where was the inner turmoil that was supposed to be a part of mental illness? Where was the bizarreness and irregularity? I failed to sense the immense suffering, the internal torment that this situation, frozen and still, kept hidden within itself.*

Depression

Most people probably feel 'depressed' at some time in their lives. Pressure of work, a domestic crisis, a bereavement—these and many other life events can make us feel as if we are not in control of our destinies, that we cannot cope with the problems or the loss. We refer to the resulting 'down' mood as depression. But this depression is a typical reaction to a particular situation and it lasts for only a few days or weeks. It is known as 'reactive' depression, and while it may give way to feelings of great sadness at a loss, or to strategies of coping with a change of job, the depression itself does not normally linger.

In some people this is not the case. They describe themselves as feeling permanently depressed even though there may have been no obvious trigger. The depression may last for months or years and this, coupled with the absence of a trigger characterizes what clinicians call 'true', 'melancholic', or 'endo-genous' depression. It is not just that people feel depressed. They become very apathetic, they are unable to function socially and have no desire to interact with other people so that they become withdrawn, lose friends, and become isolated. Their body movements and often their speech become slowed and they often lose appetite and stop eating correctly. A study of six European

* From *The Rise of Psychopharmacology* by R. Rossi, Fabre, 1998, p. 26.

countries in 1996 showed that nearly 1 in 5 people had symptoms of depression at some time during the year.

The discovery of antidepressant drugs

The first drugs able to reverse depression were discovered accidentally. In 1952 Henri Laborit in France, together with Jean Delay and Pierre Deniker, had noticed that an antihistamine, chlorpromazine, would calm schizophrenic patients. The makers, Geigy Pharmaceuticals, then modified the structure of the chlorpromazine molecule to try and eliminate its antihistamine activity (and other undesirable effects). Eventually the compound they produced was ready for testing in schizophrenic patients. Continuing from the scene referred to in the quotation which opened this Chapter, Alan Broadhurst, one of the Geigy team involved in the trial relates what happened next:*

> The whole team of medical and nursing staff waited with bated breath. At first, very little happened. Then, within a period ranging from a few days to several weeks, certain very definite results began to appear. These were not only fascinating. They were, in some patients, quite alarming. Several previously quiet patients began to deteriorate with increasing agitation. One man, in such a state, managed to get hold of a bicycle and rode in his nightshirt to a nearby village singing lustily, much to the alarm of the local inhabitants. Our disappointment was intense. The trial was abandoned.

Over the succeeding months Broadhurst and his colleagues analysed their results carefully and discussed constantly the reasons for the drug's effects. Eventually they realized that the patients who had shown the greatest development of excitement and agitation were those who had been depressed as well as schizophrenic and the idea developed of trying the new drug in patients who were only depressed. Alan Broadhurst again:

> After forty patients had been treated, it was clear that G22355 [the company's code name for the drug] was producing a dramatic, and this time beneficial, response. I had seen some seriously depressed patients, and I was all too aware of what a merciless and devastating illness severe and unremitting depression could be. The fact that we might now, for the first time ever, have an effective treatment seemed incredible. If this therapeutic effect could be repeated in larger groups of patients, then G22355 represented a major advance in medicine.

G22355 was eventually given the name imipramine, and became the forerunner of dozens of drugs, called 'tricyclic antidepressants' because the molecules all contain three rings of atoms. The trial just described was in 1955, but imipramine itself is still available and widely used for the treatment of depression.

A second drug was also discovered accidentally when doctors realized that

* In *The Rise of Psychopharmacology*, p. 73.

iproniazid, a drug being used to treat tuberculosis, caused depressed patients to feel happier.

What causes depression?

The first clue to answering this question came from a drug called reserpine, in the first half of this century. Reserpine is present in the roots of the *Rauwolfia* plant (*see* Chapter 9), and extracts of this plant had been used for at least 2000 years in the medical armouries of doctors who were using it to lower blood pressure in hypertensive patients. It does so by causing the sympathetic nerves to lose their stores of the neurotransmitter norepinephrine (noradrenaline). Normally the nerve stores norepinephrine in small packets known as vesicles which are secreted onto receptors on blood vessels when the nerves are active (*see* Chapter 1). Reserpine disrupts the vesicles so that norepinephrine can no longer be stored or released, the sympathetic stimulation of the heart and blood vessels decreases and the blood pressure falls. Doctors soon realized that some patients taking reserpine for their blood pressure became severely depressed, sometimes suicidal. This gave the first clue that depression might be caused by a reduced release of norepinephrine from nerve cells.

The drugs which had been found accidentally to benefit depressed patients also affected norepinephrine neurons in the brain. Like all other neurotransmitters the amines are secreted from nerve cells when these are active. The transmitters produce their effects by activating receptors on cell membranes as we saw in Chapter 1. But once the receptors have been activated the transmitters need to be removed so that the receptors can respond to another batch of transmitters a fraction of a second later. To do this nerve cells have a system of molecules on their endings which transport the transmitters from the region of the receptors back into the nerve cell ending (Fig. 11.1). This process of removal by transport is known as 'uptake'. Once inside the nerve cell, some of the amine transmitter molecules are used again, but some molecules are destroyed by the enzyme monoamine oxidase (MAO). Imipramine prevents nerve cells removing norepinephrine from the receptors, prolonging its effects. Iproniazid inhibits the MAO enzymes which normally break down norepinephrine. The effects of imipramine and iproniazid, therefore, are the same—to increase the amount of norepinephrine acting on its receptors. The overall effect is the opposite of the effect of reserpine.

These and related experimental observations led to a suggestion by the American pharmacologist Joseph Schildkraut in 1957 that a decrease in the function of nerve cells secreting norepinephrine in the brain causes depression whereas an increase in the activity of those neurons will reverse depression or even cause euphoria.*

* This idea became known as 'the catecholamine hypothesis of affective disorders'. The term 'affective' in this context refers to disorders in which the primary change is one of mood (affect).

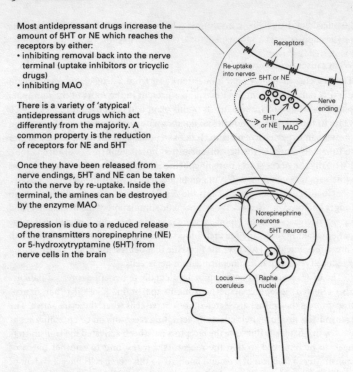

Most antidepressant drugs increase the amount of 5HT or NE which reaches the receptors by either:
• inhibiting removal back into the nerve terminal (uptake inhibitors or tricyclic drugs)
• inhibiting MAO

There is a variety of 'atypical' antidepressant drugs which act differently from the majority. A common property is the reduction of receptors for NE and 5HT

Once they have been released from nerve endings, 5HT and NE can be taken into the nerve by re-uptake. Inside the terminal, the amines can be destroyed by the enzyme MAO

Depression is due to a reduced release of the transmitters norepinephrine (NE) or 5-hydroxytryptamine (5HT) from nerve cells in the brain

Receptors
Re-uptake into nerves
5HT or NE
Nerve ending
5HT or NE
MAO
Norepinephrine neurons
5HT neurons
Locus coeruleus
Raphe nuclei

Fig. 11.1 How drugs act to reduce depression. The abbreviation MAO refers to monoamine oxidase, NE to norepinephrine, and 5HT to 5-hydroxytryptamine.

Of course, things are never as simple as they first seem. For example, drugs such as cocaine and amphetamine increase the release of norepinephrine from nerve cells in the brain. But while they produce euphoria—the sense of well-being which contributes to their addictive properties—they do not reverse depression. We also now know that several amines in the brain are involved in the control of mood, not just norepinephrine. Two other important amine transmitters are dopamine and 5-hydroxytryptamine (5HT). Reserpine can prevent the storage of all these chemicals in nerve cells, iproniazid can increase the levels of them all, and imipramine can inhibit their uptake. As a result, we believe that depression is caused by a fault in nerve cells secreting amine neurotransmitters, but which one, or ones, is still not entirely clear.

There are also nagging problems with the amine hypothesis. When imipramine or iproniazid are given to patients, their effects on amine removal or destruction by MAO enzymes occur within a few hours. Yet depressed patients show little improvement for several days, usually weeks, after treatment is started.

Drugs used to treat depression

Tricyclic antidepressants

The tricyclic antidepressants raise the amount of transmitter at the receptors by preventing their uptake into the nerve ending (Fig. 11.1). This leaves more of the amine outside the nerve cells and able to interact with the receptors. Tricyclic drugs affect mainly cells which secrete norepinephrine. They include imipramine and desipramine (Table 11.1, p. 164).

There are several related tricyclic drugs which act in exactly the same way, inhibiting amine uptake into nerve endings, but they affect cells which release a different amine: 5-hydroxytryptamine (5HT). This is also known as serotonin, because it was first extracted from serum (sero-) and found to raise the tension (-tonin) in muscle cells. This group of antidepressant drugs are, therefore, known as selective serotonin reuptake inhibitors (SSRIs), and include fluoxetine, fluvoxamine, citalopram, and sertraline (Table 11.1, p. 164). They probably work in depression because they compensate for a lower than normal amount of 5HT in some areas of the brain.

Fluoxetine (Prozac®)

Fluoxetine was introduced into the USA in 1987 with the trade name 'Prozac'. It proved so popular that by 1989 the costs of prescribing Prozac exceeded that of all antidepressants in the previous two years. The reason for its success seems to be that it is not only able to relieve depression, but it adds something extra—a general 'feel-good factor' which makes patients taking the drug assert that they have never felt better. Even healthy, non-depressed people have been using it to give them that sunnier feeling which was not produced by the older antidepressant drugs.

Animals can also apparently be made to 'feel good'. Two scientists at the Neuropsychiatric Institute of the University of California, Michael Raleigh and Michael McGuire, were trying to identify what it was that made one male monkey become dominant over a colony. They discovered that the dominant male had more 5HT in its brain than other monkeys, but that if that animal were displaced from its position of dominance, the level of 5HT fell and the animal's behaviour came to resemble that of a depressed human, with a subdued and withdrawn attitude, a slowing of movements and a loss of appetite. The researchers then found that if they removed the dominant male of a colony and administered Prozac to another animal, that monkey invariably became the new dominant one. These observations suggest that the ability to become dominant depends on the amount of 5HT in the brain. If we allow ourselves to extrapolate from monkey to Man, it is possible that the popularity of Prozac is due to its producing similar feelings of confidence and self-esteem in people.

Fortunately, Prozac is relatively safe, even in large doses: there are cases of patients taking up to 100 times the recommended dose and surviving. The side-effects are few and relatively mild in most people. It may cause headaches, insomnia, and weight loss which is often seen as an advantage by some patients. A few patients report a decrease of sexual activity. Recent research has shown that Prozac may even be effective in some psychological disorders which have not previously responded to drugs, including bulimia (eating followed by induced vomiting) and kleptomania (compulsive stealing).

Problems

Many of the tricyclics can block receptors for acetylcholine (*see* Chapter 1), producing a dry mouth due to reduced secretion of saliva, blurred vision because the eyes do not adjust for objects at different distances, and constipation because the movements of the intestine are reduced. The body usually adjusts to these effects, so that they disappear after a few weeks. A drug related to the tricyclics, trazodone, does not have these effects, which occur much less often with the newer SSRI drugs. Trazodone sometimes has the unusual side-effect of causing a persistent penile erection, a condition know as priapism which can be unpleasant and painful.

Some of the tricyclics, such as imipramine, can produce sedation and drowsiness, probably because they block receptors for acetylcholine and histamine in the brain. The SSRI drugs are much less likely to produce these effects. Amoxapine can block receptors for dopamine in the brain, leading to problems with movement similar to those in Parkinson's disease.

There is also, frequently, a tendency for the blood pressure to fall, with the risk of fainting, and occasionally changes in the rhythm of the heartbeat. These unwanted side-effects are due to the changed amounts of norepinephrine being released by the nerves to the heart and blood vessels, and the ability of these drugs, especially doxepin, to block the alpha-receptors which cause the blood vessels to contract.

One of the side-effects which most often causes patients to stop taking their antidepressant drugs is that of reduced sexual function. Substances which activate 5HT-2 receptors in the brain and spinal cord inhibit sexual activity in animals, and as the amounts of 5HT are increased by antidepressants the amine activates these receptors, causing reduced sexual drive. A few drugs such as mirtazapine can block these receptors, so that this side-effect does not occur.

Monoamine oxidase inhibitors (MAO inhibitors)

The second major group of antidepressants inhibit monoamine oxidase. This means that less amine is destroyed inside the nerve ending, leaving more available for storage and release by the nerve cell. This group includes phenelzine, tranylcypromine, and moclobemide.

Problems

As with the tricyclics, the most common side-effect of monoamine oxidase inhibitors is a fall of blood pressure and the associated risk of fainting. The reason for this is not understood. The MAO inhibitors are able to block the actions of acetylcholine to some extent, so they can produce the dry mouth, blurred vision, and constipation seen with the tricyclics.

By far the most serious complication of using MAO inhibitors is what is known as the 'cheese reaction', a phenomenon first described in 1963 by Barry Blackwell working at the Maudsley Hospital in London. Some foodstuffs, such as cheese, contain amines which are usually broken down in the body by MAO. When this enzyme is inhibited by MAO inhibitors, these amines, including tyrosine (from *tyros*, the Greek word for cheese) and tyramine, can accumulate in the blood and activate receptors for norepinephrine. The result can be a huge increase in blood pressure which, in a few people, may be enough to cause bleeding into the brain, i.e. a stroke. Patients taking MAO inhibitors, therefore, are always warned not to eat or drink several food items, some of which are listed in Table 11.2, p. 164.

Problems understanding antidepressants

Clearly, our understanding of depression and its treatment is far from complete. For one thing, it seems odd that drugs which affect two quite different transmitter systems, using norepinephrine or serotonin, should all be antidepressants. But there are other problems too. One is that there are also effective antidepressants which do not seem to affect the re-uptake of either norepinephrine or serotonin. These are known as 'atypical' antidepressants and include iprindole and mianserin.

Another problem lies in the time course of drug effects. Suppose that a depressed patient is given desipramine. The uptake of amines will be suppressed within 24 hours of starting treatment, yet it will be 2 to 4 weeks before the patient's depression starts to lift. The same problem applies to inhibitors of MAO, since the enzyme is inhibited within 24 hours with no sign of relief of depression for several weeks.

Pharmacologists are, therefore, trying to find out whether there are other actions of antidepressant drugs which the various groups have in common. Some common changes have been found on nerve cells, such as a decrease in the number of beta-receptors or a type of serotonin receptor known as 5HT-2, but there is not yet any general agreement as to whether these are the explanation for the antidepressant actions. The changes of beta-receptors and 5HT-2 receptors are very interesting, though, because they are also produced by a form of non-drug treatment for depression: electric shock treatment (also known as electroconvulsive therapy or ECT).

Electroconvulsive therapy (ECT)

About one in every four patients with depression does not respond to any of the drugs described here, but many of those resistant subjects will obtain relief from depression after a series of four or five sessions in which they are anaesthetized and the body is made to convulse by a large electric current. The treatment sounds rather unpleasant, but patients do not suffer lasting problems apart from a slight loss of memory for events shortly before the session. The treatment is very effective, and one to two weeks afterwards, the depression begins to lift, and patients may remain free from depression for years. Interestingly, ECT in animals produces exactly the same changes of beta-receptors and 5HT2 receptors which occur with antidepressant drugs, supporting the idea that these may be important common factors in the alleviation of depression.

Other antidepressants

After the non-selective amine uptake inhibitors (the tricyclics) and SSRIs, a new class of antidepressant has recently been launched—the 'serotonin and norepinephrine reuptake inhibitors' (SNRIs). Part of the reason for developing this type of drug was the discovery that depression was relieved much more rapidly—sometimes in days rather than weeks—when patients received a combination of desipramine and fluoxetine. Desipramine is particularly good at preventing the uptake into cells of norepinephrine, leading to increased levels of the amine outside cells, while fluoxetine (Prozac) is an SSRI and raises the levels of 5HT in the brain. The benefit of this drug combination, therefore, strongly suggested that increasing the amounts of both norepinephrine and 5HT might be a better strategy than increasing either one alone.

At present, the main drugs in this new class are milnacipran and venlafaxine, which are not only very effective antidepressants, but which lack many of the side-effects of the classical tricyclic drugs. For example, they do not seem to produce any block of acetylcholine, dopamine, histamine, or norepinephrine receptors. Changes of blood pressure, reduced salivation, constipation, and other autonomic side-effects noted with the older drugs are not, therefore, a problem. It seems likely that other members of this new class of drugs will appear in the near future.

Mianserin and mirtazapine

The release of neurotransmitters is partly controlled by receptors on nerve terminals. These inhibitory receptors include alpha-2 receptors for norepinephrine on the terminals of cells which release norepinephrine or 5HT. When they are activated by norepinephrine, they reduce the amount of transmitter released by the nerves.

These receptors can be blocked by two drugs, mianserin and mirtazapine. Blockade of these receptors means that more norepinephrine and 5HT will be released, increasing the amount of these amines outside the cells. The effect, therefore, is similar to that of the drugs which prevent the removal of the transmitters. All these drugs are able to relieve depression.

The antidepressant effect of 5HT released in the brain seems to involve activation of 5HT1 receptors, while activation of other 5HT receptors is responsible for many of the side-effects of drugs. However, the newer of the two alpha-receptor antagonists, mirtazapine, can block 5HT2 and 5HT3 receptors. Blockade of the 5HT2 receptors helps to reduce anxiety in patients, improve the quality of sleep, and prevent the decline of sexual activity which occurs with many of the SSRIs. Blockade of the 5HT3 receptors prevents the nausea and vomiting produced by some of the older antidepressants. Mirtazapine, therefore, seems to be a very promising new drug.

Bupropion

The pharmaceutical industry has tried many different types of chemical in an effort to find new antidepressants without the side-effects listed above. One drug, bupropion, looks very promising as it is a very effective antidepressant but does not produce any sedation (drowsiness), and does not require patients to stop taking alcohol. It can reduce all the different aspects of depression, which often include some anxiety, sleeplessness, and difficulty in thinking clearly. It is, therefore, a very effective and apparently safe drug. Since it does not affect the transmitters norepinephrine and 5HT, it also works in a new and unknown way. Unfortunately, bupropion is not available in many countries because a few patients showed serious side-effects. Nevertheless, it is a sign that better antidepressants can be produced; research continues to find similar but even safer drugs. Several such drugs, such as reboxetine, are approaching the end of clinical trials and may be available in the near future.

Bipolar or manic depression

A small number of patients have a disorder in which their mood changes in cycles between depression and its opposite—mania. The cycles may occur over a period of a few hours, although they usually take place over several days or weeks. During the manic phase, people become agitated and easily irritated, their speech and movements are rapid, their attention span is short, and they are easily distracted by fanciful ideas. They sleep less and generally show flamboyant, extrovert behaviour. Some patients may have hallucinations. It is said that van Gogh suffered mania with hallucinations of sight and hearing which caused him to mutilate himself by cutting off his ear.*

Lithium

The usual treatment for mania or manic-depression is lithium. This is a simple ion, rather than a complicated molecule, and the means by which it controls bipolar depression is not well understood. There are changes in the amine-releasing nerve cells in the brain, including those that use dopamine and serotonin, and changes in the number of receptors for these neurotransmitters. However, which, if any, of these changes is responsible for the beneficial activity of lithium is uncertain.

Problems

Lithium levels in the body must be controlled very carefully, or patients can experience side-effects. For this reason, doctors usually measure the amount of lithium in the blood regularly, and change the dose prescribed if necessary. The commonest side-effects are tremors, blurred vision, vomiting, weakness, drowsiness, and changes in thyroid and adrenal gland function.

Lithium, therefore, has disadvantages, both as a result of these side-effects, and in taking several weeks to bring mania under full control. Other drugs may be needed in some cases to help until lithium works fully.

Alternatives

Two other drugs are sometimes used to treat mania. One is carbamazepine. Better known as an anticonvulsant drug (see Chapter 12), this also seems to calm manic patients. How exactly it does this is not known, but it does block some of the ion channels for sodium in nerve cells which allow them to communicate with each other. Carbamazepine may, therefore, simply interfere with the ability of nerve cells to pass on a state of hyperexcitability to other cells.

Another alternative to lithium is sometimes used when patients are so manic that they need to be controlled rapidly, perhaps because they are becoming a danger to other people (for example by trying to drive a car). In these cases, some of the antipsychotic drugs discussed in Chapter 9, such as haloperidol, seem to be very effective in calming the patient, even though they have no such effect in normal people. It is as though the antipsychotic drugs interrupt processes in the brain which are specific to mania. They are effective within a few

---

* From *Ailments through the ages*, by R. Gordon.

hours, and can be used to control mania until lithium takes effect after a few weeks. Unfortunately, these drugs do not control mania for more than a few days or weeks, and prolonged use can result in a number of serious side-effects which are discussed in Chapter 9. They cannot, therefore, be used as a long-term substitute for lithium.

Other disorders

Antidepressant drugs are the most effective treatment for what is known as obsessive-compulsive disorder, or OCD. Patients with OCD have great difficulty in leading normal lives, because so much of their time is taken satisfying their obsessive or compulsive behaviours. For example, they may feel compelled to wash their clothes every night because they cannot bear to have dirty clothes in the basket; they may have to check a dozen times that they have switched off the oven or locked the house door. Many people find it reassuring to check doors and ovens a couple of times and such behaviour is considered normal, but when taken to extremes, carrying out such compulsions every day can consume a great deal of time. One patient could not have people in her house (she was divorced) because their presence produced dirty glasses and crockery which she then felt compelled to wash immediately.

While several antidepressants are useful in OCD, the SSRI drugs are by far the best treatments. They are also proving to be useful in a number of complex psychological disorders such as eating disorders, panic attacks, phobias, and chronic pain.

Phobias

Phobias are intense, often irrational fears which in some people give rise to profound, desparate anxiety or panic. They include conditions such as agoraphobia (a fear of open spaces which can prevent patients from ever leaving their homes) and claustrophobia (fear of enclosed spaces). Although these conditions sound like anxiety states, they can be treated with antidepressant drugs, but not anti-anxiety drugs.

Pain

The use of antidepressants in chronic, severely painful conditions reflects the idea that the intensity of pain can produce depression which in turn increases the intensity of the pain. Treating the depression, therefore, improves the patient's condition as well as allowing the dose of pain-killing drugs to be reduced.

Chronic fatigue syndrome

The condition known as chronic fatigue syndrome, postviral fatigue syndrome, Royal Free disease, or myalgic encephalomyelitis (once also cynically referred to as 'yuppie flu' as it affects primarily people in their late teens and twenties) is characterized by repeated bouts of severe fatigue with intense muscle pains and depression. The cause remains unknown, although some experts believe it can be caused by infection, while others argue that the problem is entirely psychological. Most treatments have proved ineffective, but antidepressant drugs have been among the most successful, suggesting that there is a major psychiatric component in the disorder.

Table 11.1 Antidepressant drugs

Tricyclic and related drugs	Related and ('atypical') antidepressants
amitriptyline	Bupropion (USA)
amoxapine	Iprindole
clomipramine	Maprotiline
desipramine	Mianserin
dosulepin*	Mirtazapine
dothiepin*	Reboxetine
doxepin	Trazodone
imipramine	Venlafaxine
lofepramine	Viloxazine
nortriptyline	
protriptyline	**Monoamine oxidase inhibitors (MAOIs)**
trimipramine	Isocarboxazid
	Moclobemide
Selective serotonin reuptake inhibitors (SSRIs)	Phenelzine
	Tranylcypromine
citalopram	
fluoxetine (Prozac®)	
fluvoxamine	**Drugs for mania**
nefazodone	Carbamazepine
paroxetine	Haloperidol
sertraline	Lithium carbonate
	Lithium citrate
SNRIs	
milnacipran	
venlafaxine	

* These are different names for the same drug.

Table 11.2 Food restrictions for patients taking monoamine oxidase inhibitor drugs

Avocados	Liver
Beers	Raisins
Broad beans	Sour cream
Canned meats or figs	Soy sauce
Cheeses (especially aged or blue)	Wine (especially red Chianti) and liqueurs
Chocolate	Yeast and meat extracts (Marmite, Bovril)
Coffee	Yoghurt
Herrings, sardines, anchovies	

Summary

- Depression is due to a lack of amine neurotransmitters in the brain, mainly norepinephrine and 5-hydroxytryptamine (5HT).

- Tricyclic antidepressants (such as doxepin) prevent nerve cells from removing the amines from their receptors, leading to an increased activation of those receptors in the brain.

- The MAO inhibitors inhibit the enzyme monoamine oxidase which normally destroys the amines, again resulting in an increased activation of the receptors on nerve cells.

- Mianserin and mirtazapine block $\alpha 2$-receptors on nerve terminals, causing an increased release of the amines.

- Buproprion and reboxetine are new drugs whose mechanisms are not yet fully understood.

- Bipolar or manic depression is treated with lithium, carbamazepine, or haloperidol. How they work is not fully understood, although haloperidol blocks dopamine receptors and calms over-excited patients with disorders such as schizophrenia.

- Antidepressant drugs are used to treat obsessive and compulsive disorders, panic, and phobias such as claustrophobia.

CHAPTER 12

Epilepsy

A few years ago I was sitting in the audience at a meeting of my local camera club, waiting for a visiting speaker to organize himself before showing slides of his recent visit to India. The young man seated on the end of the row in front of me raised his hand, rather slowly I thought, and ran it through his hair. He put his hand down again. Then he raised it and stroked it through his hair again. I sat while this sequence was repeated three, four, five, six times. At this point, I got out of my seat, went to the man and asked him if I could help him. As I did so, I gently took hold of his arm and eased him out of his chair. He looked at me with a totally blank expression, as if he did not know what was happening. He said nothing but slowly walked with me out of the room. I sat with him for a minute or so, during which I could see his normal movements returning to him, his blank expression disappeared, and he began to look more relaxed.

He then thanked me for helping him, explaining that he suffered from epilepsy. He did not have attacks very often, but when he did they often began with a repeated, stereotyped, and sometimes quite purposeless movement such as the stroking of his hair I had witnessed earlier. Had I not broken the chain of events, he told me, he would probably have progressed to a complete whole-body seizure.*

Epilepsy

Epilepsy has been with mankind at least as long as written records. In Rome in the fifth century BC, the 'falling sickness' as it was called was believed to be a sign of displeasure from the gods. The Greek word *epilepsia* means to take hold of, to throw down or to attack. There is a long list of people throughout history who are believed to have suffered from epilepsy, including Byron, Julius Caesar, Handel, Napoleon, Alfred Nobel, Tschaikovsky, and van Gogh.

Epilepsy can take many different forms. When most people think of epilepsy, they envisage someone falling to the ground and having a convulsion or fit, in which the arms and legs flail around dangerously, and the mouth may be

* Story related by a friend of the author.

clamped shut so tightly that parts of the tongue may be bitten off unless an object which can take the force of the bite is placed in the mouth. This form of epilepsy is known as tonic-clonic,* because the muscles are often rigid, with high tone, before they exhibit the convulsive, clonic, jerking movements of the arms and legs.

Generalized seizures

Tonic-clonic fits are one of two types of epilepsy, called generalized seizures, in which the patient loses consciousness. The other type is absence epilepsy.[†] Absence seizures usually affect children, and take the form of periods lasting from a second or so up to a minute, during which the child becomes totally unaware of their surroundings: for that period they are mentally unconscious, although they continue to sit or stand without collapsing. The seizure may interrupt an action or a sentence being read or spoken, and often the child will continue after the attack as if nothing had happened. If these fits occur frequently at school, the child must feel as if he or she is listening to a teacher talking through a microphone with a bad connection. It will be difficult to make sense of what is being said, and is extremely disruptive to the child's education.

Partial seizures

The young man—let's call him Tony—with whose story we began this chapter was suffering from a form of epilepsy called 'partial' because only a part of the body, in this case his arm, moved during the attack. Partial epilepsies may be either 'simple' in which part of the body shows twitching movements and then stops, or 'psychomotor' in which the body or a part of it shows a complex, often purposeless movement, repeated in a stereotyped fashion several times, as in Tony's case. If the patient loses consciousness, the seizure is referred to as a complex partial seizure. He or she may progress to a full tonic-clonic fit, although this is not usual. Sometimes the patient may experience, not a complex movement, but a complex aura of flashing lights, or sounds, or smells. Tony was showing the early stage of an attack of psychomotor epilepsy.

Causes of epilepsy

The cause of most epilepsies remain unknown. They may follow a head injury, or be associated with an infection or tumour in the brain. The majority are 'idiopathic'—the medical term for 'of unknown origin'. Whatever the precipitating cause, an epileptic attack begins when a group of nerve cells in the brain begin to fire their electrical impulses in an abnormally rapid fashion. This area or 'epileptic focus' of abnormally intense activity may remain

---

* Tonic-clonic seizures used to be called 'grand mal' seizures or fits.
† Absence epilepsy used to be called 'petit mal' epilepsy.

localized, causing simple twitching of one part of the body, or it may affect a wider area so that twitching in one part spreads to adjacent muscles. In some cases, the abnormal excitability spreads throughout the brain, leading to a tonic-clonic seizure of the whole body.

The seizures which involve twitching movements usually seem to start in the cerebral cortex—the outer layers of the brain, which are more highly developed in humans than in any other animal. The cortex includes areas that receive sensory information from different parts of the body. One area is concerned with vision, for example, another area with hearing, another with touch, and so on.

There are also areas which produce movement. Within one such area are groups of nerve cells which cause movements of individual parts of the body, such as a finger, or a thigh, or the lips. These areas are arranged in the same order as the body itself, so that, for example, the thumb area is next to the finger areas, which are next to the forearm area, which is next to the upper arm. Seizures involving movement usually begin in one of these areas and the spread of neuronal activity to adjacent areas is reflected in the spread of twitching to nearby parts of the body.

If the epileptic focus begins in a sensory area, the patient may experience a sensory aura, such as flashing lights if the focus is in the visual area of cortex.

Drug treatment of epilepsy

Bromide

The first two agents used to treat convulsions were used accidentally. In 1857, Sir Charles Locock (physician to Queen Victoria) argued that most cases of epilepsy were due to masturbation. Since high doses of bromide were believed to reduce sexual activity, he used it to treat several patients, all of whom improved. We now know, of course, that the effect of bromide has nothing whatever to so with sexual activity, but is the result of its depressing those nerve cells in the brain which trigger the epileptic seizure. Bromide is no longer used as the doses required to control epilepsy produce many unpleasant side-effects.

Barbiturates

The second drug discovered was phenobarbitone (phenobarbital). Several barbiturates had been produced by chemists working at the Bayer company in Germany. These were known to be sedatives (see Chapter 13). In 1911 a German doctor called Alfred Hauptmann was working and living in a hospital with a ward of epileptic patients, whose repeated fits kept him awake at night. He gave them phenobarbitone to sedate them, increase the depth of their sleep and reduce the number of fits. This approach worked, but he then noticed that the number and severity of fits declined greatly throughout the following day, even though the sedative effects had largely worn off. Hauptmann correctly guessed that the barbiturate had an anticonvulsant effect in addition to its sedative activity. Phenobarbitone is still available today for the treatment of epilepsy (Table 12.1, p. 175).

Effective though phenobarbitone was, there was clearly a need to develop drugs which did not cause sedation. In 1934 Tracy Putnam, an American physician in charge of the neurological unit at Boston City Hospital, began to test drugs related to phenobarbitone, obtained by writing to drug companies. One of these, phenytoin, looked promising when tested in animals and in 1936 Putnam and his assistant, Houston Merritt, gave it to a patient who had had a seizure every day for several years. The seizures stopped immediately and completely.

The modern drugs used to treat epilepsies include phenobarbitone and phenytoin as well as several derived from them. They either suppress the excessive excitability of nerve cells within the epileptic focus in the brain, or they stop the abnormal activity spreading to other regions of brain.

Phenytoin and carbamazepine

Phenytoin and carbamazepine act rather like local anaesthetics. The impulses produced by nerve cells are caused by the movement of sodium ions through pores, or channels, in the membranes of the cells. These channels are not holes in the membrane, but complicated molecules which can change their shape to block the passage of ions through the cell wall, or to allow them through. Phenytoin and carbamazepine, like local anaesthetics, block the sodium channels in the membranes, preventing the cells from generating impulses. This diminishes the epileptic activity, and prevents its spread away from the epileptic focus.

The question then arises of why these drugs do not stop *all* neuronal activity, causing sleep, coma, or even death? The answer is that sodium channels pass through a cycle of different physical states, being open, then closed, and then changing to a resting state before they can be opened again. Both phenytoin and carbamazepine prefer to block sodium channels when they are in the closed state immediately after being open. This means that the drugs will block channels which are excessively active (repeatedly opening and closing) much more readily than those in the resting state. They will, therefore, be much more effective in reducing neuronal activity in the highly active epileptic focus than in normal regions of the brain.

Despite the selectivity of phenytoin for those nerve cells producing a fit, it must also affect some of the other neurons in the brain. This may be why it often makes patients, especially children, tired and less able to think clearly.

One of the most common side-effects of treatment with phenytoin is very unusual. It promotes the formation of connective tissue, leading to an increased growth of body hair and gums, a condition know as 'gingival hyperplasia'.

Lamotrigine

Another drug which acts partly in the same way as phenytoin and carbamazepine, by blocking channels for sodium ions and reducing the ability of nerve cells to fire action potentials, is lamotrigine. However, it seems to show this effect more strongly at nerve endings which release the amino acid glutamate. This is the main transmitter responsible for exciting nerve cells in the brain, and it is certainly important for the spread of activity from cells in the epileptic focus to other areas of the brain. By reducing the release of glutamate, lamotrigine stops this spread of activity, and suppresses seizures.

Benzodiazepines, barbiturates

Several other drugs work by increasing the inhibitory effects of an inhibitory neurotransmitter, GABA* (Fig. 12.1). They include the group of benzodiazepines discussed in Chapter 13, phenobarbitone, vigabatrin, and valproate.

When GABA acts on its receptor, it increases the movement of chloride ions into the nerve cell. This makes the inside of the cell more negative, and the cell becomes less excitable, producing fewer impulses. Benzodiazepines interact at a different site on the GABA receptor. By themselves, they have no effect on the chloride channels, but when GABA and a benzodiazepine act at the same time, the channels open more frequently. Phenobarbitone acts in a similar way, but at a different site on the GABA receptor and its associated chloride channel, increasing the length of time that the channels are opened by GABA. In both cases, the net effect is the same: more chloride ions are allowed into the cells; the cells become inhibited and less able to indulge in the intense activity needed to trigger an epileptic attack.

As with any drug which decreases the activity of cells in the brain, these drugs tend to produce a degree of mental slowing and confusion in some patients.

Valproate and vigabatrin

The antiepileptic properties of valproate were discovered quite accidentally. In 1963, Pierre Eymard, a research student in Lyon, France, was studying the pharmacology of a substance he had made in the laboratory and which might have anticonvulsant activity. Unfortunately the compound would not dissolve in the usual solutions and he asked the advice of Professor H. Meunier in the University of Grenoble. Meunier had recently had a similar problem and had

* GABA is an abbreviation for the amino acid gamma-amino-butyric acid.

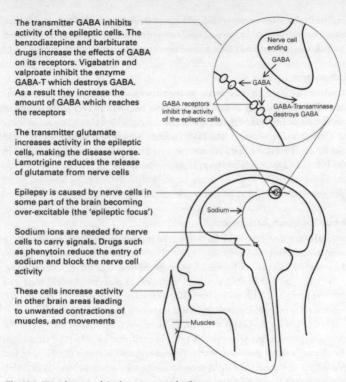

The transmitter GABA inhibits activity of the epileptic cells. The benzodiazepine and barbiturate drugs increase the effects of GABA on its receptors. Vigabatrin and valproate inhibit the enzyme GABA-T which destroys GABA. As a result they increase the amount of GABA which reaches the receptors

Nerve cell ending

GABA

← GABA

GABA receptors inhibit the activity of the epileptic cells

GABA-Transaminase destroys GABA

The transmitter glutamate increases activity in the epileptic cells, making the disease worse. Lamotrigine reduces the release of glutamate from nerve cells

Epilepsy is caused by nerve cells in some part of the brain becoming over-excitable (the 'epileptic focus')

Sodium →

Sodium ions are needed for nerve cells to carry signals. Drugs such as phenytoin reduce the entry of sodium and block the nerve cell activity

These cells increase activity in other brain areas leading to unwanted contractions of muscles, and movements

Muscles

Fig. 12.1 How drugs work in the treatment of epilepsy.

used a simple organic solvent, valproic acid, to dissolve his chemicals. Eymard followed suit and was delighted to find that his new chemical had anticonvulsant activity in animal tests. Shortly afterwards, Meunier himself tested a totally different chemical in animals, also dissolved in valproic acid, and was surprised to find that it had anticonvulsant activity very similar to that seen by Eymard. Meunier knew that it was very unusual to find substances which were so totally different chemically but with such similar biological properties. He soon realized that it was not the new substances that were responsible for the anticonvulsant behaviour, but the substance used to dissolve them—valproic acid (or valproate).

As with benzodiazepines and barbiturates, valproate and another very simple substance—vigabatrin—increase the effects of GABA, but in a different manner. When it has been released from nerve cells as a transmitter, GABA is normally removed by being absorbed back into the nerve endings, where it can be destroyed by the enzyme GABA transaminase. Vigabatrin and valproate reduce the removal of GABA into the nerve endings, and they also inhibit GABA transaminase. Once this enzyme is inhibited, the amount of GABA in the brain increases, and more may be released from the nerve endings as a neurotransmitter. The overall effect is once again to increase the inhibition of the nerve cells, suppressing the epileptic focus and preventing the spread of excitability around the brain.

In addition to these effects, valproate probably also increases the effects of GABA at its receptor but does so by acting at a site different from that of the barbiturates and benzodiazepines.

Topiramate

The new drug topiramate is a jack-of-all-trades. It blocks not only sodium channels, like phenytoin, but also receptors for glutamate, and increases the inhibitory actions of GABA. Blocking glutamate reduces the spread of excitability around the brain, as does lamotrigine, while potentiating the effects of GABA inhibits the cells in the epileptic focus.

Gabapentin

This compound was produced because it had a molecular structure similar to that of the inhibitory transmitter GABA. The idea was that by acting directly on GABA receptors in the brain, gabapentin would inhibit nerve cell activity and stop seizures. In fact, it has turned out that gabapentin does *not* stimulate GABA receptors, and at the time of writing we still have no clear idea of how it works. Nevertheless, it does help to stop seizures in some patients.

Status epilepticus

Usually a tonic-clonic fit lasts no more than a minute or two, after which the patient falls into a sleep for some time before regaining consciousness. On occasions, a fit may last very much longer: if it lasts more that about 30 minutes it is referred to as 'status epilepticus'. This is potentially dangerous since the muscles, including those of respiration, become fatigued. The intense activity of the muscles results in the accumulation of waste products which can damage tissues including the brain, and the patient may suffer from increasing lack of oxygen or carbon dioxide accumulation as a result of the abnormal breathing. It is essential, therefore, that 'status' be stopped as soon as possible, before the patient suffers serious brain damage or even death. The usual way of achieving this is to inject a benzodiazepine such as diazepam, or clomethiazole. The latter probably acts in the same way as diazepam, increasing the effects of

GABA and rapidly depressing nerve cell excitability to a level at which the seizure stops.

Absence seizures

'Absence seizures' are very different from other types of seizure, with no abnormal movement of the body. Nevertheless, the cause of these events still seems to be an abnormal epileptic focus of increased nerve cell activity, but the focus is now not in the cerebral cortex but in a part of the brain called the thalamus. This is a large and complicated region which is involved in processing sensory information on its way to the cortex. When a seizure begins in this area, the sensory input to the cortex is temporarily interrupted, resulting in the blank stare and mental 'absence' of the patient.

Absence seizures can be treated with valproate or benzodiazepines, which were described above. The drug ethosuximide can also be used, although it is of no use in any other type of epilepsy. The abnormally excitable neurons in the thalamus allow calcium ions to pass into them through special calcium channels called 'T-channels'. This entry of calcium is believed to maintain their abnormal activity. Ethosuximide can block T-channels, an effect which would reduce the nerve cell excitability and explain the anti-epileptic effect.

Eclampsia

A small proportion of pregnant women develop a condition called 'eclampsia' in the late stages of pregnancy. One of the symptoms is the occurrence of seizures. These do respond to some of the antiepileptic drugs, such as valproate, diazepam, and clomethiazole, but these present some risk to the developing embryo. One of the best and most effective treatments is to administer magnesium sulphate. Magnesium ions can substitute for sodium and calcium ions in the membranes of nerve cells, reducing both their excitability and the release of neurotransmitters. The overall result is a very effective suppression of eclamptic seizures.

Trigeminal neuralgia

Carbamazepine is the best drug for treating the condition of 'trigeminal neuralgia'. In this disorder, neurons supplying the face send their electrical messages at an excessive rate, producing severe, shooting pains down the face. The abnormal electrical activity obviously has features in common with epilepsy, and this may explain the ability of carbamazepine to be effective.

Table 12.1 Drugs used in epilepsy

Generalized epilepsies	Status epilepticus
valproate	amylobarbitone
	clomethiazole
Partial and tonic-clonic seizures	clonazepam*
carbamazepine	diazepam*
clobazam*	lorazepam*
clonazepam	
ethotoin (USA)	**Absence seizures ('petit mal')**
gabapentin	clonazepam*
lamotrigine	ethosuximide
metharbitone (USA)	methsuximide (USA)
methoin (USA)	phensuximide (USA)
methylphenobarbitone	troxidone
phenacemide (USA)	valproate
phenobarbitone (phenobarbital)	
phenytoin	**Eclampsia**
primidone (converted to phenobarbitone in the body)	magnesium Sulphate
topiramate	
valproate	
vigabatrin	

* These are all members of the class of drugs known as benzodiazepines.

Summary

- The epilepsies are a group of disorders in which an area of brain becomes abnormally excitable and triggers convulsive movements of part of the body or, in some cases, of the entire body. Seizures may involve sensory and other psychological disturbances such as visual images, and transient unconsciousness (absence seizures).

- The barbiturate and benzodiazepine drugs increase the activity of the receptors responding to the inhibitory transmitter GABA in the brain, reducing the excitability of the nerve cells.

- Carbamazepine and phenytoin block pores allowing sodium into nerve cells. This effect is similar to that of local anaesthetics and blocks nerve impulses.

- Lamotrigine inhibits the release of the excitatory transmitter glutamate from nerve cells, stopping the spread of excitation through the brain.

- Valproate and vigabatrin increase the activity of GABA partly by preventing its destruction. This depresses nerve cells and reduces the abnormal excitability of the epileptic brain.

- Topiramate has actions common to several of the other drugs.

- Status epilepticus is the condition in which a seizure continues for long enough to place the patient at risk of brain damage or death.

- Eclampsia is a condition in which seizures occur occasionally during pregnancy. They can be treated by magnesium salts.

- Trigeminal neuralgia is characterized by shooting pains in the face and is best treated by some anti-epileptic drugs, especially carbamazepine.

CHAPTER 13

Anxiety and sleep

The irrationality of anxiety is exemplified by the story of the man who became excessively anxious at the influence of terrorists on the safety of flying. When he discovered that the chances of two bombs being placed aboard a plane were several million to one, he countered his fear by taking a bomb of his own on board flights.

Most of us feel anxious about something now and then, but it is usually a short-lived anxiety related to a specific event or situation. The cause might be an interview, an examination, or making a speech. The accompanying feelings of concern and worry become worse as the appointed time approaches. Our hands may tremble, our throat and voice seem tense, there is a sensation of 'butterflies in the stomach', and we are aware of palpitations—the heart rate increases and the beat becomes stronger. We may also feel tired and sweat a great deal. These signs of anxiety are all due to the effects of epinephrine on our tissues, causing increased activity of muscle reflexes, tightening the muscles in the throat, suppressing movements of the stomach and increasing the force of the heartbeat. As soon as our ordeal is over, and often before it has finished, the epinephrine secretion from the adrenal glands diminishes and we should return to our normal state of relaxed calm.

We 'should'. For some people there is no return to normal. They are constantly worried, anxious, 'a bundle of nerves'. Often there is not even an identifiable reason for their anxiety, and yet they remain anxious for months or years, imposing great stress on themselves and on those around them. Sometimes patients worry excessively about matters which are trivial to most people, and there is probably a continuum between anxiety and so-called 'obsessive-compulsive neurosis'—the state of mind in which a person may need to check a dozen times whether they have locked the house door or turned off a tap.

What causes anxiety?

As yet, science is not able to explain why this prolonged, pointless anxiety occurs, but there are several fascinating theories. One of the transmitters in the brain is CCK (*see* Chapter 1). This same chemical is a hormone in the intestine, but it also causes animals to behave as if they were anxious. For example, rats showed less interest in their surroundings and reacted more to sudden noises.

When injected into human volunteers, CCK created feelings of intense anxiety, even panic in some subjects. These observations have led drug companies such as Parke-Davis to try to develop drugs which block the receptors for CCK. The results so far indicate that such drugs can reduce long-standing anxiety in patients. The results also raise the possibility that the cause of anxiety might be that nerve cells in the brain are producing too much CCK.

Another theory is based on the discovery, by Claus Braestrup at the drug company Ferrosan in Denmark in 1980, that the brain can produce chemicals called beta-carbolines which cause anxiety in animals or human subjects and which act on the same sites as the major anti-anxiety drugs such as diazepam. Perhaps the brains of anxious people are producing too much of these chemicals and diazepam works by blocking their effects.

Despite our poor understanding of anxiety, there are several drugs which calm patients and make them less worried and less bothered by events. They are the same drugs, in general, which help people to fall asleep, probably because a frequent reason why people do not sleep well is that they are worrying about something! Because of their dual function these drugs are known as sedatives (when used to calm, or to improve sleeping), or anxiolytics (when used specifically to treat a patient in whom anxiety is a major problem).

Anxiety and fear

Scientists sometimes discuss the relationship between anxiety and fear. In 1943, Stewart Wolf and Harold Wolff published a book called *Human gastric function* in which they described their studies of a patient, Tom. Tom had accidentally drunk some boiling soup and, as a result, his oesophagus had become closed permanently by scar tissue. An operation was performed to open an artificial tube from Tom's mouth into his stomach, a tube which also allowed his doctors to examine events in his stomach. Wolf and Wolff noticed that when Tom was afraid of something specific, the movements and blood supply of his stomach diminished, whereas when Tom simply complained of feeling anxious or worried, but about nothing in particular, his gastric movements and blood flow increased. This observation suggests that the physiological changes associated with nonspecific anxiety and specific fears are quite distinct.

The changes seen in Tom's stomach during specific fears are those which would be expected if the sympathetic nerves were active and the stomach were responding to epinephrine. This would fit with a theory proposed by the American physiologist Walter Cannon who, in the 1930s, suggested that the sympathetic nerves prepared the body for a confrontation—the 'fight or flight' reaction (see Chapter 1). We could also call this the 'fright, fight, or flight' reaction, because conflict with an adversary or predator is often preceded by pronounced fear and high levels of epinephrine.

In a related theory the American psychologist William James and the Danish physician Carl Lange, proposed that all anxiety was due to the activities of the sympathetic nerves. However, we now know that blocking almost all sympathetic responses does not remove anxiety.

Types of anxiety

The preceding summary of anxiety refers to what doctors call 'generalized anxiety', but there are other disorders which are included in a family of anxiety disorders. For example, some patients suffer from panic disorder, with brief periods of intense fear, while others suffer from social phobia, avoiding any situation in which they may be subject to criticism from others.

Drugs used to treat anxiety and sleep disorders

The first drug ever used to reduce anxiety and to promote sleep was almost certainly alcohol* but more will be said about this in Chapter 24. The first efforts to produce a specific sedative in the last twenty-five years of the nineteenth century were based around alcohol (ethanol), with drugs such as trichloro-ethanol and compounds which produced this chemical in the body, urethane and chloralose.

After carefully analysing the structures of these compounds, Josef von Mering (1849–1908) at the Universities of Strasbourg and Cologne in Germany, set out to synthesize a quite different compound, derived from barbituric acid. This had been prepared in 1864 by Adolph von Baeyer and given its name either because of his affections for a young lady called Barbara, or because it was prepared on St Barbara's day—both stories have some evidence to support them. By 1911, von Mering had produced a number of barbiturates, one of which, phenobarbitone (phenobarbital) was a very effective sedative and the first to be introduced into medicine. Over the next fifty years many different barbiturates were produced and marketed by all the major pharmaceutical companies, but by the 1950s it was clear that many people were becoming addicted. The barbiturates also depressed breathing, resulting in the deaths of several elderly patients. These problems presented a serious limitation to the usefulness of barbiturates. The search was on for new and better drugs.

In 1952 chemists at Ciba in Switzerland produced the first sedative of a different type. This was glutethimide, and it was followed by the very similar

* The term alcohol is used throughout this book to refer to ethyl alcohol, ethanol.

compounds methyprylone and thalidomide from other companies. The problems surrounding thalidomide are well known, and arose from the fact that, unlike the overwhelming majority of drugs, it is treated differently in humans and the several animal species on which it was tested. Ironically, except for the appalling defects caused by the drug in unborn babies, it was one of the safest drugs for adults ever produced: even huge doses caused few side-effects.

At about the same time B. J. Ludwig, working at the Wallace Laboratories in Cranbury, New Jersey, was searching for a drug to reduce anxiety and induce sleep. In 1950 he produced meprobamate, better known under its original trade name of Miltown. This is used much less now partly because it can produce feelings of happiness and euphoria which caused some patients to become addicted, and partly because it has been superceded by much safer drugs.

Benzodiazepines

The most common drugs in use for the treatment of anxiety and sleep disorders are the benzodiazepines (Table 13.1, p. 186). Although these are among the most widely prescribed drugs in the world, we only have them by a twist of fate. In the 1950s a Polish chemist called Leo Sternbach moved to the USA to work for the pharmaceutical company Roche, taking with him about forty chemicals he had made in Poland. Most of these were tested by Lowell Randall and other biologists at the Roche research laboratories in Nutley, New Jersey, but none showed any properties of interest. One day, thinking that all his chemicals had been tested, Sternbach began to clear his laboratory before starting to make a different set of compounds. Fortunately Earl Reeder, one of the scientists in the laboratory, noticed that one of the chemicals was still unopened in its packet. When this was tested, it was found to make animals less anxious. In addition it was safe in large doses, and also produced sedation.

Even after this lucky finding, the drug was almost thrown away a second time because the first people to whom it was given were elderly, and they behaved as if drunk: they became very confused, with slurred speech, and eventually fell asleep. We now know that older patients are very sensitive to the benzodiazepines, and the doses used must be kept low. Indeed, there are several reports in the modern medical literature of patients being considered to have Alzheimer's disease or other forms of dementia, when their only problem has been too high a dose of a benzodiazepine.

Several dozen different members of this benzodiazepine group are now used around the world. The original drug made by Sternbach was chlordiazepoxide (better known under its original trade name of Librium®), while the related drug diazepam (better known as Valium®) was introduced in 1959. The various members of the benzodiazepine group differ mainly in their strength and duration of action.

Side-effects

Benzodiazepines are relatively safe. The main side-effects include a hangover next morning, with some residual drowsiness which may affect the ability to drive or manipulate complex equipment. They also reduce reaction times, making driving even more of a danger. In general, the benzodiazepines reduce anxiety at doses that do not affect general intelligence, alertness, memory, or thought processes. Even when patients take them in large overdoses they rarely come to any great harm, usually just sleeping for a day or two and then waking with a headache.

They are, however, addictive even when taken for a short time, and they have been prescribed far too freely by doctors keen to help patients to deal with life's problems. Many patients then have great difficulty in stopping the drugs when the real need for them is over. When they do stop, the psychological need for benzodiazepines is accompanied by physical signs of withdrawal. Patients may experience rebound anxiety, depression, nausea, insomnia, loss of appetite, tremors, and headaches for several weeks if the drugs are stopped suddenly. They should not be taken for more than two weeks at a time and, as with most drugs, patients should stop taking benzodiazepines gradually.

Benzodiazepines and sleep

In addition to their use in reducing anxiety, benzodiazepines are valuable drugs for helping patients to sleep. They shorten the time taken to fall asleep, and also increase the duration of sleep.

It is still not certain why we sleep. One theory is that sleep evolved to force silence and immobility upon animals as a form of protection against predators. When we sleep, the brain cycles through several stages. As we fall asleep we enter stage one first, then a deep stage two, and finally delta sleep. After about ninety minutes the depth of sleep decreases and gives way to a period of around ten minutes during which there are rapid, flickering movements of the eyes (rapid eye movements or REM); it is during REM sleep that we dream. Everyone needs to dream to maintain good mental health. People who have been blind since birth have purely auditory dreams. Throughout the night we cycle between deep and REM sleep, and it is only when we have the correct balance of sleep that we wake feeling refreshed and ready for the next day. The switching of sleep states is determined by groups of cells in the brain including those that secrete the neurotransmitters 5HT and norepinephrine (active during waking, silent during dreaming) and those that secrete acetylcholine (active during dreaming).

One of the problems with benzodiazepines is that, while increasing total sleep, they reduce the amount of REM sleep by up to 75 per cent. When patients suddenly stop taking benzodiazepines, the brain attempts to catch up by increasing the proportion of REM sleep, with the amount of deep stage two and delta sleep being correspondingly less. As a result, sleep is restless with vivid dreams and patients are likely to wake still feeling tired and not refreshed. Patients should 'grin and bear' this for a few days until the brain has caught up with its loss of REM sleep, but some immediately resort to taking more of the drugs in order to get a better night's sleep. They are addicted, and need to be taken off the drugs gradually by taking smaller and smaller doses each night so that the 'rebound' REM sleep is kept under control.

The best way to avoid this problem of REM rebound is to take a benzodiazepine only every second or third night. This gives the patient a good night's sleep every second or third night, and also allows the brain to catch up continually on its loss of REM sleep rather than building up a huge loss over several days or weeks.

The benzodiazepines originally used to treat insomnia, such as diazepam and nitrazepam, were long-acting. This means that patients sleep soundly throughout the night and do not waken early, but also that many patients still feel drowsy the next day. Nowadays the benzodiazepines used to treat insomnia are shorter-acting compounds such as lorazepam, lormetazepam, loprazolam, and temazepam. The effects of the shortest-acting benzodiazepines, such as triazolam wear off during the night, allowing the patient to wake early.

Amnesia

Most of the benzodiazepines can produce some forgetfulness if taken in high doses and the effects of most are increased by alcohol, although some are worse than others in this respect. Flunitrazepam has recently gained a bad reputation as the 'date-rape' drug Rohypnol®. When combined with alcohol it produces a very marked sedation combined with pronounced amnesia, so that people abused while under its influence have little recollection of the circumstances surrounding the event.

How do benzodiazepines work?

Benzodiazepines work by decreasing the activity of nerve cells in the brain. This is achieved by potentiating the inhibitory effect of the neurotransmitter GABA. When GABA acts on its receptor, it increases the passage of chloride ions into the cell. This makes the inside of the cell more negative, and the cell becomes less excitable. Benzodiazepines interact at a different site on the GABA receptor. By themselves, they have no effect on the chloride channels, but when GABA and a benzodiazepine act at the same time, the channels open more frequently, allowing more chloride into the cells, and producing a greater degree of inhibition.

While this interaction with GABA is now well understood on single cells, we still do not know for certain whether there is a particular region of the brain which is most important for the sedative and anxiolytic effects of benzodiazepines. There is a small area in the lateral part of the brain called the amygdala (from the Greek word for 'almond', because of the shape of the region) which is believed to be very important, but there are other areas in the hind parts of the brain which affect anxiety in animals, and which may also be important. One area is called the locus coeruleus because it can appear bluish in colour (from the Latin *caeruleus* meaning sky-blue). If this is stimulated electrically it produces anxious behaviour in animals.* Conversely, if the area is removed the animals seem unable to show anxiety.

Zolpidem and zopiclone

These two drugs are not members of the benzodiazepine group, although they act in much the same way, increasing the effects of GABA and inhibiting the activity of nerve cells. However, their actions seem to be more selective than the benzodiazepines, with less suppression of REM sleep, so that the quality of sleep is better. In addition, there is less rebound insomnia when patients stop taking the drugs, and much less of a problem with withdrawal symptoms. Even so, these drugs should not be taken for more than a few days to ensure that patients do not become entirely dependent on them for getting to sleep.

Zaleplon is another sedative, from Wyeth, which is different from the benzodiazepines and should not have the same side-effects and problems. As yet there is little information on how it works.

Buspirone

A different type of drug was introduced into medicine in 1985. It is exemplified by buspirone, which does not interact with GABA receptors, but acts on specific receptors (called 1A receptors) for the neurotransmitter 5-hydroxytryptamine (5HT). Buspirone is an agonist (*see* Chapter 1) at these receptors, activating them and slowing the activity of nerve cells in several parts of the brain. Buspirone is quite specific as an anxiolytic drug and has several advantages over the benzodiazepines as it does not seem to cause addiction and produces almost no sedation.

Buspirone has other advantages too. It is an agonist at receptors for dopamine in the brain and increases the actions of dopamine and norepinephrine. Activity of the norepinephrine neurons helps maintain arousal and attention, so that buspirone is less likely to produce drowsiness than most other anti-anxiety drugs.

---

* Anxiety is not easy to study in animals because they cannot be asked how they are feeling. Scientists have devised some simple tests for anxiety which respond to drugs in the same way as true anxiety in humans. For example, rats prefer dark or enclosed areas, probably because they are 'afraid' of being detected by predators in brightly lit or exposed areas. Drugs which reduce human anxiety and fear induce rats to spend a higher proportion of their time in the exposed or illuminated areas of a box. There are other, more sophisticated, tests but most are based on a similar principle.

Overall, buspirone appears to be one of the most promising drugs for the treatment of anxiety.

Beta-blockers

When the main problem is the bodily symptoms produced by epinephrine, rather than mental anxiety, the most appropriate drug is a beta-blocker such as propranolol. These drugs prevent the tremor, the 'butterflies', and the palpitations due to epinephrine, and will see the patient through the immediate problem without the need for true anxiolytic drugs affecting the brain.

Barbiturates

Lastly, we should mention the barbiturates. These are the drugs whose discovery was described earlier and which doctors used to prescribe quite freely as 'sleeping tablets'. They are no longer used to treat insomnia because they are dangerous. They can easily be taken in overdose, accidentally or otherwise, when they can kill by depressing the activity of the nerve cells which control breathing. They increase the ability of the liver to break down other drugs, an interaction which can be very dangerous to an elderly patient taking other types of medication. They are also addictive.

Antihistamines

Anyone who has taken antihistamines for hay fever or travel sickness knows that many of them can cause drowsiness. Modern antihistamines have been produced without this side-effect, and can be used to help people sleep. Promethazine, for example, is available as a sedative for this purpose. It is believed to work by blocking receptors for histamine and acetylcholine in a part of the brain known as the reticular formation and which helps to maintain the balance between sleep and waking.

Clomethiazole

Clomethiazole is free of the hangover effects of some benzodiazepines, but can depress breathing, especially if taken with alcohol. It is short-acting and, therefore, valuable for use in elderly patients whose liver cannot eliminate drugs as quickly as in the young. Long-acting compounds such as some benzodiazepines and barbiturates may accumulate in the elderly and cause daytime sleepiness, confusion, and memory loss. Clomethiazole works in much the same way as the benzodiazepines, potentiating the inhibitory actions of GABA.

Hypochondria

A hypochondriac has been defined as someone preoccupied with his or her health, often characterized by a belief or fear that normal bodily sensations indicate serious disease.* The condition has many similarities with anxiety disorders, the main feature here being anxiety about the state of health. Some cases of hypochondria have been successfully treated using drugs such as pimozide, which blocks dopamine receptors in the brain and has also been used in schizophrenia (*see* Chapter 9).

Panic disorder

Panic attacks are associated with a variety of symptoms including sensations of choking, difficulty breathing, faintness, trembling, palpitations, sweating, nausea and chest discomfort, often with an overwhelming fear of imminent death. Although considered a form of anxiety disorder, panic attacks seem to be best treated by drugs which are also useful in depression (Chapter 11). These include the tricyclic antidepressants such as imipramine, desipramine, nortriptyline, and clomipramine, the monoamine oxidase inhibitors such as phenelzine and moclobemide, and the selective serotonin reuptake inhibitors such as fluoxetine and sertraline. The mechanisms of action of these drugs and their major side-effects are described in more detail in Chapter 11.

Panic disorder can also be treated with two benzodiazepines, alprazolam and clonazepam, both of which can produce some drowsiness and impair patients' memory and learning abilities.

Phobias

Phobias are a form of anxiety which are best treated, not by anti-anxiety drugs but by antidepressants. They have been discussed in Chapter 11.

---

* *Martindale's Extra Pharmacopocia*, 31st edition, 1996. The Royal Pharmaceutical Society, London, p. 672.

Table 13.1 Drugs used to treat anxiety and sleep disorders

Sedatives	Anxiolytics	Panic disorder
Benzodiazepines	*Benzodiazepines*	*TADs*
flunitrazepam	alpazolam	clomipramine
flurazepam	bromazepam	desipramine
lopazolam	chlordiazepoxide	imipramine
lormetazepam	clobazam	nortriptyline
midazolam	clorazepate	
nitrazepam	diazepam	*MAOI*
oxazepam	halazepam (USA)	moclobemide
quazepam (USA)	ketazolam	phenelzine
talbutal (USA)	loprazolam	tranylcypromine
temazepam	lorazepam	
triazolam	medazepam	*SSRI*
	oxazepam	citalopram
Other drugs	prazepam (USA)	fluoxetine
clomethiazole		fluvoxamine
dichloralphenazone (USA)	*Barbiturates*	paroxetine
ethchlorvynol (USA)	amylobarbitone	sertraline
ethinamate (USA)	aprobarbital (USA)	
glutethimide (USA)	butabarbital (USA)	*Miscellaneous antidepressants*
meprobamate	butalbital (USA)	mirtazapine
methyprylone	butobarbitone	nefazodone
zolpidem	cyclobarbitone	venlafaxine
zopiclone	pentobarbitone	
	(pentobarbital)	
	quinalbarbitone	*Benzodiazepines*
	secbutobarbitone (USA)	alprazolam
		clonazepam
	Other drugs	
	buspirone	
	chlormezanone	

Summary

- *The same groups of drugs are used to reduce anxiety (anxiolytics) and to produce sedation and sleep (sedatives).*
- *Benzodiazepines and barbiturates increase the actions of GABA at its receptors in the brain. The barbiturates are now rarely used because of the likelihood of serious side-effects and of addiction; the benzodiazepines are very safe but can produce psychological dependence.*
- *Zolpidem, zopiclone, and clomethiazole also work by increasing the effects of GABA.*
- *Buspirone activates receptors for the transmitter 5HT. It reduces anxiety without producing sedation and is not addictive.*
- *Beta-blockers prevent the autonomic signs of fear and anxiety such as a palpitating heart, sweating, and hand tremor.*
- *Antihistamines block receptors for histamine and acetylcholine in the brain and cause sedation and drowsiness.*
- *Panic disorders seem more related to depression than anxiety and are best treated by antidepressant drugs.*

CHAPTER 14

Blood: anaemia and coagulation

Blood is a very complex mixture. It consists of a watery solution (plasma) in which are suspended millions of cells. The cells are of two main types, red and white (Figs 14.1 and 14.2). The white cells remove dead and dying tissue, bacteria, and viruses, and are the lookouts and soldiers of the immune system, as described in Chapter 2.

The red blood cells (or erythrocytes, from the Greek *erythros*, red) are present in far higher numbers than the white. They contain haemoglobin, a pigment which is responsible for the overall red colour of blood and which can hold molecules of oxygen. When four of these are attached to each molecule of haemoglobin the combination is bright red; this is the normal state for most of the haemoglobin in a healthy person and is the colour of blood in the arteries carrying freshly oxygenated blood from the lungs to the various tissues of the body.

As oxygen is used by the tissues it detaches from the haemoglobin and is replaced by the waste product, carbon dioxide. Once haemoglobin has lost all

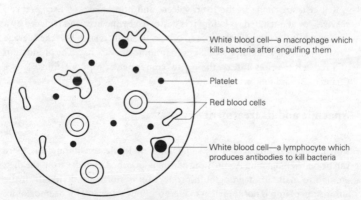

Fig. 14.1 The blood consists of a fluid (plasma) in which are red and white cells and cell fragments called platelets.

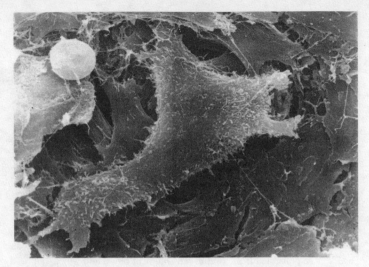

Fig. 14.2 Section through a small blood vessel showing a single red blood cell (top left) and a large white cell, magnified about 2000 times. (Professor A P Payne)

its oxygen and is carrying carbon dioxide instead, it is no longer bright red but more purple. This is why people suffering from a serious lack of oxygen, after nearly drowning or suffocating, for example, have a bluish-purple colour in their lips and fingers, a condition known as cyanosis.

Red cells are made in the liver, spleen, and bone marrow. Each red cell survives for about 120 days before it is destroyed by the liver and replaced by a new one, but the total number of red cells in the body is such that the average person makes two million new cells every minute of every day. The production of a red cell requires at least three vital components: iron, vitamin B_{12} (*see* Chapter 22), and folic acid.

Anaemia and its treatment

Iron

Iron atoms make up part of the haemoglobin molecule, so without iron, there can be no haemoglobin. About 1 mg of iron is absorbed each day from the diet, enough to maintain haemoglobin production in normal individuals. If the absorption of iron is not sufficient to meet the body's demand for haemoglobin, people become anaemic (deficient in haemoglobin), new red cells are smaller than normal (microcytic), and contain less haemoglobin. As a result, the tissues are not supplied with enough oxygen so that some cells may die and most will not work efficiently. The individual may begin to tire very easily when performing simple physical tasks. He or she also feels breathless as the rate of breathing increases to try to pull more oxygen into the blood.

This situation may occur after a serious accident and haemorrhage, in any circumstances in which blood loss is excessive, and in women during pregnancy. If, for example, a woman's iron is being used by the growing foetus or is being lost during menstruation, she may become anaemic unless the iron is replaced artificially.

In most cases, iron can be given in the form of tablets of ferrous* salts such as ferrous citrate, ferrous gluconate, ferrous sulphate, or ferrous fumarate, which are absorbed readily in the intestine. Some people experience irritation of the gut with these tablets at the usual doses of 200–600 mg per day, with abdominal pain, nausea, and diarrhoea or constipation. These can usually be reduced by lowering the dose.

Vitamin B_{12} (hydroxocobalamin)

In addition to iron, red cell formation needs vitamin B_{12}. The vitamin is essential for the activity of enzymes involved in the metabolism of DNA, fat, and carbohydrate and a deficiency will slow the formation of new cells.

Sometimes known as hydroxocobalamin, vitamin B_{12} is present in meat, fish, eggs, and milk but not plants. Strict vegetarians are, therefore, at risk of developing a deficiency. Vitamin B_{12} is not usually destroyed by cooking and, after absorption from food, is stored in the liver.

Pernicious anaemia

During digestion, the vitamin binds to two proteins: 'intrinsic factor' and 'R-binder'. Intrinsic factor is produced by cells in the stomach, and vitamin B_{12} can only be absorbed from the intestine when it is bound to this protein. A frequent cause of vitamin B_{12} deficiency is a lack of intrinsic factor. This may occur because the body produces antibodies which destroy intrinsic factor, or because the cells which secrete it have died. The loss of intrinsic factor results in a type of anaemia known as 'pernicious anaemia', and the only way to correct it is to treat with injections of vitamin B_{12}. Usually injections are given once a month, using a solution from which the vitamin is absorbed slowly over the next four weeks.

Effects and treatment of B_{12} deficiency

It is essential to treat vitamin B_{12} deficiency as early as possible because the molecule is used not only for the synthesis of red blood cells, but also for other

* Iron can exist in two forms—ferrous (iron II, or Fe^{++}) and ferric (iron III or Fe^{+++}). Only the former should be used to replace the body's iron stores.

enzyme reactions. In the absence of vitamin B_{12}, one of these enzymes* produces unusual and abnormal fatty chemicals which can become incorporated into the fatty membranes of nerve cells. This can result in serious disturbances of the function of the nervous system, with abnormal sensations such as 'pins and needles' in the fingers and toes, loss of position sense, weakness and difficulty in walking in a straight line. (This condition is known as sub-acute combined degeneration of the spinal cord.) In the most serious cases, when more nerve cells are affected, paralysis, dementia, and blindness may also occur. These can all be avoided if the vitamin is replaced before serious neurological damage has occurred.

Folic acid (folate)

Green vegetables such as spinach and broccoli, and visceral organs such as liver and kidney are rich sources of folic acid. Cooking destroys 60–90 per cent of the folate and, unlike vitamin B_{12}, the body stores of folate are relatively low and need to be replaced continuously. A poor diet can result in folate deficiency in a few weeks and folate intake may need to be increased during pregnancy when some of the mother's stores are being used by the developing embryo.

Folic acid is needed for cells to make new DNA, an essential step before cells divide. The result of a deficiency is that the liver and bone marrow produce fewer red cells. These are large and relatively fragile, leading to anaemia because the overall amount of haemoglobin in the blood is reduced. The condition is called a 'macrocytic' or 'megaloblastic' anaemia in recognition of the enlarged red cells. It can be treated by taking tablets containing folic acid, which is absorbed readily in the intestine.

It is important to make sure that folate and not vitamin B_{12} deficiency is responsible for any anaemia. If it is due to B_{12} deficiency, but is treated incorrectly with folic acid, the lack of B_{12} could lead to the very serious nervous system disorders described above.

Erythropoietin (epoetin)

The manufacture of red blood cells is regulated by a protein hormone, erythropoietin or epoetin, secreted mainly by cells in the kidney. If a person develops anaemia or hypoxia (too little oxygen in the blood) at high altitude, the kidneys produce more epoetin in an attempt to increase the formation of more red cells.

In the presence of kidney disease the amounts of epoetin in the body may decline, resulting in a fall in red cell production and anaemia. This type of anaemia used to be extremely difficult to treat, since epoetin had to be isolated and purified from large amounts of animal tissue. As a result, it was not only

* Methylmalonyl-coenzyme A mutase.

exceedingly hard to obtain but was also exceptionally expensive. Nowadays, molecular biologists can insert the gene which produces epoetin into cells which can be grown artificially in vast quantities. The hormone is then extracted and purified so that it is identical to the natural substance. Although the hormone produced by this means is still rather expensive, it is at least available relatively freely, and in quantities which mean that a person requiring it does not live in fear that one day his or her supply may come to an end.

Blood clotting

Bleeding

When a blood vessel is cut or damaged, we bleed. Most of us take it for granted that the bleeding will soon stop, without realizing the enormous complexity of the processes which cause blood clotting. Exposure of blood to air, or contact with a foreign surface, triggers a cascade sequence of about ten chemical reactions in the blood involving over a dozen 'clotting factors', which clot the blood within one or two minutes. If one of the clotting factors is absent clotting may take very much longer, to the extent that a person may lose large amounts of blood from a small cut. The best known example is haemophilia, in which patients lack clotting factor VIII. Any injury has to be avoided or the patient may be in danger of bleeding to death.

Clotting

For most people, however, the major source of concern is not bleeding, but the opposite—blood clotting (haemostasis or thrombosis) in the blood vessels. Blood clots form not only when blood vessels on the skin are damaged and we can see the clot, but also if there is damage inside a vessel, particularly if fatty material has been deposited on the lining of the vessel, a condition known as atherosclerosis. This narrows the diameter of the blood vessel and makes thrombosis and blockage more likely. In addition to the red and white cells, blood contains small fragments of cells called platelets (Fig. 14.1). These can attach to an area of damaged vessel wall or fatty deposit and secrete chemicals which act on other platelets to make them sticky. The growing number of sticky platelets clump together, a process known as 'aggregation', and start the cascade sequence described above and which leads to clotting (Figs 14.3 and 14.4). The result is a jelly-like blood clot which can partly or completely block the inside of the vessel.

Normally, during movement, muscles contract and continually squeeze the veins, keeping blood flowing freely. Without those contractions blood moves more slowly. Blood clots are more likely to occur in blood vessels in which blood is moving sluggishly. They are most common in the veins of patients who are

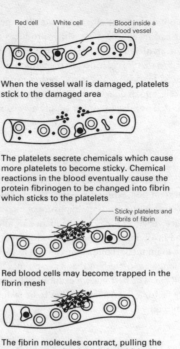

When the vessel wall is damaged, platelets stick to the damaged area

The platelets secrete chemicals which cause more platelets to become sticky. Chemical reactions in the blood eventually cause the protein fibrinogen to be changed into fibrin which sticks to the platelets

Red blood cells may become trapped in the fibrin mesh

The fibrin molecules contract, pulling the aggregate together into a clot which prevents dirt and bacteria entering the blood

Fig. 14.3 The sequence of events in the formation of a blood clot.

bedridden or who are lying down for long periods such as after major surgery. In these cases, the platelets are more sticky than normal as a result of the surgery, and post-operative patients are often treated with drugs such as heparin to prevent clotting.

Heart attacks and strokes
If blood does clot within a blood vessel the flow of blood will be blocked; the cells and tissues receiving blood from that vessel become starved of oxygen and may die. The most feared examples of this are heart attacks, when a blood clot forms within one of the coronary arteries supplying blood and oxygen to the heart itself, and strokes, in which a clot (thrombus) forms in an artery supplying

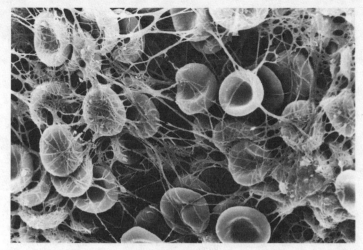

Fig. 14.4 The formation of a blood clot. The photograph, magnified about 4000 times, shows red cells becoming entangled in strands of fibrin, at the start of the process of clotting. (Wellcome Photo Library)

part of the brain. In the former case, the heart may no longer be able to pump blood efficiently so that tissues become damaged from a lack of blood; the patient may die in severe cases. In the case of a stroke caused by a clot, the region of brain deprived of blood may die, leaving the patient partially paralysed, or without the ability to speak.

Emboli

Blood clots themselves are not the only problem. Once a clot has formed, a new series of reactions come into play which, over a period of time, gradually dissolve and remove the clot. During this time, however, there is a real danger that part of the clot, an embolus, may break away and be carried in the blood to another part of the body, where it may block another, smaller, vessel. The blockage is called an embolism.

Blood in the veins moves along larger and larger veins to the heart, so that the clot fragment meets smaller vessels only when the blood is pumped to the lungs. If it becomes lodged in a vessel there, the embolus may cut off the blood supply to part of the lungs, reducing the amount of oxygen which can be absorbed into the blood. The rate and depth of breathing, and often the heart rate too, increase to compensate for this. If the area of lung damaged is large, the patient may be in very serious danger.

Emboli may also be thrown off from a clot lining the inside of the heart, particularly in patients with irregular heart rhythms such as atrial fibrillation (see Chapter 16). Such patients are usually treated with anticoagulants to protect against emboli.

Anticoagulant drugs

To prevent blood from clotting, doctors use anticoagulant drugs (Fig. 14.5 and Table 14.1, p. 201). One of the main problems of these drugs is that the dose must be carefully adjusted. Enough must be given to prevent the formation of unwanted clots, but too much may produce bleeding.

Heparin

Heparin is a natural chemical present in greatest amounts in the lungs and liver, from which it can be extracted and purified (hence the name, from the Latin *hepar* meaning liver). It was first obtained in a relatively pure form in 1922 by William Howell, Professor of Physiology at the Johns Hopkins University in Baltimore, after a medical student working in his laboratory, Jay MacLean, noticed the presence of anticoagulant activity in tissue extracts. In addition to

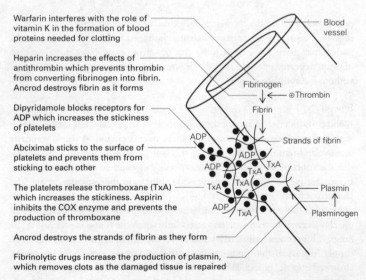

Fig. 14.5 Drugs which affect blood clotting. The abbreviation ADP refers to adenosine diphosphate and COX to cyclo-oxygenase.

heparin itself, various fragments of the whole molecule, such as dalteparin, are also now used.

How does heparin work?

The final stage in the cascade process of blood clotting is that an enzyme, thrombin, converts the protein fibrinogen into fibrin (Figs 14.3 and 14.5). The molecules of fibrin then bind together, forming a mesh of fibres which trap red blood cells and platelets. The whole complex gradually contracts, squeezing out fluid (serum), and becoming a fully formed clot.

Blood also contains antithrombin, molecules of which inhibit the action of thrombin. Heparin greatly increases the effect of antithrombin, preventing thrombin from converting fibrinogen into fibrin. The net effect is a very efficient inhibition of blood clotting by heparin.

Heparin must be given by injection as it is a polysaccharide (made up of sugar-like molecules) and would be destroyed in the stomach. It is used whenever a thrombus is suspected or, in low doses, to patients undergoing major surgery. Low molecular weight heparins, such as tinzaparin, have a long-lasting effect and, since they can be given as a once-daily injection under the skin, they are convenient to use. Patients can often be treated in their own homes instead of needing admission to hospital.

Warfarin

In the early years of the twentieth century attempts were made to improve the use of land in parts of North America. Sweet clover was introduced into several areas of poor land quality where more conventional crops would not survive. In 1922, a veterinary physician at the Ontario Veterinary College in Alberta, F. W. Schofield, described a new disorder of cattle in which the primary problem was excessive bleeding. Over the next few years, the chemical responsible for this haemorrhagic disease was extracted from clover and identified as dicoumarol, one of a group of compounds called coumarins. The only one in regular use today is nicoumalone.

Following this lead, several similar chemicals were manufactured to improve their effectiveness and safety. The best was named warfarin* but it was still thought to be too toxic to give to humans. It was, therefore, introduced as pest control, rapidly becoming the world's best selling and most effective rat poison.

In 1951, a new recruit to the American army tried to commit suicide by taking large amounts of warfarin on several occasions. Since the man survived, doctors realized for the first time that warfarin was in fact very safe in humans. This experience prompted serious clinical trials of warfarin for use in

---

* An acronym for the group holding the patent rights— the Wisconsin Alumni Research Foundation—plus the ending of the chemical group name—coumARIN.

preventing clotting disorders in people, and the drug was finally introduced into medicine in 1959. Since these drugs can be given by mouth, in contrast to the heparins, they are often known as the oral anticoagulants.

How do warfarin and coumarins work?

Warfarin works by interfering with the normal functions of vitamin K.* This is normally obtained in the diet from leaves and vegetable oils, although it is also synthesized by bacteria living in the intestine (*see* Chapter 22, Table 22.5). It is essential for blood clotting since the liver needs it to make several of the clotting factors mentioned above (II, VII, IX, and X). Warfarin is a chemical with a molecular structure very similar to vitamin K so that it competes with vitamin K for enzymes. Its presence means that the liver cannot complete its manufacture of the various clotting factors, greatly reducing the ability of the blood to clot.

Warfarin is taken as tablets, but two or three days are needed for it to be fully effective, since it has to stop the production of new protein clotting factors and does not affect the activity of those already in the blood.

Nicoumalone and phenindione are drugs which have the same action as warfarin.

Aspirin

Blood platelets are important in clotting. As they become entrapped in the fibrin mesh, or come into contact with air or foreign matter, they begin to release several chemicals, one of which is thromboxane-A2. As the name implies, this promotes thrombus (clot) formation by causing platelets to stick together (aggregation). Aspirin slows the formation of thromboxane by inhibiting the COX enzyme which produces it and can, therefore, reduce the likelihood of clot formation. In this way, low doses of aspirin reduce the chance of a second heart attack, and doses of about 75 mg daily are now recommended routinely to people who have had one heart attack. This topic is quite complex and is discussed in more detail in Chapter 6.

Once aspirin has interacted with COX, the enzyme is unable to recover. Even a single dose of aspirin, therefore, can inhibit blood clotting for several days. Only when new platelets, containing fresh enzyme, are produced does clotting gradually return to normal. Reduced clotting of the blood can be detected for up to about two weeks after one 300 mg tablet of aspirin.

Dipyridamole

Another of the substances which increases the stickiness of platelets in the early phases of aggregation, is adenosine diphosphate (ADP). Its effects are inhibited

* Also known as phytomenadione.

by the presence of another substance, adenosine. Dipyridamole slows down the removal of adenosine from the blood by stopping its uptake into cells. As the amount of adenosine in the blood rises, it blocks the effects of ADP, and aggregation is suppressed.

Abciximab

Abciximab is a portion of an antibody which interacts with proteins on the surface of platelets. When platelets come into contact with damaged tissue some of the proteins on their surface change shape to interact with other platelets and trigger the clotting process. Abciximab binds to those proteins as soon as they have changed shape and before they can interact with anything else, preventing platelet aggregation and clot formation. Abciximab should be used only once, because the body produces antibodies to it after the first exposure and a second dose may provoke an immune response (an 'anaphylactic shock', similar to an allergic reaction). The drug is usually given by experienced physicians to high-risk patients who are having a coronary angioplasty—a minor surgical procedure undertaken to unblock a coronary artery. There are now several other drugs which act in the same way, including lamifban, tirofiban, and eptifibatide. These cost much less than the £1500 per patient needed for abciximab.

A new drug, ticlopidine, works in a similar way, but prevents the platelet proteins changing their shape in the first place. It also prevents the clotting which occurs in response to ADP.

Ancrod

Ancrod is an enzyme from the venom of the Malayan pit-viper. It destroys tiny particles of fibrin as they are formed normally in the blood and this causes more fibrinogen to convert into fibrin. The enzyme thus sets in motion a chain reaction which lowers fibrin levels in the blood. The overall effect is to reduce the likelihood of a clot forming within a blood vessel.

Fibrinolytic drugs

Small blood clots are being formed naturally all the time in response to tissue damage which may be obvious, as it is in the skin, or hidden if it occurs within a vessel deep inside the body. Once a clot has formed, whatever the cause, a series of chemical reactions is initiated which clear the clot from the blood as the tissue damage is repaired. The final stage of clot removal is the conversion of the protein plasminogen into plasmin. Plasmin gradually breaks down the mesh of fibrin molecules, allowing the clot to be slowly dissolved over a period of time.

If a thrombus occurs where it might be dangerous, as in the heart or lungs, it is important to remove the clot more quickly than would occur naturally. In these cases, several drugs are available to hasten the breakdown of the fibrin mesh which is formed early in the development of a clot. These are known as fibrinolytic or thrombolytic drugs or, sometimes, as 'clot-busters'.

Streptokinase is a protein extracted from bacteria. It forms a complex with plasminogen, which then converts more plasminogen into plasmin.

Urokinase is an enzyme which itself converts plasminogen into plasmin, allowing removal of the clot. It was originally discovered in human urine, hence the name. Produced naturally by the kidney, it is now manufactured using cultured kidney cells from which the enzyme can be isolated.

Anistreplase is a ready-formed complex of streptokinase and plasminogen, but the complex is made inactive by chemists adding a special group of atoms (an anisoyl group) onto the molecule. When anistreplase is injected into the blood, enzymes gradually remove the anisoyl atoms, producing a steady level of active plasminogen in the blood for several hours.

Alteplase is a form of the natural hormone called tissue plasminogen activator. It acts directly on plasminogen to activate it and increase the formation of plasmin. The increased level of plasmin can then remove the clot within minutes or hours, depending on its size, rather than several days. Alteplase activates only the plasminogen which is bound to fibrin, so that its effects are confined to a developing clot and do not affect the general circulation.

Fibrinolytic drugs have been extremely valuable in saving the lives of patients with coronary thrombosis or embolism in the lungs, although they cannot be used in patients with disorders of blood clotting, a peptic ulcer, signs of bleeding, or after recent surgery, since it is essential that clotting is helped in these cases, not hindered.

Drugs of the future

One of the chemicals which promotes platelet aggregation is ADP. The process of ADP-induced clotting is prevented by drugs such as clopidogrel, although it is not yet certain how this drug works. Clinical trials have shown that clopidogrel is more effective than aspirin in preventing heart attacks and strokes.

One of the most exciting developments in the pharmacology of blood clotting is the discovery of several compounds such as sulotroban, which can prevent the effects of thomboxane A2. These drugs should, therefore, be most active only in situations where clotting is occurring and thromboxane is being produced: they should have no effect in normal blood. As a result, they may be safer than existing drugs, and the results of toxicity studies and clinical trials are eagerly awaited. Related drugs are being developed which prevent the formation of thromboxane by the platelets.

The stickiness of platelets is reduced when the amounts of a chemical called cyclic AMP* are increased inside them. Cilostazol is a new drug which inhibits an enzyme—phosphodiesterase III—which breaks down cyclic AMP. As the levels of cyclic AMP increase, the rate of blood clotting is reduced.

We have seen in Chapter 6 that the pro-clotting effects of thromboxane are opposed by the related hormone prostacyclin, which reduces platelet stickiness and increases the flow of blood through blood vessels. Taprostene is a new drug which acts on the prostacyclin receptors, that is, it is a prostacyclin receptor agonist. It mimics the effects of prostacyclin itself and reduces platelet stickiness when this is raised by substances such as thromboxane, ADP, norepinephrine, or thrombin.

In addition to these approaches, several companies are developing drugs to inhibit directly the enzymes and factors involved in the clotting cascade.

Table 14.1 Drugs which affect blood clotting

Anticoagulants	Inhibitors of platelet aggregation
heparin and its components:	abciximab
—certoparin	aspirin
—dalteparin	dipyridamole
—enoxaparin	ticlopidine (USA)
—nadroparin	
—parnaparin	**Fibrinolytic drugs**
—reviparin	alteplase
—tinzaparin	anistreplase
danaparoid	streptokinase
	urokinase
Oral anticoagulants	
anisindione (USA)	
nicoumalone	
phenindione	
warfarin	

* An abbreviation for Cyclic Adenosine 3'5'-MonoPhosphate.

Summary

- *Blood contains red cells with haemoglobin, the red pigment which carries oxygen around the body. A deficiency of iron slows the production of haemoglobin, causing anaemia.*
- *The formation of new cells also needs vitamin B_{12}. An intrinsic factor from the stomach is needed to absorb vitamin B_{12}, so a deficiency can occur if this factor is lacking, resulting in 'pernicious anaemia'.*
- *A deficiency of folic acid can occur in pregnant mothers, also leading to anaemia.*
- *Epoetin can be used to stimulate red cell formation.*
- *Anticoagulant drugs are used to prevent blood clotting, for example when there is a danger of thrombosis caused by blood clotting in the leg or pelvic blood vessels following hip replacement.*
- *Heparin prevents the formation of fibrin and stops blood clotting.*
- *Warfarin and the coumarins block the synthesis of vitamin K, an essential factor in red cell formation.*
- *Aspirin and related drugs inhibit the formation of hormones such as thromboxane which promote blood clotting and prostacyclin which stops it. In small doses their overall effect is to slow clotting, so they are used to prevent heart attacks.*
- *Dipyridamole slows clotting by blocking the effects of ADP.*
- *Abciximab interacts with proteins on the surface of platelets to stop their aggregation.*
- *Streptokinase, urokinase, and anistreplase increase the activity of the body's own system for dissolving and removing clots.*

CHAPTER 15

Blood pressure

Until about 1600, it was believed that blood was made continuously in the liver. This idea was only replaced as a result of studies by a British physician, William Harvey, born in Folkestone. In 1628 Harvey published a book, *De motu cordis*, in which he described the pumping action of the heart. Careful study of different animals, including demonstrations on humans, led him to propose that the blood circulated around the body, propelled by the heart acting as a pump.

Harvey showed, for example, that the volume of blood leaving the heart every minute was far greater than the total amount in the body, so it could not possibly be made afresh at that rate; the same blood must travel around the blood vessels again and again.

Another of his experiments can be performed on anyone with reasonably prominent veins, say on the surface of the forearm. There are valves every few centimetres along the veins, usually visible as swellings along the vein. If gentle pressure is applied to one of these, using a finger, and another finger is then stroked towards the heart for several inches, the vein becomes emptied of blood and does not refill until the finger pressure over the valve is removed, allowing blood through from the hand. If the second finger is now stroked from its new position towards the hand, the vein does not empty but in fact becomes engorged and swollen as the valve prevents blood from travelling towards the hand. This experiment helped Harvey to conclude that the veins carry blood towards the heart, and that veins contain valves which stop it from flowing backwards. Arteries, on the other hand, carry blood from the heart to the tissues.

What is meant by 'blood pressure'?

The heart (*see* Chapter 16) has two main tasks. Firstly, it has to push blood upwards, against the force of gravity, into the head and that most important of organs—the brain. (This is a problem for any animal which walks upright on two legs, and particularly for a giraffe.)

Secondly, the further away the blood travels from the heart, the narrower are the blood vessels. The smallest of these—the capillaries—are only a fraction of the diameter of a hair, but there are miles and miles of them. If all the blood vessels from an adult person were placed end to end, they would stretch for about 25 000 miles—the circumference of the Earth. The heart has to push very hard indeed to force the blood through all of them and the force it exerts is measured as 'blood pressure'.

If we were to connect one end of a tube into a large blood vessel such as an artery near the heart or at the wrist, then every time the heart contracted it would force blood up the tube for a distance of about 5 feet. The heart could also push a column of mercury about 5 inches, or 120 millimetres at each contraction, the height of the column falling to about 80 millimetres between contractions.* This is why doctors refer to normal blood pressure as 120/80 (spoken as '120 over 80'). The higher figure, generated when the heart contracts, is the 'systolic' pressure. The lower figure, between contractions, is the 'diastolic' pressure. This is precisely how blood pressure was first measured by an English clergyman, Stephen Hales, in 1733, using a long glass tube inserted into an artery of a live horse (Figure 15.1).

How is blood pressure controlled?

Blood pressure is regulated by the interplay of several different mechanisms (Fig. 15.2). A change in one is usually compensated by adjustments in others so that blood pressure remains fairly constant. Let us consider some of these mechanisms in turn.

The heart

The heart itself has a major influence on blood pressure. If it beats more strongly or at a faster rate, it pushes more blood into the vessels and this tends to increase pressure in those vessels. These parameters—the rate and force of the heart's contractions—are controlled primarily by two chemicals. The first is the hormone epinephrine, secreted by the adrenal glands in response to stress, anxiety, or exercise (see Chapter 1). The second is the transmitter norepinephrine, secreted by nerves supplying the heart. Stress and exercise increase the activity of these nerves and, therefore, the secretion of norepinephrine.

Both epinephrine and norepinephrine make the heart beat more strongly and more quickly by activating beta-receptors (see Chapter 1) in the walls of the heart (Fig. 1.4). This is why we are often aware of our heartbeat in a stressful or anxious situation. Activating beta-receptors increases the amount of a

---

* Blood pressure is measured in terms of the distance a column of mercury can be pushed up a glass tube—millimeters of mercury, often abbreviated to 'mm Hg' using the chemical symbol Hg for mercury.

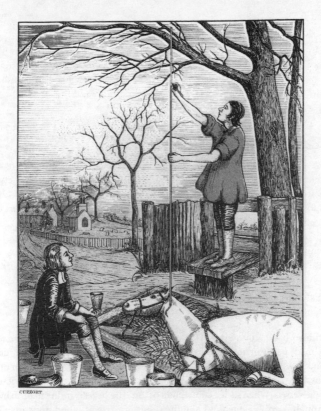

Experiment III

Fig. 15.1 An etching illustrating the first measurement of blood pressure by the Reverend Stephen Hales in 1733. (Wellcome Photo Library)

chemical, cyclic adenosine monophosphate (AMP), inside the cells and this, in turn, increases the movement of calcium into the cells. Because the contraction of all muscle cells, including those of the heart, depends on the amount of calcium present, this movement of calcium allows the heart to contract more strongly and more quickly.

Blood vessels

A second important factor regulating blood pressure is the diameter of the blood vessels. Imagine a piece of soft tubing or a rolled up sheet of paper with

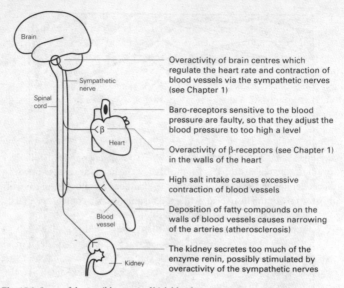

Overactivity of brain centres which regulate the heart rate and contraction of blood vessels via the sympathetic nerves (see Chapter 1)

Baro-receptors sensitive to the blood pressure are faulty, so that they adjust the blood pressure to too high a level

Overactivity of β-receptors (see Chapter 1) in the walls of the heart

High salt intake causes excessive contraction of blood vessels

Deposition of fatty compounds on the walls of blood vessels causes narrowing of the arteries (atherosclerosis)

The kidney secretes too much of the enzyme renin, possibly stimulated by overactivity of the sympathetic nerves

Fig. 15.2 Some of the possible causes of high blood pressure.

a rubber band around it. This is a model of a blood vessel in which the walls are made partly of muscle cells—the rubber band. If we now tighten the rubber band, it will cause a narrowing of the tube. In the same way, contraction of the muscle cells in the walls of arteries and veins causes narrowing (constriction) of the vessels. When such a contraction occurs, the heart is trying to push blood through narrower openings and the result is a rise of blood pressure. Conversely, if the muscle cells in the vessel walls (the vascular muscle cells) relax, decreasing resistance to the movement of blood, the pressure in the vessels will fall.

The diameter of the blood vessels is, like the heart, regulated mainly by norepinephrine released by nerves. The norepinephrine can act on alpha (α) and beta (β) receptors (*see* Chapter 1). If the alpha receptors are activated, this makes the muscle in the blood vessel walls contract and raises blood pressure. Activation of beta-receptors has the opposite effect on some vessels, causing them to relax.

This rather complex situation has probably evolved as part of an emergency system called the 'fight or flight' response by the American physiologist Walter Cannon (*see* Chapter 1). In an emergency, such as confrontation by an aggressor or predator, when an animal needs to prepare to fight or flee in order to survive, it makes sense to reduce blood supply to organs which are not immediately important and to divert blood to organs which are. Activation of the motor nerves, and the secretion of epinephrine, contract blood vessels in non-essential organs such as the intestine and skin by activating alpha-receptors. At the same time, they act on beta-receptors to increase blood flow to those voluntary muscles in the arms and legs needed for fighting or fleeing. The predominant effect is that of activating alpha-receptors, so that blood pressure normally rises in this situation.

The brain

The changes in epinephrine secretion and nervous activity are controlled by the brain. In the posterior parts (at the back of the head) are areas known as cardioaccelerator and vasomotor centres. The cardioaccelerator centre controls mainly the rate of the heartbeat, while the vasomotor area controls primarily the state of contraction or relaxation of the blood vessels.

Both contraction and relaxation are produced by altering the amount of activity in the nerves which release norepinephrine to stimulate the heart or to contract blood vessels.* These two control centres receive information from pressure-sensitive receptors in the vessels and adjust the activity of the sympathetic nerves to try to maintain blood pressure at a constant level. If pressure falls, they increase nerve activity to contract the blood vessels and stimulate the heart. If blood pressure rises, they reduce the nerve activity.

What is 'high' blood pressure (hypertension)?

As we get older the blood vessels become harder and less flexible and the complex interactions between tissues, hormones, and the nervous system, which regulate blood pressure, begin to fail. Blood pressure may then tend to rise. In some people, however, it rises to high levels even when they are relatively young, in their thirties and forties. The levels of blood pressure considered desirable for optimal health have been somewhat controversial in the past, since too great a reduction may compromise blood supply to the brain. The current consensus is that a target of 140/80 to 140/85 is appropriate, with diabetic patients (see Chapter 3) at the lower end of this range in view of their greater cardiovascular risk.

Blood pressure can definitely be called abnormal when it is associated with ill-health and an increased risk of death. This level varies with age, sex, race, and country, but for life assurance purposes a level of 160/100 millimetres of mercury (mm Hg) in a young adult is definitely hypertensive, and a diastolic pressure over 95 mm Hg is probably hypertensive. The World Health

* The 'sympathetic' nerves (see Chapter 1).

Organisation (WHO) defines hypertension as 160/95 mm Hg. The medical debate about a correct definition of hypertension arises because these levels of blood pressure are not at all uncommon, particularly over the age of 65.

The reason why doctors are concerned about high blood pressure is that it increases the risk of heart failure and strokes, which are among the modern world's major killers. High blood pressure can damage the delicate endothelial cells lining the inside of blood vessels. If this happens, white cells in the blood are attracted to the damaged area and stick there. This can start the build-up of a layer of tissue which grows, over the years, as fats from the blood are deposited there, leading to atherosclerosis and narrowing the diameter of the vessels.

High blood pressure may cause weak blood vessels to leak or burst. If this happens in the brain, the result is a stroke, with the potential for damage to a part of the brain as a result of the lack of blood flow and oxygen. If hypertension is maintained for several years the heart, which is then pumping blood against abnormally high resistance, begins to weaken, leading to heart failure.

What are the major causes of hypertension?

Occasionally high blood pressure is the result of a known medical problem such as poor kidney function, or excessive production of steroid hormones. However, in 90 per cent of cases it is idiopathic—of unknown cause. High blood pressure of unknown cause is often called 'essential hypertension' because at one time doctors believed that the increased pressure developed in people as an essential means of adequately supplying blood to their tissues. This does not seem to be correct, because the tissues appear to receive a perfectly adequate supply of blood in such people, even when their blood pressure has been lowered by drugs to 'normal' levels. The term 'essential' is, therefore, inappropriate and misleading.

Salt

Despite the lack of certainty, there is no shortage of ideas as to the cause of hypertension. One is that it results from an imbalance of sodium, because there is some association between the intake of sodium and the development of hypertension. The body has several mechanisms to regulate the amount of sodium in the tissues, but a large intake over many years (particularly in the form of common salt, sodium chloride) may induce a small, gradual shift in the level of sodium which the body tries to maintain.

Any increase in the amount of sodium inside the muscle cells of the blood vessels will increase their tendency to contract by making them more excitable and will, therefore, raise blood pressure. Since a diet lacking salt is rather unpalatable, this is no longer considered to be necessary in hypertensive patients, although they are advised to eliminate as much salt as possible from their diet.

The brain

Another possible cause of hypertension is a gradual change in the level at which the brain tries to maintain blood pressure. Normally the pressure is measured by specialized receptor cells called 'baroreceptors' (meaning pressure receptors), in the large blood vessels near the heart.

If the blood pressure tends to rise, these sensors are normally activated to send impulses along their sensory nerves into the brain. There, the nerve impulses act upon brain cells in the vasomotor and cardioaccelerator centres which reduce the activity of the sympathetic nerves. The result is relaxation of blood vessels and a slowing of the heart rate, with a lowering of blood pressure towards normal within a few seconds. There is a theory that, if blood pressure is frequently and repeatedly raised in some people (for example by stress, anxiety, or anger), the baroreceptors or the brain centres on which they act adjust the level at which the pressure is regulated. Over several years this could lead to a gradual increase in the blood pressure.

Atherosclerosis

Another theory is that fatty materials (cholesterol, triglycerides; see later) are gradually laid down in the walls of the blood vessels. Over a number of years this causes narrowing of the arteries (atherosclerosis or arteriosclerosis) and reduces their ability to contract and relax, causing blood pressure to rise. The same thickening or 'hardening' process reduces the sensitivity of the baroreceptors to changes of blood pressure and make it more difficult for them to respond to and to correct high levels of blood pressure.

The kidney

A fourth idea is that hypertension in some people results from abnormalities in the kidney, which has several functions in addition to producing urine. One of these is to regulate blood volume. If the volume of blood in the body falls, for example after a haemorrhage, specialized cells in the kidney* release an enzyme called renin.† This acts on a protein in the blood to change it into a substance—angiotensin 1—which is rapidly converted into angiotensin-2 (AT2). Angiotensin 2 has several effects, all of which are designed to compensate for the loss of blood which triggered the production of renin. Firstly, it is a powerful constrictor of blood vessels and directly causes a rise of blood pressure

---

* The juxtaglomerular cells.
† Pronounced 'reenin' and very different from the enzyme called rennin which aids the digestion of milk in the stomach.

which preserves blood flow to the vital organs. Secondly, it makes the kidney produce less urine, thus conserving water, some of which remains in the blood and increases the volume of blood. Thirdly, AT2 acts on the brain to stimulate drinking, and some of this additional water intake again remains in the blood. These three factors together tend to increase blood pressure. If the kidney produces too much renin, one consequence is a rise in blood pressure.

Other factors

Many other factors contribute to the development of high blood pressure. Smoking, for example, produces chemicals called 'free radicals' (*see* Chapter 22) which damage blood vessel walls and speed up the development of atherosclerosis. In obesity the body has to grow many additional miles of vessels to take blood to all the new fat cells. In order to pump blood to all the cells, the heart has to work harder and the pressure in the large vessels has to increase.

Controlling blood pressure

The effective control of blood pressure in middle-aged and elderly patients (and probably also in young adults) reduces the frequency of strokes, heart attacks, and death from cardiovascular disease. The aim of treatment is usually to lower diastolic blood pressure to a level of 80–90 mm of mercury (mm Hg).

Recent surveys from the United States, however, suggest that there is considerable room for improvement in treatment: about 35 per cent of people with high blood pressure are undetected, 50 per cent of those detected are not being treated, and 80 per cent of those being treated for their high blood pressure still have pressures over 140/90 mm Hg. Over 50 per cent of people over the age of 65 have high blood pressure (over 140/80).

Only about half of the patients treated for high blood pressure continue to take their drugs for more than six months, primarily because most do not realize that when the drugs are stopped, blood pressure will return to its previous high level. The risk of heart attacks and strokes caused by high blood pressure then also increases again to dangerous levels. Blood pressure should be checked regularly and at least every three months to make sure that it is being controlled satisfactorily.

Drugs used to treat hypertension

Hypertension should never be diagnosed on finding one high blood pressure reading, since blood pressure goes up and down from hour to hour and day to day under the influence of stress, exercise, and other factors. Even walking quickly to see the doctor can raise it by 20 mm Hg. Some control of blood

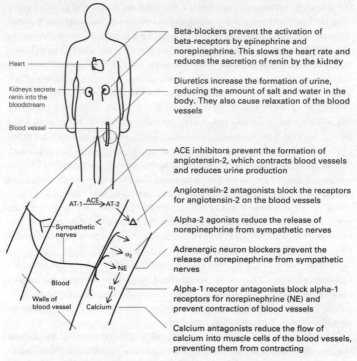

Beta-blockers prevent the activation of beta-receptors by epinephrine and norepinephrine. This slows the heart rate and reduces the secretion of renin by the kidney

Diuretics increase the formation of urine, reducing the amount of salt and water in the body. They also cause relaxation of the blood vessels

ACE inhibitors prevent the formation of angiotensin-2, which contracts blood vessels and reduces urine production

Angiotensin-2 antagonists block the receptors for angiotensin-2 on the blood vessels

Alpha-2 agonists reduce the release of norepinephrine from sympathetic nerves

Adrenergic neuron blockers prevent the release of norepinephrine from sympathetic nerves

Alpha-1 receptor antagonists block alpha-1 receptors for norepinephrine (NE) and prevent contraction of blood vessels

Calcium antagonists reduce the flow of calcium into muscle cells of the blood vessels, preventing them from contracting

Fig. 15.3 The actions of drugs which are used to lower a high blood pressure.

pressure can be achieved by reducing weight, stress, salt, and alcohol intake (to less than two or three units a day*) with regular exercise.

When these are not effective by themselves, there is a wide range of drugs which can be used for treatment, separately or in combination (Fig. 15.3). Combinations have the advantage that lower doses of the different drugs can often be used, reducing the probability of side-effects.

Diuretics (water tablets)

The first drugs to be tried are usually those which increase the formation of urine by the kidney. These are the diuretic drugs described in more detail in Chapter 5. Those used to treat high blood pressure usually belong to a group called the

---

* One unit is roughly equivalent to a half pint of beer, a glass of wine, or a single measure of spirits. The recommended safe limits of drinking are 14 units per week for women and 21 per week for men.

thiazides. The increased production of urine results in a loss of salt and water from the body and reduces the volume of blood which the heart has to pump through the tissues. The body will compensate for this over a period of days or weeks by, for example, increasing the production of renin. The thiazides have a second mechanism of reducing blood pressure, since they act directly on blood vessels to relax their muscle cells. The vessels do not compensate for this effect, so this action of the thiazides lasts as long as the drugs are being taken.

Thiazides are not only very mild drugs, but are also considered to be very safe and are usually the first group of drugs to be used for hypertension. Their main side-effect is the lowering of potassium levels in the body, which can result in muscle cramps, weakness, and changes in the rhythm of the heartbeat. Potassium supplements may be needed in some patients (see Chapter 5).

These drugs can also cause impotence and loss of libido in some men. They should not be used in diabetic patients because they may raise blood sugar levels, or in patients with gout (see Chapter 20) because they can reduce the removal of uric acid from the body. Thiazides may also cause dizziness and may make the skin unusually sensitive to light, with a tendency to burn more quickly and seriously on exposure to the sun or to ultraviolet light.

As with many drugs, it may be dangerous to stop taking the thiazides suddenly since, once the body has adjusted to their presence, their sudden removal may result in a rebound increase in blood pressure. Particularly in elderly patients, this may be sufficiently severe that blood vessels may be damaged or even burst, resulting in a stroke.

Other diuretics are equally effective in lowering blood pressure and include the so-called 'loop diuretics' such as frusemide and bumetanide (see Chapter 5). These are more powerful than the thiazides and are normally used when a stronger drug is required because of impaired heart or kidney function.

Beta-blockers

The discovery of beta-blockers

The idea that epinephrine and norepinephrine can act on alpha and beta receptors originated with Raymond Ahlquist, Professor of Pharmacology at the Medical College of Georgia in Atlanta, in 1948. At that time the chemicals available blocked only alpha receptors and did not block the effects of epinephrine at beta-receptors in the heart (see Chapter 1). It was another ten years before Irwin Slater, working for the pharmaceutical company Eli Lilly in Indianapolis, produced the first compound to do this. However, it was too toxic to use in medicine and had many side-effects, but its discovery gave James Whyte Black and his team at ICI in England the idea that useful drugs might also be made with the opposite effect, acting selectively on beta receptors (see Chapter 2).

By 1960, the team had produced pronethalol, the first drug able to block only the beta-receptors in the heart with no effects on other receptors. Its potential value to medicine was shown in a clinical trial by Tony Dornhorst and Brian Robinson at St. George's Hospital in London when they found that it greatly reduced angina in patients. Unfortunately, this pioneering drug was soon found to cause cancer in mice and the first beta-blocker to be introduced into widespread use was a similar drug, propranolol. This is more powerful than pronethalol, it has few side-effects, produces no risk of cancer, and is still widely used today.

Beta-blockers in hypertension

Beta-blockers are popular treatments in patients with hypertension (Table 15.1, p. 222). They interact with the beta-receptors which mediate some of the effects of epinephrine and the sympathetic nerve transmitter norepinephrine (*see* Chapter 1). Activation of the beta-receptors increases the rate and force of the heart's contraction, the release of norepinephrine from the nerves, and the secretion of renin from the kidney. Beta-blocker drugs prevent all these effects and, therefore, reduce heart rate and force, the nerve-induced contraction of blood vessels, and the formation of AT2 in the blood. The overall effect is to lower blood pressure.

Side-effects

Several of the beta-blockers can enter the brain, and this may result in disturbed sleep at night, sometimes with vivid dreams.

Another problem follows from the fact that epinephrine and norepinephrine act on alpha-receptors as well as beta-receptors. The two families usually have opposing effects in the tissues, maintaining an overall, long-term balance of function. Blockage of the beta-receptors means that epinephrine and norepinephrine can act without opposition on the alpha-receptors. Since alpha-receptors cause contraction of blood vessels, this can result in narrowing of vessels in the hands and feet, with unpleasant feelings of coldness in the fingers and toes as the blood flow declines, and painful sensations as the blood vessels later dilate. These effects may be worse if the patient is stressed, and is secreting large quantities of epinephrine and norepinephrine. Alpha-receptor activity, unopposed by beta-receptors, may also lead to an excessive, potentially dangerous rise of blood pressure under stress or during exercise.

In fact, blockade of beta-receptors in the heart means that this organ cannot increase its activity with exercise, and cannot pump enough blood to the muscles. It is, therefore, difficult and possibly dangerous to take anything more than the mildest exercise when taking beta-blockers: too much exercise may produce feelings of weakness with muscle pains and cramps.

As with other drugs used to combat hypertension, patients should not stop taking beta-blockers suddenly because the blood pressure may rebound to levels higher than before starting the drugs. This may result in a bleed or haemorrhage because the blood vessels cannot cope with the high pressure and may burst.

Beta-blockers and asthma

Although safe, beta-blockers should be used only with great care by asthmatic patients because beta-receptors relax the airways (*see* Chapter 2) and limit their constriction during an asthmatic attack. If beta-blockers are taken by an asthmatic patient, a trigger stimulus is likely to produce a much greater contraction of the airways.

Fortunately, some beta-blockers are far less likely to affect the airways than others. An American group at Stearns, led by Al Lands, discovered in 1967 that beta-receptors exist in at least two varieties. The beta-1 type is found on the heart, and the beta-2 type in the airways. Some beta-blockers are selective blockers of only one type. The beta-1 blockers, for example, such as atenolol and metoprolol, have most of their effect on the heart. They should, therefore, be safer for asthmatic patients to use since they have less tendency to block beta-2 receptors in the lungs. In practice, since all beta-blockers affect all beta-receptors to some extent, they are probably best avoided for asthmatic patients.

ACE inhibitors

We have already seen that AT2 powerfully contracts blood vessel walls and has other actions leading to an increase of blood pressure. In some people AT2 contributes to the development of high blood pressure, so that drugs which prevent the formation of AT2 should help to lower it.

Angiotensin converting enzyme, or ACE, is the enzyme which produces AT2 in the blood. The original idea for using ACE inhibitors to control blood pressure arose from a discovery in 1965 by a Brazilian scientist, Sergio Ferreira. He found that the venom of the Brazilian viper, which induces a profound drop of blood pressure, contained a substance which inhibited ACE. After a long period of research, David Cushman and his team at the Squibb Institute in Princeton produced the first artificial drug to inhibit the enzyme. This was captopril, introduced into medicine in 1977.

Several similar drugs are now available, the most commonly used of which are captopril, enalapril, and lisinopril. They work well as antihypertensive drugs. Apart from the side-effects common to many drugs, such as occasional dizziness and headaches, they have the more unusual side-effect of producing a dry cough in some patients. This is because ACE inhibitors prevent the destruction of a peptide called bradykinin which can stimulate sensory receptors in the airways. These receptors normally respond to irritating chemicals in the atmosphere (smoke, for example) and trigger coughing as a means of eliminating them from the lungs. By raising the levels of bradykinin, the ACE inhibitors also stimulate the irritant receptors and produce a dry cough which may be such a nuisance that treatment with these drugs has to be stopped.

In fact, bradykinin is a potent dilator of blood vessels and can produce a large drop in blood pressure. The increase in bradykinin levels produced in the blood by ACE inhibitors, therefore, probably accounts for part of the success of these drugs in treating hypertension.

ACE inhibitor plus . . .

One drug which is soon to become available is sampatrilat. This is also an ACE inhibitor, but has another very important property. There is a peptide hormone called 'atrial natriuretic factor' (ANF). As its name suggests, this hormone is produced by cells in the atria of the heart and its main effect is to increase the loss of water and sodium (Greek *natrium*) in the urine: it is the body's natural diuretic hormone.

Atrial natriuretic factor is normally destroyed by an enzyme called 'endopeptidase' and this is inhibited by sampatrilat. The result is that ANF lasts longer in the body, causing a greater loss of water and salt. As the volume of water and blood in the body falls, the blood pressure also falls. The combination of ACE inhibition and ANF potentiation makes sampatrilat valuable in patients who do not respond well to the ACE inhibitors alone.

Angiotensin antagonists

A group of drugs, such as losartan, block the receptors for AT2. They therefore prevent all the effects of AT2 and are almost as effective as the ACE inhibitors at reducing high blood pressure in some patients. Since they do not inhibit ACE or increase the levels of bradykinin, they do not cause the irritating cough which ACE inhibitors can produce.

Alpha-receptor blockers

Since activation of alpha-receptors (*see* Chapter 1) regulates the degree of contraction of the blood vessels, another method of controlling high blood pressure is to block the alpha-receptors by drugs such as prazosin or terazosin. When these drugs are taken, the blood vessels cannot contract as much as normally, and blood pressure falls.

When the alpha-receptors are blocked, however, epinephrine and norepine-phrine will still act on the beta-receptors, with unpredictable effects on blood pressure. Some drugs, such as labetalol and carvedilol, reduce this problem by blocking both alpha and beta-receptors.

Postural hypotension

These drugs are certainly effective, but their side-effects can be troublesome. One of the main problems is that some patients feel faint when they stand up suddenly. This is known as 'postural hypotension' and is particularly noticeable after the first few doses of drug. It happens because changes of posture, such as standing from a sitting or lying position, tend to cause a brief drop in blood pressure as gravity pulls blood towards the legs and away from the heart and brain.

The body normally deals with this problem by the 'baroreceptor reflex' described earlier. Pressure-sensitive detectors in the walls of large blood vessels detect the fall in pressure and correct it by making the veins in the legs contract. Because the alpha-blockers prevent the blood vessels from responding to norepinephrine released from the sympathetic nerves, this reflex contraction cannot occur. The fall in blood pressure on standing therefore reduces blood flow to the brain, leading to dizziness and fainting.

Other side-effects

The block of alpha-receptors on blood vessels in the nose results in dilation of these vessels and nasal congestion (*see* Chapter 2). Alpha-receptors are also responsible for the contraction of the vasa deferentia (the tubes which produce ejaculation in the male and which are tied off in a vasectomy operation). Alpha-receptor blockers may, therefore, interfere with ejaculation and may even cause impotence.

Alpha-2 receptor agonists

Alpha-receptors can be divided into two subtypes, alpha-1 and alpha-2. Most of the drugs described in the previous section block only alpha-1 receptors.

Alpha-2 receptors do occur on blood vessels, but the drugs used to combat hypertension seem to affect mainly those in the brain. Alpha-2 receptors exist in those parts of the brain, such as the vasomotor centre, which control nerves acting on the heart and blood vessels. When these are stimulated by drugs such as clonidine (Table 15.1, p. 222) the activity of the nerves declines, relaxing blood vessels and causing a fall of blood pressure.

These are useful drugs for the long-term control of blood pressure, although they can produce tiredness by affecting parts of the brain in addition to the cardiovascular control centres, as well as a dry mouth by preventing the secretion of saliva. They may also produce impotence.

One member of this group, alpha-methyldopa, was once frequently prescribed but is now rarely used since it can produce many side-effects including depression, the development of breasts in males, and disorders of sexual function, nightmares, and abnormal movements. These are due to the stimulation of receptors for the transmitter dopamine in the brain.

Adrenergic neuron blockers

An alternative to blocking the receptors for epinephrine and norepinephrine to reduce the contraction of blood vessels by the sympathetic nerves, is to stop the nerves from releasing norepinephrine. This can be achieved by using drugs such as guanethidine. Unfortunately, these suffer from many of the same side-effects and problems as the alpha-receptor antagonists.

Calcium antagonists

One of the most important steps in the contraction of any muscle, including those which make up the walls of blood vessels, is the movement of calcium ions into the cells. The discovery of compounds able to block this movement of calcium was made by the German scientist Albrecht Fleckenstein at the University of Freiburg and the Belgian pharmacologist Theophile Godfraind at the University of Louvain in the 1960s. All of these 'calcium antagonists', including nifedipine, verapamil, and diltiazem can reduce contraction of the blood vessels and lower blood pressure. Drugs similar to nifedipine are among the most useful and effective. Their side-effects in a few people can include generalized flushing, dizziness, headache, and disturbances of the digestive system, all of which are due to interference with the movement of calcium ions into muscle cells in different tissues.

5HT2 antagonists

In addition to receptors for norepinephrine, blood vessels also possess receptors for 5-hydroxytryptamine (5HT) which cause contraction and raise blood pressure. One drug, ketanserin, blocks these receptors and restores a raised blood pressure towards normal.

Potassium channel openers

Finally there are drugs which make the muscle cells of the blood vessels less excitable and, therefore, less able to respond to transmitters such as norepinephrine which make them contract.

The excitability of cells depends on an electrical potential across their walls. This potential depends partly on the high amount of potassium inside the cells, compared with the much smaller amount present in blood. Drugs such as cromakalim increase the permeability of the cell walls to potassium so that some leaks out and reduces the potential across the cell wall. The result is a reduced excitability, relaxation of the vascular muscle cells, and a lowering of blood pressure.

Hydralazine and minoxidil

It is rare for a patient not to respond to one or other of the groups of drugs described above, but everyone is different, and such cases do occur. One solution may be to use a combination since two drugs, acting by different mechanisms, may work together to produce an effect which is much greater than either drug alone. Another solution is to use drugs which are less effective but which have side-effects which are less serious than the dangers of hypertension. Hydralazine and minoxidil are two such drugs. Both act directly on blood vessels to relax the muscle cells in their walls and reduce pressure. Hydralazine, however, can trigger an allergic reaction and minoxidil attracted attention when it was introduced into medicine, as it induces a marked growth of hair. This aroused the interest of men seeking a possible cure for baldness, but the hair growth on the face, arms, back, and chest is less welcome to some people, especially women.

Minoxidil and hair growth

Hairs are produced by pockets of tissue called hair follicles. Each follicle lives for between two and six years, after which it dies and is normally replaced by a new one. As we (especially men), get older, follicles become smaller, produce smaller and smaller hairs, and live for a shorter time. The result is a tendency for normal hair to be replaced by a covering of very tiny hairs called velus hairs.

Since the follicles are not dead, however, they can be stimulated to produce larger hairs and thus restore, at least partially, the original head of hair. This seems to be the effect of minoxidil, which boosts blood flow to the hair follicles, increases the rate of hair formation, and extends the life span of each follicle.

After careful trials and the examination of side-effects, minoxidil was finally given official approval for use in the treatment of male pattern baldness (alopecia), in 1989. It is the first and so far only drug for this condition.

Cholesterol and atherosclerosis

One cause of high blood pressure is the gradual narrowing of blood vessels by deposits of fatty substances on the walls. The process is known as atherosclerosis and the increasing resistance to the flow of blood will slowly raise the blood pressure. As first described by the American physician James B. Herrick in 1912, atherosclerosis may also block important arteries such as those in the heart, leading to a shortage of blood, the formation of blood clots, and a heart attack.

The main fatty substances in the blood are cholesterol and triglycerides (so called because they are a complex of a molecule of glycerol with three molecules of fatty acids). Cholesterol is an important chemical which is used to make the walls of cells and the fatty layers surrounding nerve cells. It is also the starting material from which the body makes steroid hormones and bile salts.

The amount of cholesterol in the blood tends to increase with age so that more becomes deposited in the blood vessels. People with a blood cholesterol level of more than 2.45 g per litre (6.4 mmols per litre)* have a three- to four-fold greater risk of heart disease than those with less than 1.8 g per litre (4.7 mmols per litre). In people with high levels, some protection against athero-sclerosis and heart attacks can be given, therefore, by lowering the levels of cholesterol and triglycerides.

'Good' and 'bad' cholesterol

This phrase refers to the fact that cholesterol in the blood is bound to other molecules called lipoproteins (part fat, part protein). The low-density lipo-proteins (LDL) are combined with larger amounts of cholesterol than high-density lipoproteins (HDL). The LDL-cholesterol mixture is more likely to deposit cholesterol in blood vessels and is, therefore, sometimes known as 'bad' cholesterol. The HDL-cholesterol complex is referred to as 'good' cholesterol since it can remove cholesterol from blood vessels and carry it to the liver, thereby protecting against vascular damage.

Control of cholesterol levels

Some cholesterol comes from food, especially meats, liver, eggs, and dairy products, and the simplest way of lowering cholesterol levels is to reduce the consumption of these. However, around 90 per cent of the cholesterol in our blood is produced by our own livers. Cholesterol is used to strengthen the walls of cells throughout the body, it is the basic chemical from which the steroid hormones (*see* Chapter 19) are made, and it is used by the liver to make bile salts which assist in the digestion of food. Only the last of these can be modified by drugs.

Inhibitors of cholesterol absorption

Bile salts are produced in the liver from cholesterol and are then secreted into the intestine where they aid digestion. Normally, some of the bile salts are reabsorbed from the intestine and the cholesterol is reused in the liver. The drugs cholestyramine and colestipol combine with the bile salts in the intestine so that they cannot be reabsorbed and are lost in the faeces. This means that the liver has to use more cholesterol from the blood to make more bile salts. These two effects result in a fall in the amount of cholesterol in the blood. As a bonus the liver, in making more cholesterol, uses up some of the LDL in the

* These are different ways of expressing the weight of a chemical. 1 millimole (mmol) of cholesterol weighs 0.386 grams (g).

blood so that the largest change in the blood is a drop in the amount of LDL-(bad)cholesterol.

Ispaghula husk, a form of soluble dietary fibre, also combines with the bile salts in the intestine and can be used to produce the same effects as these drugs. Soluble fibre is also found in oats and baked beans and, when included in the diet, this will combine with cholesterol in the intestine, preventing its absorption and lowering blood cholesterol levels by about 10 per cent.

The main drawback with these drugs is that they can combine with some vitamins such as A, D, and K, which dissolve in fat, so these may need to be replaced if the drugs are taken for long periods. They can also increase the amounts of the triglycerides in the blood which can lead to inflammation of the pancreas (pancreatitis).

Fibrates

The fibrates are a different group of drugs which lower blood cholesterol in several ways. Firstly, they increase the secretion of bile salts by the liver, and increase the amount of cholesterol excreted from the body. Secondly, they increase the activity of an enzyme called lipoprotein lipase which helps to destroy some of the fatty substances in the blood. This results in a change in the balance between lipoproteins such that the amounts of LDL-cholesterol are lowered, and those of HDL-cholesterol are raised. Thirdly, the fibrates make it easier for the lipoproteins to pass into cells from the blood, so that more is destroyed by the cells. Overall, these drugs lower blood cholesterol and triglycerides.

Statins

Since the liver produces most of the cholesterol in blood, the most effective way to reduce cholesterol levels is to stop that production. The statins are drugs which inhibit one of the main enzymes which make cholesterol.* Not only does this reduce the production of new cholesterol, but the liver also has to take from the blood more of the cholesterol which is absorbed from food. The net result is a marked fall in the amount of LDL-cholesterol and an increase in HDL-cholesterol.

Nicotinic acid, acipimox, and probucol

It was discovered accidentally in the 1950s that nicotinic acid could decrease the formation of cholesterol in the liver. It also increases the amount of HDL-cholesterol and decreases LDL-cholesterol and triglycerides. The main problem with this substance is that it relaxes blood vessels, resulting in unpleasant

---

* The enzyme is called 3-hydroxy-3-methylglutaryl coenzyme A reductase (HMG-CoA reductase).

flushing of the skin. The related drug acipimox is less likely to cause flushing and is usually preferred.

Probucol increases the rate at which the LDL are broken down in the liver, causing more to be removed from the blood for the manufacture of bile salts and steroid hormones.

Drugs of the future

Researchers in universities and the pharmaceutical industry are developing other types of drug for the treatment of hypertension which are more effective than those currently available, safer (having fewer side-effects), or which may be effective in those patients who do not respond to existing drugs. For example, there is interest in the hormone endothelin, which contracts blood vessels very powerfully, and which may have some role in establishing high blood pressure. Research is aimed at finding antagonist drugs able to block endothelin receptors on the vessels.

Low blood pressure: shock

Low blood pressure is not a problem for most people, but can become so if a patient loses a great deal of blood. It can also be dangerous after injuries which do not themselves involve a loss of blood but which cause the body to lose control of blood vessel size.

If all the vessels were fully open at the same time, they could contain many times the volume of blood in an average adult (usually about 5 litres or 8 pints). Most vessels are maintained in a state of partial contraction which can be modified on demand. For example, after a meal, blood vessels to the stomach and intestine open to help with the digestion and absorption of food. In a hot environment vessels in the skin open to facilitate sweating and allow more heat to be lost, and during exercise, vessels in the muscles open to allow delivery of more oxygen and glucose for the muscle activity. The balance between open and partially closed vessels is determined largely by the nervous system, which can secrete more or less norepinephrine (see Chapter 1).

A traumatic life event, such as an accident or a close bereavement, can lead to a temporary loss of the nervous control of blood vessel size, and a profound drop in blood pressure. This is why people may faint under such circumstances, and is the reason for the usual advice: 'I think you should sit down . . .'. It is almost as if, in the face of serious emotional stress, the brain 'forgets' to support the blood pressure. Such a state of abnormally low blood pressure is medically called 'shock'.

The drop in blood pressure means that parts of many tissues do not receive enough blood to survive, and the cells begin to die. As they do so, they leak chemicals into their surroundings which damage other cells and cause a further drop in blood pressure. This chain of events can rapidly deteriorate into a state of irreversible shock from which it may be impossible to recover and death may follow.

The best treatment for shock is to give the patient, as soon as possible, a transfusion of blood or of fluids which 'expand' the blood volume and maintain pressure. Doctors now prefer to use drugs very cautiously during shock and only when absolutely necessary. The drugs most commonly used include dobutamine, a beta-1 receptor stimulant which increases activity of the heart to raise blood pressure without constricting blood vessels, and steroids which seem to protect tissues from the damaging effects of low blood pressure and poor oxygen supply.

Table 15.1 **Drugs used to control hypertension**

Thiazide diuretics	Potassium-sparing diuretics	Beta-blockers.
bendrofluazide	amiloride	(Selective for the heart)
benzthiazide	triamterene	acebutolol
chlorothiazide	potassium canrenoate	atenolol
chlorthalidone	spironolactone	betaxolol
clopamide		bisoprolol
cyclopenthiazide	**Alpha-blockers**	celiprolol
hydrochlorothiazide	alfuzosin	esmolol
hydroflumethiazide	doxasosin	labetalol
indapamide	indoramin	metoprolol
mefruside	phenoxybenzamine	nadolol
methyclothiazide (USA)	phentolamine	oxprenolol
metolazone	prazosin	
polythiazide	terazosin	**Beta-blockers (not selective)**
quinethazone (USA)		carteolol
trichlormethiazole (USA)	**Alpha-2-agonists**	nadolol
xipamide	apraclonidine	penbutolol
	clonidine	pindolol
	guanabenz (USA)	propranolol
Loop diuretics	guanfacine (USA)	sotalol
frusemide	methyldopa	timolol
bumetanide		
ethacrynic acid		**Alpha + Beta-blocker**
piretanide		carvedilol
torasemide		labetalol

Table 15.1 *Continued*

Adrenergic neuron blockers	Calcium blockers	Direct vasodilators
bethanidine	diltiazem	glyceryl trinitrate
bretylium	verapamil	hydralazine
debrisoquine	nifedipine group	minoxidil
guanadrel (USA)	—amlodipine	nitroprusside
guanethidine	—bepridil (USA)	
	—felodipine	**Cholesterol-lowering drugs**
ACE inhibitors	—isradipine	Inhibitors of bile absorption:
benazepril (USA)	—lacidipine	cholestyramine
captopril	—lercanidipine	colestipol
cilazapril	—nicardipine	ispaghula
enalapril	—nifedipine	
fosinopril	—nimodipine	**Fibrates**
lisinopril	—nisoldipine	bezafibrate
moexipril	—nitrendipine	ciprofibrate
perindopril		clofibrate
quinapril	**Potassium channel openers**	fenofibrate
ramipril	cromakalim	gemfibrozil
sampatrilat*	diazoxide	
spirapril (USA)	levcromakalin	**Statins**
trandolapril	nicorandil	atorvastatin
		fluvastatin
Angiotensin antagonists	**5HT2 antagonist**	lovastatin
candisartin	ketanserin	pravastatin
eprosartan		simvastatin
losartan	**Reserpine and related drugs**	
saralasin	Rauwolfia serpentina (USA)	**Other drugs**
tasosartan	rescinnamine (USA)	acipimox
telmisartan	reserpine (USA)	nicotinic acid
valsartan		probucol

* Sampatrilat also increases the actions of ANF. It should become available during 2000.

Summary

- *High blood pressure (hypertension) increases the chances of heart damage and stroke.*
- *Drugs can be used to lower blood pressure by:*
  - *increasing the loss of water in the urine (diuretic drugs)*
  - *blocking beta-receptors which respond to epinephrine and norepinephrine. This reduces the rate and force of the heart beat*
  - *inhibiting the enzyme which produces angiotensin (ACE), a hormone which contracts blood vessels and increases salt and water reabsorption in the kidney*
  - *blocking the receptors for angiotensin on blood vessels*
  - *blocking alpha-receptors for norepinephrine which contract blood vessels*
  - *activating alpha-2 receptors for norepinephrine, receptors which reduce norepinephrine release from sympathetic nerves*
  - *blocking the release of norepinephrine from sympathetic nerves*
  - *preventing the influx of calcium needed for contraction of blood vessels*
  - *blocking 5HT2 receptors which respond to 5HT by contracting blood vessels*
  - *direct relaxation of the muscle cells in blood vessel walls, for example by drugs releasing nitric oxide.*
- *Cholesterol is carried in the blood attached to fatty chemicals which can be deposited on blood vessels walls (atherosclerosis), making the vessels narrower and stiffer, and raising blood pressure.*
- *Most cholesterol is made in the liver. Cholesterol levels in the blood can be lowered by the statins, drugs which reduce the synthesis of new cholesterol.*
- *The fibrates increase the secretion and destruction of cholesterol.*
- *Bile salts are made from cholesterol and are secreted into the intestine to break down fats for absorption. Cholestyramine and colestipol combine with bile salts, preventing their reabsorption so the cholesterol cannot be re-used by the body.*
- *Nicotinic acid, acipimox, and probucol decrease the manufacture of cholesterol in the liver.*

CHAPTER 16

The heart

David was just 65. He had retired earlier in the year and was now enjoying his daily brisk walk around the park with Jack, his Scottish terrier. Suddenly he became aware of a tight, constricted feeling in his chest. He felt as though he wanted to take deeper breaths, but the tightness prevented him from doing so. He slowed his walking and when he came to a park bench he sat down for a few minutes. Slowly the tightness went away and David was able to breathe more easily. He then carried on his walk, slowly at first, but was soon back up to his usual speed. David thought nothing more about this incident, as he had no more immediate problems, and he soon forgot the episode entirely.

It was about five years later, after several walks during a particularly cold winter, that David began to feel short of breath even when he was not walking, but just sitting at home. In fact he now walked much more slowly, and had to pause for a minute or two when climbing stairs. His doctor sent him for a check-up and, after that, for an angiogram test. In this test, a dye was injected into his heart so that doctors could watch the movement of the dye through the coronary arteries using an X-ray machine. The results showed two things.

Firstly, two of the blood vessels in David's heart were partly blocked, so that the heart muscle was not being supplied with enough oxygen to work properly. Secondly, part of the heart was not contracting at all. This was an area damaged when David had already had a heart attack without realizing it—the episode in the park five years earlier.

David's recent breathlessness was because his heart was too weak to pump enough blood to the lungs to take up the amount of oxygen his body needed. When the amount of carbon dioxide in the blood is too high, or oxygen is too low, specialized receptor cells in the brain detect this and increase the activity of the nerves responsible for breathing. David's body was trying to cope with the problems with his heart by increasing the rate of breathing to increase the removal of carbon dioxide from the lungs and replace it with oxygen.

The example reveals several points. Firstly, it is possible to have a very mild heart attack which may damage or kill part of the heart, without realizing it.

Secondly, as David's heart became progressively weaker from a combination of the heart attack and partly blocked blood vessels, his heart would be working harder and harder to pump blood to the lungs. During the cold winter, an additional strain would be placed on his heart, as his body metabolism increased to generate extra body heat. It was only at this stage that David became aware of his more rapid breathing.

The heart

The heart is a pump, made of muscle and about the size of a clenched male fist. Its job is to pump blood—about 5 litres or 1 gallon of it every minute—around the body, and it beats every second from well before birth until death, a total of around 36 million times a year or 2.5 billion times in a life spanning 70 years. If the heart stops, and the flow of blood to the brain is interrupted for more than about four minutes, then death will usually occur from irreversible brain damage.

The heart is divided into four chambers, first described by a French professor of anatomy, Raymond de Vieussens, at the University of Montpellier, in 1705. There are two atria and two ventricles separated by valves (Fig. 16.1). Blood returning from the tissues, where it has given up most of its oxygen, contains little oxygen and much carbon dioxide. This blood enters the atrium on the right side of the heart and then passes into the right ventricle. From here it is pumped to the lungs, where it loses carbon dioxide and picks up oxygen, before returning to the left atrium and ventricle. From the left ventricle, which has a very powerful, muscular wall, the oxygenated blood is pumped to all parts of the body to deliver its life-sustaining cargo of oxygen to the various organs and tissues.

Control of the heartbeat

The heart – always drawn as if facing a person, with the left side on the right of the drawing

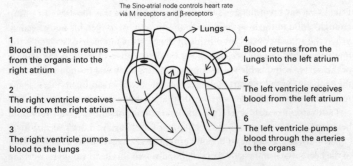

The Sino-atrial node controls heart rate via M receptors and β-receptors

→ Lungs

1
Blood in the veins returns from the organs into the right atrium

2
The right ventricle receives blood from the right atrium

3
The right ventricle pumps blood to the lungs

4
Blood returns from the lungs into the left atrium

5
The left ventricle receives blood from the left atrium

6
The left ventricle pumps blood through the arteries to the organs

Fig. 16.1 The structure of the heart.

Perhaps because it is so critically important to life, the heart does not depend on any other part of the body for its activity. If a normal, healthy heart is removed from the body and placed into a solution similar to blood, with oxygen and the same major ions as blood (sodium, potassium, calcium, magnesium, chloride, phosphate, and bicarbonate) at normal body temperature (37°C), then it will continue to beat on its own for many, many hours.

Inside the body, however, the rate and force of the heartbeat is affected by a number of factors including nerves and hormones. The sympathetic nerves, for example, secrete norepinephrine, and the adrenal glands secrete epinephrine, both of which stimulate the heart to beat more strongly and more quickly. They do this by acting on specialized molecules called beta-receptors (see Chapter 1) on the heart muscle itself and on specialized cells in areas known as the sinoatrial node (SA node) and the atrioventricular node (AV node). Activation of these nerves releases norepinephrine which acts on the beta-receptors to increase the rate and force of the heartbeat.

Angina

The word 'angina' has the same origin as the word 'anguish' (from the Latin *angustia*), and means tightness, distress, or suffocation. This is appropriate since angina (or 'angina pectoris' to give it its full name) refers to feelings of pain, distress, tightness, and choking in the chest. Like other tissues, the heart requires its own supply of blood, and angina occurs when it is forced to pump too vigorously for its blood and oxygen supply to keep up.

The most common form of angina is described as 'stable' because the attacks generally occur under predictable circumstances. The cause of stable angina is that one or more of the blood vessels supplying the heart with blood (the coronary arteries; Fig. 16.2) have become narrow or even blocked by fatty deposits (atheroma) (Fig. 16.3) or by a blood clot (thrombosis) (Fig. 16.4). Part of the heart will be receiving too little blood and oxygen, and as soon as any extra demand is placed upon it, by exercise for example, the heart cells are unable to meet that demand. Efforts by the heart to work without enough oxygen result in the formation of acidic chemicals which stimulate nerve endings and give rise to the sensations of pain, tightness, and pressure. The pain may be felt only in the chest, or may spread to the shoulders (usually the left), the arms, back, or lower jaw.

Angina afflicts one in every five people over the age of 65, and half of all people over 60 years of age in the 'developed' countries have narrowing of the coronary arteries. Several factors encourage the development of angina and some of these are summarized in Table 16.1, p. 230.

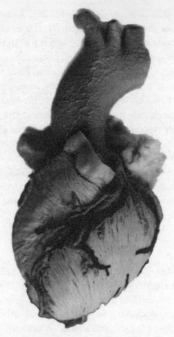

Fig. 16.2 The heart, showing the coronary arteries (light-coloured) and coronary veins (dark-coloured) on the surface of the heart. The coronary vessels penetrate into the heart muscle to supply the entire organ with blood. The heart pumps blood out into the aorta (top of picture) from where arterial branches carry the blood to all organs of the body. (From a specimen held in the Pathology Museum, International Centre for Health Sciences, Manipal, India, by permission of Dr D Murthy.)

Treatment

There are several ways to treat stable angina. Firstly, patients should not expose themselves to undue or sudden exercise or stress, and should never exercise in spite of chest pain. Doing so would risk serious damage to the heart. Instead, patients should rest as soon as the angina begins and allow the pain to subside as the demands made on the heart fall back to levels with which it can cope. Some patients, particularly those with mild angina, can and do control their symptoms simply by pacing themselves so that they never take exercise hard enough to bring on the symptoms.

For those with more severe angina, however, this is not a practical way of controlling symptoms, and pain cannot be avoided simply by limiting exercise. It is for these patients that drugs may be required.

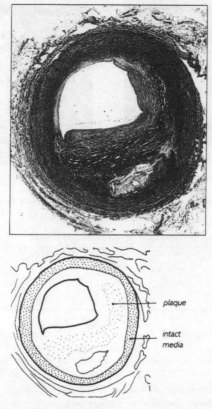

Fig. 16.3 An example of atherosclerosis. The upper photograph shows a section through a real coronary artery, revealing how the lumen has been reduced by the presence of a fatty deposit (atherosclerotic plaque) on the vessel wall. (Professor R H Anderson.)

There are two main ways to treat angina with drugs. One is to reduce the demands made upon the heart, and the other is to increase the blood supply to the heart to enable it to cope with the work it has to do.

Drugs used to treat angina

Beta-blockers

Beta-blockers (*see* Chapter 15) such as atenolol, metoprolol, and propranolol reduce the demand made on the heart by blocking the stimulant actions of

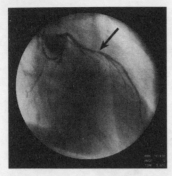 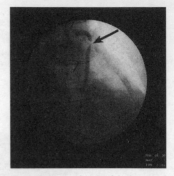

Fig. 16.4 An angiogram, obtained by injecting a dye into the circulation of the heart and observing the heart using X-rays. The picture reveals a blood vessel which is almost blocked, either by a blood clot or from the presence of fatty plaque laid down on the inside of the vessel (*see also* Fig. 16.3).

Table 16.1 Risk factors for coronary artery disease including angina

Age
Male
Family history
Strong association
Diabetes mellitus
High blood pressure
Cigarette smoking
Weak association
Obesity
Type A personality (competitive, ambitious)
Alcohol (over 14 units per week for women, 21 for men)*
Gout
Soft water intake
Lack of exercise
Contraceptive pill

* One unit is approximately equivalent to one half pint of beer, one glass of wine or one measure of spirits.

epinephrine and norepinephrine. They thereby prevent activation of the heart by stress or exercise (Fig. 16.5). They are useful and effective drugs, but patients should always remember that when they stop taking them they should do so gradually, reducing the dose each day for several days. If the drugs are stopped suddenly, there is a danger of a rebound increase in the number and severity of anginal attacks.

(a)

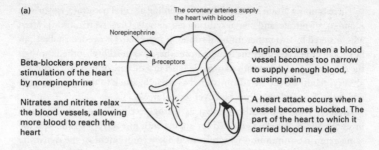

The coronary arteries supply the heart with blood

Norepinephrine

β-receptors

Beta-blockers prevent stimulation of the heart by norepinephrine

Nitrates and nitrites relax the blood vessels, allowing more blood to reach the heart

Angina occurs when a blood vessel becomes too narrow to supply enough blood, causing pain

A heart attack occurs when a vessel becomes blocked. The part of the heart to which it carried blood may die

(b) heart failure occurs when the heart is not pumping blood efficiently around the body

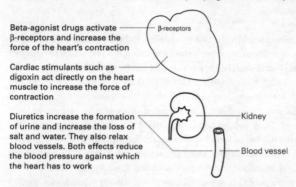

Beta-agonist drugs activate β-receptors and increase the force of the heart's contraction

β-receptors

Cardiac stimulants such as digoxin act directly on the heart muscle to increase the force of contraction

Diuretics increase the formation of urine and increase the loss of salt and water. They also relax blood vessels. Both effects reduce the blood pressure against which the heart has to work

Kidney

Blood vessel

Fig.16.5 Drugs used in the treatment of angina (a) and heart failure (b).

Beta-blockers may, in some people, provoke asthma or heart failure, so any shortness of breath should be reported immediately to the doctor. In general, however, beta-blockers are very safe drugs.

Nitrates and nitrites

Credit for the first use of nitrites in the treatment of angina goes to a Scottish doctor, Thomas Lauder Brunton, born in 1844. He was concerned at the pain and death rate of patients who developed pain in the chest and arms, and speculated that these symptoms might involve changes in the blood supply to the heart. Brunton knew of previous work in animals showing that amyl nitrite could relax blood vessel walls and lower blood pressure and he resolved to try it in patients. No doubt to his great satisfaction, the symptoms that we now recognize as angina disappeared almost immediately when his patients breathed amyl nitrite vapour.

There is now a group of 'nitro' drugs, including glyceryl trinitrate, isosorbide mono- or di-nitrate, and pentaerythritol tetranitrate. Glyceryl trinitrate is often administered by two rather unusual routes. If rapid relief is needed a tablet can be sucked or placed under the tongue from where it is quickly absorbed through the membranes of the mouth to provide relief in a minute or two. Alternatively, glyceryl trinitrate can be administered as a patch, stuck to the skin, through which the drug is slowly absorbed over several weeks.

Glyceryl trinitrate is also known as nitroglycerin. Indeed, the Swedish inventor Alfred Nobel was treated for angina with nitroglycerin. This was the same explosive compound which formed a key component of the dynamite which he invented and which made him rich enough to establish the Nobel Prize foundation.

How do nitrates work?

In 1978 a technician working in pharmacologist Robert Furchgott's laboratory in the State University of New York was examining the responses to drugs of strips of animal blood vessels. He became puzzled by the fact that some strips responded to acetylcholine with a strong relaxation, while others did not respond at all. After months of detective work, the researchers realized that those which did not respond had been prepared in a way which damaged their internal linings. They subsequently published their observation with the proposal that the linings of blood vessels normally responded to acetylcholine by secreting a hormone which caused the relaxation. When the vessel lining was damaged, the hormone was not produced and there was no relaxation.

There followed a period of great excitement while many laboratories tried to identify the new hormone. Among the first to do so was Dr Salvador Moncada and his team at the Wellcome Research Laboratories in Beckenham, England. In 1987 they identified the mysterious agent as nitric oxide.*

Since then nitric oxide has been shown to have dozens if not hundreds of actions and seems to be involved in many physiological processes and diseases. We also now recognize that the nitrates and nitrites relax blood vessels by being converted into nitric oxide in the blood and tissues. In 1998, the Nobel prize was awarded to three scientists who had played major roles in developing the nitric oxide story—Robert Furchgott (State University of New York), Louis Ignarro (University of California), and Ferid Murad (University of Texas).

In low doses, nitrates affect mainly veins bringing blood back to the heart from the tissues. This reduces the pressure of blood entering the heart, in turn

* Although in its natural state nitric oxide (one atom of nitrogen combined with one of oxygen— chemical formula NO) is a gas, it is very different from nitrous oxide (two atoms of nitrogen and one oxygen—N_2O). Nitrous oxide is the gaseous anaesthetic used by dentists some years ago, and which has been used to reduce the pain during childbirth. It is this gas, *nitrous* oxide which is popularly known as 'laughing gas'.

reducing the work the heart has to perform. Nitrates also dilate vessels in the heart to move blood from those well supplied with blood, to areas which are relatively starved of blood. All areas then receive a more equal distribution of blood and the heart is better able to work without producing angina.

Side-effects

Side-effects of nitrates include headaches which can be reduced by lowering the dose or by changing the type of nitrate. They can usually also be avoided by spitting out the tablet as soon as it has been sucked for long enough to stop the angina.

Nitrates may become less effective if used for a long time, but this 'tolerance' can be avoided if dosage programmes include 8 to 12 hours a day free from these drugs. There is a well-known story about munitions workers who, during the war, worked with explosive nitrites. Every Monday morning almost everyone developed a severe headache as they were exposed to the nitrites, which would relax blood vessels to the head and lead to a painful, pulsating headache. By Friday everyone would have become tolerant to these effects and was free of headache, only to recover over the weekend and experience a new headache on Monday.

Calcium antagonists

All muscle cells, including the heart muscle, must have calcium in order to contract. The calcium antagonists are drugs which reduce the movement of calcium into the cells of the heart and blood vessels. The effect on the heart is to reduce its response to demand—it cannot beat as strongly or as rapidly in response to epinephrine and less strain is placed upon it.

Calcium antagonists also slow the movement of calcium into the muscle cells which make up the walls of blood vessels. This makes these cells contract less strongly, causing dilation, reducing blood pressure and increasing blood flow to the heart through the coronary arteries. The various calcium antagonists have different profiles of activity. Nifedipine has its greatest effects on the blood vessels, while verapamil has its greatest effect on the heart itself.

Variant angina

The drugs described above work well in what is known as 'angina of effort'—angina brought on by exercise, stress, or anger. But there is also a form of angina in which exercise is not involved. This is 'unstable' angina, of which one type is known as variant angina (or Prinzmetal's angina, after the American cardiologist Myron Prinzmetal (1908–87) who first described the condition in 1959). It occurs in some patients even while resting, and is often a result of unnecessary and spontaneous contractions of the coronary blood vessels. These contractions narrow the vessels and reduce the amount of blood reaching the heart muscle. The nitrates and nitrites are particularly effective in this condition, because they act best on blood vessels which are actively contracting.

Unstable angina can also be caused by blood clots forming in the coronary vessels and blocking the supply of blood to the heart. This can occur at any time, even at rest, and if not treated may progress to a more serious heart attack.

It is important not to take beta-blockers for variant angina, because beta-receptors for epinephrine and norepinephrine normally relax blood vessels and oppose the contractile effects of alpha-receptors (*see* Chapter 1). Beta-blockers, therefore, leave alpha-activity unopposed, and this may increase vessel contraction, reduce blood flow to the heart and cause more severe angina.

Dysrhythmias

Contraction of the heart

The rhythm of the heartbeat is normally remarkably constant. The cells of the sinoatrial node, in the right atrium of the heart, control the rate of the heartbeat. These cells send an electrical impulse across the heart causing, first, contraction of the atria. This pushes blood into the ventricles and, a fraction of a second later, the ventricles also receive the electrical command to contract and push the blood into the arteries and to the tissues.

This sequence gives the heart a regular rhythm which we can hear best through a stethoscope (invented in 1816 by a French physician, Rene Laennec).

Heart rhythms

When the heart is damaged, the rhythm of the heartbeat may be disturbed. Several types of abnormal rhythm, or dysrhythmias, are known. Among the simplest are those in which part of the heart begins to beat at a faster rate than usual (a 'tachycardia' from the Greek words *takhus* meaning fast, and *kardia* meaning heart) and palpitations.

If the electrical command does not pass normally from the atria to the ventricles, the atria and ventricles beat independently of each other. This is known as heart block. If there is a complete block of the passage of signals, the heart beats very slowly as the ventricles begin beating at their own slow rate. An artificial pacemaker may be needed to control the heart rhythm.

Sometimes the heart may seem to miss a beat. This feeling usually occurs when the heart is more excitable than usual. As a result, the ventricles beat twice, one beat very quickly following another. This dual beat forces most of the blood out of the heart, so there is a long pause while the heart fills with enough blood to contract again. It is this pause which gives us the sensation of a missed beat.

The feeling of missed beats can be worrying, but is quite common. As long as they occur only occasionally and are otherwise asymptomatic, for example, not associated with pain or feeling faint or dizzy, then they are not likely to indicate that anything is wrong. They usually occur when the ventricles are more excitable than normal because of stress (which increases the amount of epinephrine in the blood), alcohol, or excessive drinking of stimulants such as tea, coffee, or chocolate.

Flutter and fibrillation

In some patients the atria (the upper chambers of the heart), begin to exceed the usual 60 to 80 beats per minute. The term atrial 'flutter' is used for rates of around 200 beats per minute while atrial 'fibrillation' refers to an abnormal, rapid, irregular rhythm of 400–600 beats per minute. When beating this rapidly, the atria no longer act efficiently as a pump, but a greater problem is the effect of the electrical impulses from the rapidly beating atria on the ventricles. They are unable to respond to all of the impulses pouring down from the atria, and so they beat more rapidly than normal, often at around 150 beats per minute, and more irregularly. As a result, the pumping of blood from the ventricles into the arteries is less efficient than normal and patients may find exercise difficult, with periods of shortness of breath, palpitations, and dizziness and fainting as a result of poor blood supply to the brain.

Richard Gordon* has described how Charles Dickens:

> In 1866 ... suffered attacks of palpitations and faintness, diagnosed as 'great irritability of the heart'. This was atrial fibrillation, bursts of irregular rhythm in the heart and upper chambers.

More serious are the problems caused when a small area of a ventricle is damaged and begins to generate its own rhythm. Such localized cardiac damage may follow a small heart attack (of which the patient may not even be aware). Electrical impulses spread out from the new generator, and compete with the impulses coming from the atria. The result can be a disorganized contraction of the heart which does not pump blood efficiently around the body.

Damage to the heart may also cause localized circuits of contraction to form, in which excitation and contraction occur around the damaged area at a rate which is independent of the rest of the heart. The damaged area does not then contribute to the organized contraction of the heart, so the heart functions much less efficiently than normal. If the patient is to carry on a normal life, with a normal heart rhythm which can respond properly to stress and exercise, it is important to use drugs which eliminate or control the abnormal excitability of the damaged heart.

* In his book *Ailments through the ages*.

Treatment

The drugs which can be used to suppress cardiac dysrhythmias fall into four main groups; sodium channel blockers, beta blockers, amiodarone, and calcium antagonists.

Sodium channel blockers

The excitability and contraction of muscle cells depends on the movement of sodium into the cells from the blood. Drugs which reduce this can reduce cell excitability to the point at which abnormally excitable circuits of cells are broken. Drugs of this type include flecainide, quinidine, procainamide, and disopyramide.

One of the earliest indications that blockers of sodium channels could be beneficial in treating abnormal heart rhythms came when a cardiologist, Karel Wenckebach, was told by a patient that his irregular heartbeat became normal when he went abroad and took quinine for protection against malaria. One of the properties of quinine is to block the movement of sodium into cells.

Since the movement of sodium is also important for the transmission of impulses in nerves, these drugs can also interfere with the excitability of nervous tissue as well as of the heart. As a result, they disrupt the nervous control of fine muscle movements and a common side-effect is a disturbance of vision because the fine muscular control needed for focussing is upset.

Beta-blockers

Activation of beta-receptors in the heart, by epinephrine or norepinephrine, increases the excitability of cells, increases the conduction of electrical impulses from atria to ventricles, and reduces the length of time it takes for a cell to become active again after the last heartbeat. All these effects can induce, or help to maintain, abnormal heart rhythms. By blocking the beta receptors, beta-blockers produce the opposite effects and can suppress some dysrhythmias, especially an abnormally high heart rate (tachycardia). The effects and side-effects of beta-blockers have been discussed in Chapter 15.

Amiodarone

A third group of antidysrhythmic drugs includes amiodarone. When a muscle or nerve cell has been active for a fraction of a second, it enters the so-called 'refractory period', during which it cannot become active again. Drugs such as amiodarone increase the length of this period in heart cells, making it more difficult for cells in damaged heart muscle to beat excessively quickly. The result is to calm the overactive areas of heart muscle, to break any abnormal circuits of activity, and to return the heart rhythm to the control of the sinoatrial node.

Calcium antagonists

Muscle cells must have calcium in order to contract. The calcium antagonists already discussed in Chapter 15 block the movement of calcium into the heart muscle cells, reducing their ability to contract.

Calcium ions are also needed for the propagation of electrical activity across the atria and to the ventricles. Calcium antagonists, therefore, reduce the excitability of the cells and slow the rate at which electrical activity is conducted around the heart. These effects tend to reduce or even to prevent the development of areas of damaged heart muscle which can function independently of the normal pacemaker and reduce the efficiency of the heart as a pump.

Cardiac glycosides

The cardiac glycosides are a group of drugs such as digoxin, which are usually used to increase the strength of contraction of the heart. It was a Scottish physician, James Mackenzie, working in Lancashire around 1900, who first realized that crude preparations of foxglove, which contains digoxin, could reduce the transmission of electrical activity from the atria to the ventricles. This meant that when the atria were contracting very rapidly, for example in a condition known as atrial flutter, the ventricles were not stimulated to contract after every contraction. They then had more time between contractions to fill with blood, and were able to contract more regularly and forcibly.

Depending on the amount of damage to the heart and the size of the area of abnormally functioning heart tissue, it may be necessary to take these antidysrhythmic drugs for several months or even years.

Potassium channel blocker

One drug about to be launched into the clinic is dofetilide, made by the Pfizer company. It prevents potassium ions from leaking out of heart muscle cells, slowing the rate at which the cells recover from a contraction, making them less able to contract again and reducing the overall rate of fibrillation.

Heart attacks

Heart disease causes about 25 per cent of all deaths. The term 'heart attack' covers a number of different conditions including clots (thromboses) which block the coronary arteries. A coronary thrombosis often results from atherosclerosis, the narrowing of the artery as a result of the slow accumulation of fatty deposits on the inside of the vessel, first described by James Herrick in 1912 (see Chapter 15). A clot or thrombus eventually forms, blocking the narrowed blood vessel.

A heart attack may be brought on by exertion, cold, or stress, and usually results in the death of that part of the heart supplied by the blocked coronary artery since it is starved of oxygen. The heart damage is called a *myocardial infarction* and is experienced as severe pain or tightness in the chest, accompanied by sweating, shortness of breath, and sometimes nausea. The pain may radiate to the arms, back, neck, or lower jaw.

In most cases enough of the heart is able to function that patients do not die from a first attack, and treatment can be instituted to reduce the presence of fatty deposits by appropriate dieting and fat-lowering drugs (*see* Chapter 15). As patients recover, any abnormal heart rhythms will be treated as they occur. Advice will also be given on weight loss, a low fat diet, fat-lowering drugs, vitamin E and fish oil supplements (which help to prevent further heart attacks), and a controlled exercise programme.

The electrocardiogram (ECG)

An electrocardiogram (ECG) should always be taken after a suspected heart attack—the ECG is a recording of the electrical activity of the heart monitored by electrodes placed on the surface of the body. The impulses or 'messages' which cause the heart to contract normally produce a consistent pattern of electrical changes at these electrodes, and a damaged area of heart will alter the electrical pattern. A trained observer can interpret the pattern to give valuable information about the site and extent of heart damage.

Treatment

'Clot-busters'

Aspirin

Immediate, 'first aid' treatment for a heart attack is to give the patient one aspirin, preferably in soluble form, without delay since speed is essential. Aspirin is used for its ability to reduce the stickiness of platelets—those cell fragments which stick together to help to make blood clot (*see* Chapter 14). A drug such as aspirin, which reduces platelet stickiness, has a 'clot busting' effect which can sometimes prevent a coronary thrombosis from forming at all, or at least can limit its size and severity. Patients are more likely to survive after a heart attack if aspirin is given up to 24 hours afterwards.

How does aspirin stop blood clotting? As we have seen in Chapters 6 and 14, many different chemicals in the blood are involved in clotting, including two members of the prostaglandin family of hormones—prostacyclin and thromboxane. If a blood vessel is damaged, platelets begin to release histamine, thromboxane, and other compounds which initiate clotting. The platelets clump together, cause red cells to do the same, and trigger the formation of sticky protein clots around the clumps. Aspirin prevents the formation of thromboxane, along with all other prostaglandins, so that blood takes considerably longer than normal to clot.

Aspirin prevents the formation, not only of thromboxane, but also of prostacyclin, a prostaglandin released by the blood vessels themselves and which prevents blood clotting. In other words thromboxane and prostacyclin have opposite effects and clotting occurs only when the amounts of thromboxane and other clotting activators exceed the amounts of prostacyclin and other clotting inhibitors. Because aspirin blocks the formation of both thromboxane and prostacyclin, high doses will have rather unpredictable effects on clotting.

Fortunately, blood vessels are continually making new COX enzyme and, thus, prostacyclin. In contrast, platelets are not complete cells (they have no nucleus), and they cannot produce new COX or thromboxane. It is possible, therefore, to find doses of aspirin which abolish thromboxane production with much less effect on prostacyclin formation, and thus shift the balance between these different prostaglandins so that clotting is inhibited and not encouraged.

This ability of aspirin to inhibit blood clotting has received a great deal of attention in recent years because of the high incidence of deaths from coronary thromboses. If a blood clot (thrombosis) occurs in a coronary blood vessel (which carries blood to the heart), then a heart attack may occur—the heart can no longer pump blood efficiently and the patient may die. This subject was discussed in detail in Chapter 14.

Other 'clot-busters'

Other 'clot-busting' drugs (see Chapter 14) have become widely used in acute coronary thromboses to break down clots in the arteries and thus limit the damage they produce. Those which reduce mortality in these circumstances are streptokinase (from some bacteria), alteplase, and anistreplase. The earlier these drugs can be given the better, to prevent damage as the clot forms in the artery. The drugs are of greatest value if given in the first 12 hours after symptoms begin. They are discussed more fully in Chapter 14.

Are clot-busting drugs a good idea?

There is a small risk in using these drugs immediately after a heart attack because the heart seems to be damaged, not as a result of the cessation of blood flow and oxygen supply, but as a result of the *restoration* of blood flow after-wards. The explanation is that during a period without blood (ischaemia) cells become so damaged that they cannot cope with the flood of substances, particularly calcium, which are introduced when blood flow is restored. This flood of calcium is then sufficient to kill many of the cells or to produce abnormal heart rhythms which can be dangerous. By removing a clot and restoring blood flow, the clot-busters, paradoxically, may be promoting damage rather than protecting the heart.

Because of these various factors, the decision by doctors of whether to use clot-busting drugs is made on the basis of the age and health of the individual patient and the extent of damage to the heart.

Ventricular fibrillation

Heart attack victims often require a strong painkiller (analgesic) such as diamorphine (heroin) which also stops the reflex secretion of epinephrine by the adrenal glands in response to the stress of pain. This is important since epinephrine, acting on beta-receptors, increases the excitability of the heart. This may lead to abnormal heart rhythms, including potentially fatal ventricular fibrillation.

In ventricular fibrillation the many heart muscle cells in the ventricles are converted into a disorganized, quivering mass of cells, unable to contract uniformly in response to impulses reaching them from the atria. The ventricles are, therefore, unable to pump blood into the arteries and death can follow in a few minutes. Fibrillation is usually stopped by placing high voltage electrodes across the chest and delivering such a high intensity electric shock that all the cells in the ventricles are forced to contract at the same time. After the shock, the ventricles should continue to contract as a unit, as in a normal heart. Ventricular fibrillation is a major cause of death after a heart attack.

Beta-blockers

Some patients may be treated with beta-blockers. By acting against the tendency of epinephrine and norepinephrine to produce abnormal heart rhythms, they will reduce by 25 per cent the risk of ventricular fibrillation. Since they also lower the rate and force of the heart contraction, they also reduce the work demand made on the heart. After a heart attack, heart cells do not die immediately, but only over a period of several hours, during which the eventual extent of damage to the heart will be determined by its activity and the amount of oxygen reaching it. If treatment with beta-blockers is started early enough, their action in reducing the heart's activity can limit the final damage. (An important rule is that the sooner a heart attack victim can be given professional attention to lower cardiac activity and prevent fibrillation, the more likely he or she is to survive.)

Nitrites and nitrates

Another early step is to administer drugs which dilate the blood vessels. Nitrates and nitrites (*see* Chapter 15) are particularly useful because they work throughout the body and lower both the blood pressure and the work demanded by the heart to pump against that pressure. They also dilate veins and so reduce the pressure of blood returning to the heart. Finally, they dilate the coronary vessels, increasing blood flow to the damaged heart tissue.

Some drugs such as glyceryl trinitrate are better than others such as nitroprusside: the latter mainly dilates the coronary arteries, which can divert blood away from damaged tissue towards healthy tissue, a phenomenon known as 'coronary steal'.

Nitrates can be used in long-lasting and slow-release preparations and two of them, isosorbide mono- and di-nitrate, can be used to prevent chest pain. They may be taken as tablets, by absorption under the tongue, as a spray, or as a patch on the skin. Some patients on long-acting nitrates or nitrites absorbed through the skin develop tolerance, decreasing the drugs' effectiveness. This can usually be avoided if the levels of nitrate or nitrite in the blood are allowed to fall to low levels for four to eight hours each day (see Chapter 15).

Heart failure

The heart fails when it is unable to pump enough blood to meet the demands of the body and is a common cause of death in old age. Some causes of heart failure (sometimes known as 'congestive' heart failure) are shown in Table 16.2. After many years of pumping blood quietly and efficiently, the heart eventually starts to weaken. This may be precipitated by other disorders of old age including decreased kidney and liver function, which can raise blood pressure and increase the demands placed upon the heart. It may also be a consequence of raised blood pressure over several years.

The most common cause of heart failure is damage to the heart caused by a heart attack, which causes scarring of the tissue and prevents it from contributing to normal cardiac function. As the heart becomes less and less able to pump out the blood which it is receiving through the veins, the pressure in these vessels starts to increase. Two things happen as a result.

Table 16.2 Causes of heart failure

- Abnormal function of the heart muscle
- Volume overload—sometimes from heart valve disease
- Obstruction to outflow from the heart—sometimes from heart valve disease
- A need for high output from the heart, e.g. in severe anaemia, untreated overactive thyroid disease
- Poor filling of the ventricles, e.g. when the outer covering of the heart is too tight to let the heart expand on filling—constrictive pericarditis
- Abnormal heart rhythm, e.g. untreated severe atrial fibrillation.

Firstly, the increase in pressure starts to force fluid through the walls of the veins into the tissues. Secondly, as the heart becomes less efficient, the blood pressure falls, leading to the secretion of aldosterone by the adrenal glands and the retention of salt and water in the kidney. Together, these two processes cause marked swelling (oedema*), particularly of the legs and feet, where blood pressure in the veins is greatest.

If untreated, the pressure in the blood vessels of the legs continues to rise, while that in the head and lungs falls as the weakening heart is unable to sustain the pressure in these organs. The patient becomes light-headed and dizzy as blood flow to the brain falls, and breathless as blood flow to the lungs declines. As the heart becomes progressively weaker, tissues begin to die as they receive insufficient blood and it becomes essential to initiate treatment before death ensues.

Treatment

Patients may feel rather anxious when they hear the word heart 'failure' since the heart is such a vitally important organ in the body and 'failure' seems to be a very final word. In practice, however, heart failure can usually be treated very effectively with a range of drugs.

Any problem which may be producing the heart failure, such as heart valve disease, thyroid disease, or severe anaemia should itself be treated. Rest will reduce the demands made upon the heart but if it is too prolonged clots may develop deep in the veins; these may be avoided by leg exercises, low-dose heparin, and elastic support stockings. Large meals should be avoided, as should salt. Overweight patients should lose weight. The drugs taken to combat heart failure dilate blood vessels, strengthen the contraction of heart muscle, or control abnormal heart rhythms.

Diuretics

Diuretics (see Chapter 5) increase the amount of urine formed in the kidney and increase the loss of water and sodium from the body. This is turn reduces the amount of blood which the heart must pump. The danger of using diuretics lies in the risk of losing excessive quantities of fluid and salts, especially sodium and potassium, which may lead to feelings of extreme tiredness and sometimes to dangerous, abnormal heart rhythms.

Vasodilators

Drugs which dilate blood vessels, vasodilators, are useful since in the process of heart failure the pressure in the circulation increases in both the vessels entering

* Oedema used to be known as dropsy.

and leaving the heart. Relaxing blood vessels restores blood pressure to normal and helps to prevent any worsening of heart failure. The vasodilator drugs include nitroprusside, glyceryl trinitrate, isosorbide mono- and di-nitrate, prazosin, ACE inhibitors, hydralazine, and calcium antagonists, all of which have been described in detail in Chapter 15. Drugs which make heart muscles contract more powerfully include digitalis, dopamine, and dobutamine.

Cardiac stimulants

Digoxin is one of a group of drugs known as the cardiac glycosides, all related to compounds in the foxglove plant *Digitalis* (Fig. 16.6). The English physician William Withering is credited with the first scientific study of the foxglove. His interest in plants is said to have been aroused by the almost daily consultations of an attractive young woman, Helena, whose passion was painting flowers. When she was not consulting him, he visited her, taking a different variety of local flowers when he could.

Withering's newfound interest in botany was of value when he heard a colleague say that a friend in Oxford had been cured of the dropsy by a preparation of the foxglove plant. This prompted Withering to seek out an elderly woman known locally as 'the old woman of Shropshire' who had been reported to cure several people of dropsy. He persuaded her to give him samples of the preparations she used and began painstakingly examining the various

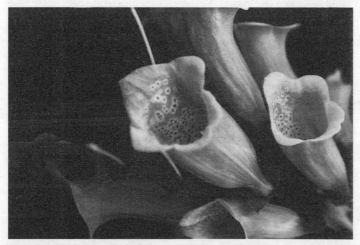

Fig. 16.6 The foxglove *Digitalis purpurea*, from which the cardiac stimulant drugs digoxin and digitoxin are obtained.

plant fragments under a microscope. Sure enough, he found fragments of foxglove leaves among them all and proceeded to carry out a careful scientific study of the effects of foxglove on his patients with dropsy. Of his first fifty patients, all were relieved of their symptoms—swollen legs and ankles and breathlessness—leading him to write up his findings in a classic book *The foxglove and an account of its medical properties* in 1776.

How do digoxin and the cardiac glycosides work?

The cardiac glycosides act in much the same way as epinephrine, increasing the flow of calcium into the cardiac cells, but their effects do not involve beta-receptors. The inflow of calcium allows the heart to beat more strongly and to pump out the blood which returns through the veins. It is often necessary to continue treatment with these drugs for life to support the heart and to prevent a recurrence of heart failure. They are of most benefit in heart failure associated with atrial fibrillation when the heart fails because its contractions cannot keep pace with the rapidly beating atria.

Side-effects

The value of these drugs is limited because they must be used very carefully to avoid side-effects, mainly nausea, loss of appetite, visual changes, and abnormal heart rhythms.

The increased inflow of calcium into heart cells can make them beat twice in rapid succession (ventricular extrasystoles), or to beat at a high rate in some parts of the heart independently of the others. In the worst cases, ventricular fibrillation may be induced, resulting in death within a few minutes, though this is very unusual.

Besides increasing contraction strength, these drugs also slow the spread of the electrical impulses from the atria to the ventricles. In susceptible patients, this can result in the ventricles beating independently of the atria. This 'heart block' is not normally a serious problem in younger subjects, but could be a significant complication in elderly patients with other cardiac disorders.

Amrinone and milrinone

These drugs mimic the action of epinephrine in activating beta-receptors and stimulating heart action by increasing both the flow of calcium into heart cells, and increasing the strength of the heart's contraction and thus helping it to pump more efficiently. But unlike epinephrine and norepinephrine these drugs bypass the beta-receptors. Normally when epinephrine activates beta-receptors it activates an enzyme, adenyl cyclase, which stimulates the formation of a chemical, cyclic adenosine monophosphate (cyclic AMP), in the cells. This increases the influx of calcium in response to epinephrine. The cyclic AMP is eventually broken down by another enzyme, phosphodiesterase. Amrinone and milrinone act by inhibiting the phosphodiesterase. Consequently, cyclic AMP inside the cells is not destroyed and the levels increase. The overall effect of promoting cyclic AMP and calcium inflow is the same as with epinephrine, but beta-receptors have not been affected.

Beta-agonists

Other drugs mimic directly the effects of epinephrine and norepinephrine by activating the beta receptors in the heart cells. These include dobutamine and xamoterol.

Other drugs

If none of the above drugs proves to be effective, it is possible to use vasodilator drugs such as ACE inhibitors, alpha antagonists, and alpha-2 agonists (*see* Chapter 15) which lower blood pressure and thus reduce the amount of work being asked of the heart.

Stroke

The term 'stroke' refers to the loss of blood flow to part of the brain. The result is often a degree of brain damage. In approximately 80 per cent of patients strokes are caused by a clot inside a vessel, while in approximately 20 per cent the stroke is due to bleeding from a vessel. The brain deficits can range from dizziness, loss of speech or paralysis of a limb, to total paralysis of all four limbs (tetraplegia). Strokes occur more often in subjects with high blood pressure (the major reason for trying to lower abnormally high blood pressure) and cardiac disorders. Other well-recognized risk factors predisposing to strokes are age (over 55), gender (males are more susceptible than females), race (black are more susceptible than white), diabetes, cigarette smoking, and high alcohol intake (over 50 grammes per day) (Table 16.3).

Unfortunately, there is little to say in a book on drugs, because there are none of much use in the treatment or prevention of strokes. Administration of low-dose aspirin (*see* Chapter 6) and dipyridamole may help to prevent second or later strokes.

Treatment

Treatment of strokes varies according to their cause but, for most patients, includes immediate supportive management, diagnosis, and treatment of underlying risk factors. Much of the management and treatment of stroke requires not drugs but dedicated caring nursing, physiotherapy, occupational therapy, speech therapy, and sometimes art and/or music therapy.

Blood pressure should be lowered by drugs, but slowly to ensure that the

Table 16.3 Risk factors for stroke

- High blood pressure—the main reason for trying to lower abnormally high blood pressure
- Heart disease, e.g. disease of a heart valve
- Diabetes mellitus—sugary, fatty blood in uncontrolled diabetes tends to encourage blood clots
- Obesity
- Family history
- Cigarette smoking
- High blood fat levels
- Oral contraceptives—'the pill' The risk is however very small unless accompanied by other risk factors (over 40 years old, smoking, high blood pressure)
- High alcohol intake—more than 50 grammes per day
- Age—increasingly common after 50 years of age
- Gender—men affected more often than women
- Race—black races more susceptible than white, particularly when blood pressure is high

brain remains well supplied with blood. Anticoagulants may be needed to thin the blood, to reduce blood clotting, and to prevent clots from being thrown into the blood vessels from the heart when heart rhythm changes occur. Their use must be delayed until the stroke has been shown by a brain scan not to be the result of a haemorrhage, to reduce the risk of bleeding into the brain.

Aspirin and the new drug clopidogrel (*see* Chapter 14) are used in patients who have suffered from a 'transient ischaemic attack' (TIA). These are small strokes usually caused by a piece of a blood clot becoming lodged in an artery of the brain and impairing some functions of the brain for a few minutes or hours until the clot disappears. Dickens appears to have suffered from these:

> ... In April 1869 ... he became giddy, with weakness in his left hand and leg. It was the first of his TIAs, transient ischaemic attacks, the passing strokes sprung by the clots from his heart.*

In these cases, early administration of drugs such as aspirin and clopidogrel may prevent a full stroke by reducing the stickiness of blood platelets.

A new development for stroke patients is the investigation of 'clot-busting' drugs (*see* Chapter 14) which can prevent damage from strokes as they occur. These drugs, such as rt-PA, tissue-type plasminogen activator, must be used within a few hours of the beginning of symptoms to prevent irreversible damage and cannot treat all strokes, particularly those caused by bleeding into the brain.

Fits occurring with a stroke may need to be controlled with antiepileptic drugs and some severe spastic symptoms after a stroke may be helped by baclofen, dantrolene sodium, or diazepam.

* R. Gordon, *Ailments through the ages.*

Drugs of the future

There is a vast amount of research in progress to develop drugs for use in stroke. During the stroke and for several hours afterwards, nerve and glial cells in the brain release amino acids such as glutamate. High concentrations of glutamate cause an influx of calcium into cells and this, it appears, is the main reason why nerve cells die after a stroke. Drugs which stop the release of glutamate or prevent its stimulation of calcium movements seem to be promising agents for limiting the amount of brain damage after a stroke. Many of the drugs now being developed are related to a molecule which exists naturally in the brain, kynurenic acid. Trevor Stone, (co-author of this book), then working at St. George's Hospital Medical School in London in 1982 discovered that this compound would block glutamate receptors in the brain, and most of the drugs now in development and clinical trials for the treatment of stroke are based on its molecular structure.

Drugs are also being developed which can help cells to regenerate after a stroke and thus restore normal function to the damaged area of brain. These include growth factors and chemicals called gangliosides. Some of the calcium antagonists such as nimodipine should also prove useful by blocking the inflow of calcium which triggers the death of many nerve cells after a stroke.

Table 16.4 Drugs used in disorders of the heart

For dysrhythmias:	For heart failure:	For angina:
Group 1	**Cardiac glycosides:**	**Nitro drugs**
bretylium	deslanoside (USA)	Glyceryl trinitrate
disopyramide	digoxin	Isosorbide mononitrate
flecainide	digitoxin	Isosorbide dinitrate
lignocaine	lanatoside	Pentaerythritol tetranitrate
mexiletine	medigoxin	
moracizine		**Calcium antagonists**
phenytoin	**β-receptor stimulants**	amlodipine
procainamide	dobutamine	diltiazem
propafenone	dopexamine	nicardipine
quinidine	isoprenaline (isoproterenol)	nicorandil
tocainide	xamoterol	nifedipine
		verapamil
Group 2	**Phosphodiesterase inhibitors:**	
acebutolol	amrinone	**β-blockers**
atenolol	milrinone	similar to Group 2
betaxolol	enoximone	drugs for dysrhythmias
bisoprolol		
carteolol		
carvedilol	**Diuretics:**	
celiprolol	amiloride	
esmolol	bendrofluazide	
labetalol	bumetanide	
metoprolol	chlorothiazide	
nadolol	chlorthalidone	
oxprenolol	clopamide	
penbutolol (USA)	cyclopenthiazide	
pindolol	ethacrynic acid	
propranolol	frusemide	
sotalol	hydrochlorothiazide	
timolol	hydroflumethiazide	
	indapamide	
Group 3	mefruside	
amiodarone	metolazone	
	piretanide	
Group 4	polythiazide	
bepridil (USA)	spironolactone	
diltiazem	torasemide	
verapamil	triamterene	
	xipamide	
	ACE inhibitors:	
	captopril	
	enalapril	
	lisinopril	
	quinapril	
	ramipril	

Summary

- The heart is a muscle which pumps blood round the body. Its blood supply can be reduced if the coronary arteries become blocked by fatty deposits.
- This increases the risk of the blood clotting (coronary thrombosis), causing a heart attack in which parts of the heart are deprived of blood and may be damaged (myocardial infarction).
- As soon as a heart attack occurs, aspirin should be used to reduce the occurrence of blood clots.
- Beta-blockers reduce the heart's actvity and reduce the demand on the heart.
- The restricted blood flow can also cause pain (angina) when the heart's activity is increased by cold or exercise.
- Angina can be treated by drugs which reduce the heart's activity (beta-blockers), or dilate the blood vessels (nitrate, nitrites, and calcium antagonists).
- Abnormal heart rhythms (dysrhythmias) often reduce the efficiency of the heart to pump blood. They are often due to local areas of the heart becoming over-excitable.
- Dysrhythmias can be treated by drugs which
    - block sodium channels, stopping the passage of electrical activity around the heart
    - block beta-receptors, reducing the excitability of the heart muscle
    - increase the time during which the heart does not respond to new electrical impulses
    - reduce the movement of calcium into the heart cells, reducing their excitability and contractions.
- Heart failure refers to the situation in which the heart is becoming too weak to pump blood as effectively as normal. The lower blood supply to the body, brain, and lungs leads to tiredness and breathlessness.
- Heart failure can be helped by diuretic drugs which increase the loss of salt and water in the urine, reducing the volume of blood in the body, and lowering the blood pressure.
- The blood supply to the heart can be increased by agents dilating the blood vessels, such as nitrites.
- The strength of the heartbeat can be increased by cardiac glycosides such as digitoxin, by beta-receptor agonists such as epinephrine or dobutamine, or by drugs preventing the breakdown of cyclic AMP in the heart cells.

CHAPTER 17

Infections and infestations

Microbes—tiny, unseen bacteria, viruses, fungi, and protozoa—pervade every aspect of human society and of the natural world. They provide all of our daily food; they were the original source of the world's abundant oil supplies; their presence in soil is essential to the existence of life itself. They also cause horrendous epidemics, from the plague and smallpox of past centuries to the continuing pandemics of cholera and today's growing AIDS crisis.*

Of the 50 million deaths in the world in 1998, 20 million were the result of microbial infectious diseases. About 5 million of these deaths were caused by respiratory disease, 2 million by malaria, 3 million by tuberculosis, and 3 million by diarrhoeal diseases. In 1999, one person dies of malaria every 12 seconds, and more people will have died from tuberculosis than in any year in history.

The statistics of human death and suffering caused by micro-organisms are startling enough in our own time, but in previous centuries they were even worse. Even the smallest tissue damage, cut, or pin-prick could lead to a generalized infection (blood poisoning) and end in death. The seventeenth-century French composer and conductor Jean-Baptiste Lully (1632–1687) died from this cause after accidentally banging his toe with the cane he was using to conduct a concert. In 1920, the life expectancy of the American male was 54 years. In 1998, it was 76 years—22 years longer. It has been estimated that at least ten years of these extra years are due to the use of antibiotics.

The animal body, human or not, can be invaded by many varieties of foreign organisms, including bacteria, viruses, fungi (moulds and yeasts), and other single-celled organisms responsible for diseases such as malaria. In most cases, especially when the invasion is relatively mild and the body that of a healthy adult, the immune system can cope and kill the offending cells. When an infection is severe, or the patient is very young or old, however, the body may need help. The drugs which provide that help include the antibiotics† to deal

---

* From *Power unseen* by B. Dixon, Oxford University Press, 1994.
† Strictly speaking the term 'antibacterial' is sometimes preferred, with the word 'antibiotic' being reserved for drugs which are produced by living organisms. In practice, the word antibiotic is usually used for any drug active against bacteria.

with bacteria, antiviral drugs to deal with viruses, antifungals to treat fungal infections (mycoses), and antiprotozoal drugs to deal with malaria and similar infestations.

Bacterial infections

Humans have probably been using chemicals to kill bacteria for thousands of years without realizing it. Saffron oil, obtained from the dried stigmas of the saffron crocus *Crocus sativa*, contains a mixture of chemicals, several of which can kill bacteria. Myrrh, a resin from the bark of the tree *Balsamodendron myrrha,* stops bacteria from multiplying. The ancient Greeks and Romans used both these preparations to promote the healing of wounds. A mixture of saffron oil, myrrh, and opium was also placed into the ear to treat what we now recognize as ear infections.

The discovery of bacteria

Over a century before the invention of the microscope and at a time when tiny, invisible life forms was completely unknown, a Venetian, Girolamo Fracastoro (1478–1553), wrote an amazing book. In it, he suggested that diseases such as those which we now call typhus and tuberculosis could be transmitted between people. Even more astonishingly, his work implied that the agents of transmission were living organisms which might grow and reproduce—a prescient view of bacteria and other micro-organisms which was not to be considered again for over 300 years.

Antonie van Leeuwenhoek was a Dutch draper with a passion for making and grinding lenses in his spare time and, in 1676, he invented a simple microscope. Robert Hooke (1635–1703), a physicist and Fellow of the Royal Society in London, had made a more powerful microscope ten years before, but van Leeuwenhoek was the first person who seems to have looked at a drop of water under his microscope. What he saw astonished him—millions of tiny living organisms, which he called 'animalcules', quite invisible to the naked eye. We now recognize an enormous variety of these miniature, microscopic, animals and plants, many of them consisting only of a single cell and including thousands of different types of bacteria. Despite the ideas of Fracastoro some 300 years earlier, it was not until long after van Leeuwenhoek, indeed not until the middle of the nineteenth century, that people began seriously to link these micro-organisms with disease.

Two of the most important figures in developing the concept that disease could be spread from person to person were the American Oliver Wendell Holmes (1809–1894) working at Harvard Medical School, and Philip Semmelweis, a Hungarian physician. Holmes concluded that the deaths of women in his maternity ward in Philadelphia were due to contamination carried on the hands of physicians. In 1844, Semmelweis became similarly concerned at the number of deaths of women on the maternity ward in a Vienna hospital. Thirty-six women became seriously ill and many died in his first month at the hospital. The crucial clue to the cause came when a friend of Semmelweis showed the same symptoms of illness after receiving an accidental cut during an autopsy. Semmelweis realized that doctors were often going straight from the mortuary to the labour ward, and reasoned that something was being carried over—a micro-organism or poisonous chemical—that produced the devastating results on the ward. Against much opposition and ridicule, he persuaded his medical colleagues to wash their hands after handling corpses, with the result that the death rate among women dropped dramatically within weeks. The controversy he had started, however, still cost him his job.

The first people to obtain strong evidence that diseases could be caused and spread by something passing from person to person were John Snow (1813–1858) in Westminster, London and William Budd (1811–1880) in Bristol. Around 1854, both realized that cholera was being spread through water supplies which were contaminated by sewage. John Snow was so convinced that the cholera infection in the area of Broad Street was coming from the pump which provided water for the area that he persuaded the authorities to remove the handle, making it unusable. The cholera epidemic stopped within six weeks. An investigation initiated by a clergyman, Henry Whitehead (1825–1896) showed that contaminated water was leaking from an open sewer, three feet away from the pump, into the water supply of the pump itself.

The discovery of antibacterial drugs

Paul Ehrlich was born in Germany in 1854. Despite a chequered academic start, he obtained a degree in medicine at Leipzig, but retained a fascination for organic chemistry, especially that of dyes and stains. He found a number of substances which stained different types of cells in the body, including bacteria of various shapes and sizes. As a result he made one of the most far-reaching speculations in biology: if chemicals could be found which bound selectively to bacteria and not to normal human cells, then a toxic substance, such as a metal molecule, could be attached to the chemical so that the bacteria, but not the human cells, would be killed.

This concept, of 'targetting' a drug at a select population of cells by interacting with specific sites* in the cell, is the basis of most current pharmacological research. The idea of killing cells as a therapy for disease, using specific chemicals, is known as chemotherapy, and Ehrlich is often regarded as the 'father of chemotherapy'. However, his ideas were not limited to suggestions

* Ehrlich called these sites 'receptive substance' but we now call them 'receptors' (see Chapter 1).

and hypotheses. A donation from a rich friend allowed him to set up a laboratory in which he tested hundreds of chemicals for activity against a major infection of the time—syphilis.* The 606th compound he tested was arsphenamine—a chemical containing atoms of arsenic. When he tested it on cultured cells, it failed to kill *Treponema pallidum*, the organism responsible for syphilis, and it was almost discarded.

Fortunately a Japanese bacteriologist, Sahachiro Hata, had joined Ehrlich's team and had devised a means of infecting rabbits with *Treponema*. In 1909 Hata found that arsphenamine was changed in the rabbit body to another chemical which did kill the organisms. Marketed under the trade name 'Salvarsan', arsphenamine was soon shown to have a similar effect in humans and became a life-saving drug for many of those afflicted by syphilis. Even so, it had its drawbacks. It was such a toxic drug that it could only be taken once a week. It also had to be dissolved in a pint of water and injected intravenously.

Ehrlich's primary interest, like that of most chemists up to the early twentieth century, had been in producing new dyes for clothing. Hence his discovery of the selective staining properties of bacteria. Enterprising companies, however, began to examine some of their thousands of chemicals as antibacterial drugs. In 1935 Gerhard Domagk, a bacteriologist working for the Bayer company in Wuppertal-Eberfeld, Germany, discovered a dye called Prontosil Red which he administered to mice infected with streptococci—bacteria which can cause throat infections, meningitis, and pneumonia. The dye killed the bacteria without harming the mice, just as Ehrlich had predicted. In the light of this success, Prontosil was used to treat Domagk's ten-month-old baby daughter, Hildegarde, who was suffering from an overwhelming streptococcal infection. She turned bright red because of the dye, but was saved from almost certain death. Domagk was awarded the Nobel Prize for Medicine in 1939.

In 1935, shortly after this experiment, a group of scientists led by Ernest Fourneau and Jacques Trefouel at the Pasteur Institute in France discovered that only one part of the prontosil molecule was necessary to kill the bacteria. The active portion was named sulphanilamide and became the first of the 'sulpha-drugs'.

About the same time that Domagk was working in Germany, Alexander Fleming (1881–1955) was busy in London, trying to identify antibacterial activity in bodily fluids such as sweat and tears. In 1928, having just returned from holiday, Fleming picked up several plates of bacteria to show them to his assistant before placing them in a bath of cleaning fluid. In doing so, he noticed that some of the culture plates had become contaminated by a mould. The

---

* Syphilis was the name of the shepherd hero of a mediaeval poem by Girolamo Fracastoro which described the symptoms of the disease so clearly that the disease has been known by his name ever since.

bacterial colonies around the mould had all died, and Fleming realised that the mould must have been producing a chemical which killed them. The mould was later identified as *Penicillium notatum*. Consequently Fleming called the antibacterial chemical penicillin. It was left to other scientists—Howard Florey, Norman Heatley, and Ernst Chain—over ten years later, to isolate and purify penicillin in sufficient quantity to use it by injection into human patients. The frustration of having only limited quantities available is illustrated by the treatment of a patient in Oxford.

On 12 February 1941 Charles Fletcher, a doctor at the Radcliffe Infirmary in Oxford, was faced with a patient at the point of death from an overwhelming bacterial infection which affected his upper body, face, and lungs. The patient's left eye had had to be removed the previous week. Fletcher injected several doses of the purified penicillin and found that the patient, a policeman called Albert Alexander, began to make an astonishing recovery. Unfortunately, the supply of penicillin was very limited and was soon used up. Alexander succumbed once more to the infection and died on 15 March.

However, within a couple of years of Fleming's original report of penicillin as an antibacterial, there were other, less dramatic but very effective uses of penicillin. One of the students from St Mary's Hospital, Cecil Paine, had received lectures from Fleming ('a shocking lecturer, the worst you could possibly imagine'*) and from whom he had heard about penicillin. When he began his first medical job at the Royal Infirmary, Sheffield, Paine resolved to try it in patients. Having obtained a sample of the *Penicillium* mould from Fleming, Paine grew enough of this to extract some penicillin. With the help of colleagues at the hospital, he then treated patients with eye infections, including a miner with a severe infection by *Pneumococcus* which would normally have necessitated removal of the eye, and babies whose eyes were infected with *Neisseria* from mothers with gonorrhoea. Several of these cases were cured completely and permanently, representing the first ever cures of human disease with an antibiotic.

The story of the discovery of penicillin has been told many times, with Fleming as the hero for discovering, accidentally or otherwise, the antibacterial activity of the *Penicillium* mould (see, for example, the book by Milton Wainwright). Indeed, many of the most pivotal discoveries in biology have been made accidentally by people with open minds. However, what is not usually appreciated is that Fleming was only one of a long line of scientists to have noticed these properties of *Penicillium*. The first to have done so seems to have been John Burdon-Sanderson in 1870, nearly sixty years before Fleming's discovery.

Burton-Sanderson was, strangely enough, a lecturer at St Mary's hospital in

* Paine, quoted in Miracle Cure by Milton Wainwright. Blackwell, 1990, p. 40.

Paddington, London: the same institution where Fleming was to 'rediscover' *Penicillium* sixty years later. His observation was almost identical to that of Fleming, that cultured bacteria did not grow in a solution contaminated by the *Penicillium* mould. Many others subsequently made similar observations, including Joseph Lister, one of the pioneers of bacteriology, who actually treated a wounded patient with *Penicillium*. An Italian scientist, Vicenzo Tiberio, treated infected rabbits with the mould in 1895, and similar observations were made by Ernest Duchesne at the University of Lyon in France in 1896.

The twist in the tale, however, is that these earlier strains of *Penicillium* do not produce penicillin, and their antibacterial activity is due to an entirely different chemical, mycophenolic acid. The strain which eventually fell almost literally into Fleming's lap was a rare strain which does produce large amounts of penicillin.

In fact, there is a long history of folk medicine recipes in which moulds have been used as important ingredients of healing mixtures. Some date back to ancient China 3000 years ago. More recently, there are very clear and specific prescriptions for using mouldy bread to treat infections in the 1600s, and scientists had known for years that many bacteria and moulds (fungi) could inhibit the growth of other bacteria. There are even many documented cases of micro-organisms being used in modern times to treat illness. Stanley Chambers and Fred Weidman, for example, dermatologists working at the University of Pennsylvania, used cultures of a bacterium, *Bacillus subtilis*, to treat fungal infections of the skin such as ringworm.* That was in 1927, the year before *Penicillium* landed on Fleming's plate. It was Fleming, however, who is credited with the train of events which led to this phenomenon being turned into a life-saving series of drugs.

Drugs used to treat bacterial infections (Table 17.2, p. 276)

Bacteria are single-celled organisms in which many of the important bio-chemical reactions differ from those in animals. This allows drugs to be de-veloped which can, in principle, attack the bacteria selectively without damaging the cells of the host animals. Drugs may be either bacteriostatic, stopping the growth of bacteria and allowing the body's own defence systems to attack and kill the invaders, or bactericidal, killing the bacteria directly (Fig. 17.1).

The names of some of the more important bacteria, written by convention in *italics*, are included in the sections that follow. Although some names may look complicated, many have arisen logically. *Salmonella*, for example, was named after Daniel Salmon, an American scientist who developed a vaccine

* These and many other examples of the use of micro-organisms in medicine are given by Milton Wainwright in his book *Miracle cure*.

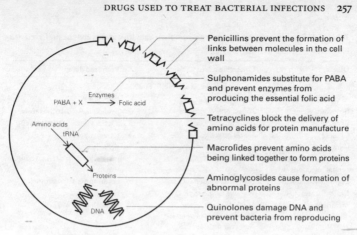

Fig. 17.1 How do antibiotics work?

against one type of the bacterium. *Yersinia*, the bacterium which causes plague, was named after its discoverer—Alexandre Yersin.

Penicillins and cephalosporins

Penicillins are effective against bacteria responsible for diseases such as pneumonia (*Streptococcus pneumoniae*), gonorrhoea (*Neisseria gonorrhoea*), and syphilis (*Treponema pallidum*) (Table 17.1, p. 258).

How do they work?

Many bacteria make their cell walls by linking together chains of molecules to form a strong network. The links include a pair of amino acids (the building blocks from which proteins are made) called D-alanine. The molecules of penicillin have a very similar structure to this pairing and can interact with the enzymes involved in wall formation, inhibiting them and disrupting the formation and maintenance of the cell wall (Fig. 17.1). New cells are unable to make a wall at all, while fully formed cells cannot repair their walls and soon die. Because mammalian cell walls are completely different from those of bacteria, the penicillins do not harm them. In other words, they show 'selective toxicity' towards the bacteria.

There are many different drugs related to the original penicillin molecule. Within about ten years of Paine's first treatments of patients in Sheffield, the first strains of bacteria were found which were resistant to penicillin. They had become resistant by producing an enzyme, penicillinase, which destroys the antibiotic by breaking open a ring of atoms called a beta-lactam ring

Table 17.1 Examples of major disease groups, their causative agents and the preferred drug treatments

Disease*	Causative agent*	Preferred drug*
BACTERIAL INFECTIONS		
Abscesses	*Staphylococcus aureus*	penicillins
Bronchitis	*Haemophilus influenzae*	penicillins + co-trimoxazole
Brucellosis	*Brucella*	a tetracycline + streptomycin
Cholera	*Vibrio cholerae*	tetracyclines
Gangrene	*Clostridium perfingens*	penicillins
Gonorrhoea and other genital infections	*Neissseria gonorrhoeae*	penicillins with a tetracycline
Legionnaires' disease	*Legionella pneumophilia*	erythromycin + rifampicin
Lyme disease	*Borrelia burgdorferi*	tetracyclines
Meninigitis	*Staphylococcus aureus; Streptococcus pneumoniae; Neisseria meningitidis*	penicillins
Meninigitis	*Flavobacterium meningosepticum Haemophilus influenzae*	erythromycin + rifampicin
Plague	*Yersinia pestis*	streptomycin + a tetracycline
Pneumonia	*Staphylococcus aureus; Streptococcus pneumoniae; Streptococcus pyogenes*	penicillins
Pneumonia	*Klebsiella pneumoniae*	cephalosporins + an aminoglycoside
Psittacosis	*Chlamydia psittaci*	tetracyclines
Scarlet fever	*Streptococcus pyogenes*	penicillins
Sinusitis	*Haemophilus influenzae*	penicillins + co-trimoxazole
Syphilis	*Treponema pallidum*	penicillins
Tetanus	*Clostridium tetani*	penicillins
Typhoid fever	*Salmonella*	chloramphenicol + co-trimoxazole
Urinary tract infections	*Escherichia coli*	penicillins + aminoglycoside + sulphonamide
Food poisoning (see Chapter 4)	*Campylobacter E. coli, Salmonella, Shigella*	various
FUNGAL INFECTIONS		
Meningitis	*Cryptococcus neoformans*	amphotericin + flucytosine
Skin and other surface infections	*Candida*	ketoconazole nystatin clotrimazole
Urinary tract infections	*Candida*	flucytosine amphotericin
VIRAL INFECTIONS		
Genital infections	*Herpes simplex*	acyclovir
Encephalitis	*Herpes simplex*	vidarabine
Influenza	*Influenza A*	amantadine or rimantadine

E. coli was named after Theodor Escherich (1857–1911) who first described the bacterium in 1886.

* Some diseases can be caused by several different organisms.

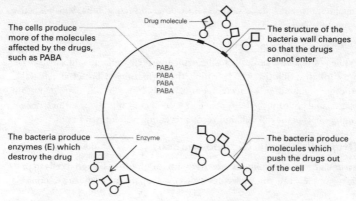

Fig. 17.2 The mechanisms by which bacteria can become resistant to drugs.

(penicillinase is also known as beta-lactamase). By modifying the penicillin molecule, chemists discovered that they could produce molecules which were not affected by penicillinase, but which could still kill the bacteria. These drugs include flucloxacillin and methicillin, although some bacteria are becoming resistant even to these.

An alternative way to attack bacteria is to use drugs such as clavulanic acid, sulbactam, and tazobactam which inhibit the activity of the bacterial penicillinase. This means that penicillins cannot be destroyed by the bacteria and so are made much more effective.

In an effort to overcome the destruction of penicillins by bacterial penicillinase, scientists developed another series of drugs which were similar to the penicillins but which were resistant to the enzyme. They include imipenem and aztreonam.

Some penicillins, such as piperacillin, azlocillin, and ticarcillin, are particularly effective against a bacterium which can cause pneumonia and septicaemia —*Pseudomonas aeruginosa*.

Cephalosporins

Following in the footsteps of Fleming, many scientists tried to find other species of bacteria or fungi which might produce antibiotics. In 1948 Giuseppe Brotzu at the University of Cagliari, Italy, found a mould, near a sewage outlet, which inhibited the growth of bacteria. This was the first of a series of antibiotics called cephalosporins whose molecules resembled the penicillins but which were not destroyed by bacterial enzymes and which killed a wider range of bacteria. They stop the formation of cell walls in the same way as the penicillins. The cephalosporins include cefadroxil, cefuroxime, and ceftazidime (which is active against *Ps. aeruginosa*).

Other drugs affecting the cell wall

While not related chemically to the penicillins, teichoplanin and vancomycin are similar antibiotics which inhibit the formation of bacterial cell walls. Another compound, bacitracin (so-called because it was extracted from bacteria taken from a patient called Tracy) blocks the enzymes which deliver components of the cell wall, indirectly preventing wall formation.

Drugs affecting nucleic acid synthesis

Several groups of antibiotics interfere with the ability of bacterial cells to produce nucleic acids—the molecules which make up the genes and are responsible for protein synthesis.

Sulphonamides

The discovery of the sulphonamides (sulpha-drugs) was described on page 254. They are active against a range of bacteria including those causing cystitis (usually *Escherichia coli,* named after Theodor Escherich, the Austrian paediatrician and bacteriologist who first described it in 1886). The sulphonamides exploit an important difference between bacteria and mammals in the way they obtain their supply of an essential vitamin—folic acid. Like most vitamins (*see* Chapter 22) folic acid is needed for many biochemical reactions inside cells, especially those which make the genetic materials DNA and RNA.

Mammals absorb enough folic acid from their food to meet those needs, but bacteria are not able to absorb enough from their environment, so they are forced to make it themselves. This they do by linking together two molecules, one of which is known as para-aminobenzoic acid (PABA).* The two molecules are joined by two enzymes (Fig. 17.1).† The molecules of the sulphonamides are very similar in structure to PABA and enzyme A is fooled into interacting with the drug rather than PABA. The drug, however, stops the enzyme from working, so that the formation of folic acid ceases and the bacteria cannot reproduce.

A related drug, trimethoprim, inhibits enzyme B with the same net effect. The combination of one of the sulphonamide drugs, sulphamethoxazole, with trimethoprim is known as cotrimoxazole. It is much more potent than either of the individual drugs on its own.

Precautions

Sulphonamides are very valuable and safe bacteriostatic drugs, but should not be taken by pregnant women. Bilirubin, produced by the liver, is normally

* The other chemical used to make folic acid is a pteridine (the 'p' is silent).
† Enzyme A is dihydropteroate synthetase and B is dihydrofolate reductase.

attached to proteins in the blood, which hold it in the bloodstream. Sulphon-amides can displace bilirubin from these proteins and it can then pass across the placenta into the developing baby, where it can affect growth and cause brain damage.

In humans, sulphonamides are inactivated by 'acetylator' enzymes in the liver which add a chemical acetyl portion onto the molecule. Humans fall into two groups, about half being able to perform this reaction relatively quickly (fast acetylators) and about half more slowly (slow acetylators). In the latter group, therefore, the amount of sulphonamides in the body remains high for longer, so less is needed.

Tetracyclines and related antibiotics

Like most of the antibiotics now available, with the exception of the sulphon-amides developed from Prontosil Red, the tetracyclines and aminoglycosides have been developed from chemicals first isolated from micro-organisms. Originally both tetracycline itself and the first aminoglycoside, streptomycin, were isolated from yeasts.

The tetracyclines stop cells from making the proteins they need. The fundamental processes by which all cells, bacterial and animal, make proteins are the same. Enzymes 'read' the DNA of the genes and make similar molecules called RNA* (a process known as 'translation'). One type of RNA is messenger RNA (mRNA) and this attaches to a large molecule called a ribosome. A different type of RNA ('transfer' RNA, or tRNA) carries amino acids to the ribosome, where the mRNA determines the sequence in which they are linked together to form proteins.

The ribosomes are different in bacteria and mammals, and the tetracyclines prevent tRNA from bringing amino acids to the bacterial ribosome (see Fig. 18.1). The aminoglycosides such as streptomycin have a similar effect, but they also prevent ribosome from linking amino acids in the correct order. As a result, the bacteria produce much less protein than normal, and that which is produced is incorrect.

The macrolide antibiotics, erythromycin, clindamycin, clarithromycin, and azithromycin, as well as the unrelated drug chloramphenicol also interfere with the ability of bacteria to synthesize proteins. As the new protein chain grows, it is moved around on the ribosome with the aid of a series of enzymes. The macrolides and chloramphenicol inhibit these enzymes so that more amino acids cannot be added to the growing protein.

Since the formation of new proteins is essential to life, all these drugs are bactericidal. The tetracyclines are active in Lyme disease, some forms of

* DNA is an abbreviation for DeoxyriboNucleic Acid, and RNA for RiboNucleic Acid.

pneumonia, cholera, and Rocky mountain spotted fever. Aminoglycosides are effective against bacteria such as *E. coli* causing urinary tract infections, and some of those, such as Klebsiella *pneumoniae,* which can cause pneumonia. Erythromycin is useful in the treatment of syphilis (caused by *Treponema pallidum*) and legionnaire's disease (caused by *Legionella pneumophilia*) (Table 17.1, p. 258).

Side-effects

While these drugs cause few side-effects in most people, the tetracyclines tend to discolour the teeth in children. The aminoglycosides can very occasionally damage the kidney and the nerves of the inner ear, leading to problems with hearing or balance. Some antibiotics can kill bacteria which normally live in our bodies and which restrain the growth of fungi such as *Candida.* The use of these drugs may, therefore, allow *Candida* to grow unchecked, causing thrush in the mouth, intestine, or vagina.

Antibiotics causing disruption of the genes

The genes, present in all cells and responsible for directing all their activities, are made of DNA. This is an extremely long and complex molecule which is normally kept folded by means of an enzyme called DNA gyrase. The 4-quinolone group of drugs (ciprofloxacin, norfloxacin, and nalidixic acid) inhibit this enzyme in bacteria so that the DNA unwinds and becomes useless. The bacterial cells die as a result. Metronidazole binds directly to the molecules of DNA, preventing its replication and thus stopping the bacteria from reproducing.

Although generally quite safe, the quinolones may precipitate fits in patients with epilepsy. They also slow the production of bone and cartilage and should not be used for long periods in children or during pregnancy.

Drugs used in tuberculosis

According to Bernard Dixon,* tuberculosis has claimed the lives of a thousand million humans over the centuries. It is caused by an unusual type of bacterium called *Mycobacterium tuberculosis.* Mycobacteria have a higher fat content than most bacteria, as well as several less obvious differences in structure and biochemistry.

The first drug able to kill these organisms was streptomycin. The details of discovery are still the subject of heated debate, with the credit being given by some to Albert Schatz, an American born in Norwich, Connecticut in 1920, and by some to Selman Waksman, a Russian Jew born in 1888 and who

* In his book: *Power unseen: how microbes rule the world.*

emigrated to the USA. Schatz worked for several years as a student and later an independent research worker in Waksman's laboratory at Rutgers University. Whether credit should go to Schatz, who performed the tedious and difficult task of extracting and isolating streptomycin, or mainly to Waksman who provided the conditions, facilities, and encouragement, will probably always remain contentious, even though the patent on streptomycin was in their joint names, as was the scientific report on the discovery of this antibiotic in 1944. It was Waksman who was awarded the Nobel Prize in 1952. It was certainly Waksman who devoted most of his life to the concept that micro-organisms from soil could produce chemicals which inhibited the growth of others.

Streptomycin works by preventing the synthesis of new protein as described in the section on tetracyclines. However, bacteria rapidly become resistant to streptomycin and it must be used in combination with other antibiotics.

In about 1948, research at the Lederle pharmaceutical laboratories suggested that one of the B vitamins, nicotinamide, had a weak ability to kill mycobacteria. This soon led to one of the main drugs still used to treat tuberculosis: isoniazid, synthesized by Harry Yale at the Squibb Institute in New Brunswick, New Jersey, in 1951. This drug prevents the formation of a group of chemicals called mycolic acids which are needed for the synthesis of cell walls. Another drug, cycloserine also prevents cell wall formation by inhibiting enzymes involved in their synthesis.

Rifampicin inhibits one of the enzymes involved in the synthesis of RNA, so that the bacteria cannot synthesize new protein. Its most notable side-effect is to cause urine and bodily fluids, such as tears and saliva, to turn orange. Resistance may develop as bacteria produce a different form of the enzyme which is not inhibited by rifampicin. Ethambutol and pyrazinamide can also be used, although we do not understand how they work. Ethambutol probably interferes with the incorporation of mycolic acids into bacterial cell walls.

Resistance to antibiotics

> In several areas, the development of new drugs is no longer keeping pace with accumulating resistance.*

A major problem confronting mankind is the consequence of microbial adaptation to antibiotics. Doctors come under great pressure to provide drugs which will help patients to recover more quickly from an infection as no-one enjoys being ill and there is often a strong desire or financial need to return to work as soon as possible. Antibiotics have also been used in vast quantities to prevent infections in cattle and other farm animals.

The problem now being faced arises from the fact that bacteria reproduce

* Drug and Therapeutics Bulletin, 1999, vol. 37, pp. 9–16.

very rapidly, some of them every few minutes. There is, therefore, a real possibility that among the countless millions of bacteria being born around the world, there will be at least one which is different from the rest, perhaps with a genetic mutation which changes one of the enzymes or other molecules in the cell. If that mutation affects one of the molecular targets of antibiotic drugs, that cell may be resistant to a group of drugs and all the bacteria which arise from the reproduction of that cell will also be resistant. This is known as 'acquired resistance'. Paul Ehrlich, the 'father of chemotherapy', was one of the first to recognize that the development of new drugs to treat infections was likely to be met by the growing resistance of the invading cells. Resistance, he predicted, would follow drug development 'like a faithful shadow'.

The situation, of course, is the basic principle of evolution. The bacterial environment is changing in that it now frequently contains antibiotics, and we could say that bacteria simply evolve rapidly to deal with that change.

To make matters very much worse than either Darwin or Ehrlich could have predicted, the altered genes responsible for drug resistance can be transferred between bacteria. A relatively harmless type of bacterium could, therefore, develop resistance to a drug and then some of its descendants could transfer it to a more dangerous, disease-producing type.

It is to reduce the development of resistance that patients are strongly recommended to take the whole of a course of antibacterial therapy in the doses stated. The doses normally prescribed should kill the invading cells as quickly as possible without harming the patient, giving the bacteria minimal chance to become resistant. If only part of the prescribed course is taken, or if it is taken over a longer time period, the bacteria may develop resistance and the patient may be faced with a more serious infection which cannot be controlled by drugs.

But the most important step in combating bacterial resistance is for doctors to stop prescribing antibiotics for trivial disorders which would clear up spontaneously within a few days, and not to prescribe them for diseases caused by viruses (which are not affected by antibiotics).

How do organisms become resistant?

Bacteria can become resistant to drugs in several ways (Fig. 17.2):

1. One is by producing enzymes which destroys the antibiotic. Some bacteria produce a β-lactamase enzyme, penicillinase, which breaks open the molecules of penicillins. Some bacteria make enzymes which inactivate the amino-glycoside antibiotics.

2. Bacteria may begin to produce more of those cell components which oppose the effect of the antibiotic. For example, some may produce more PABA, reducing the effectiveness of the sulphonamides.

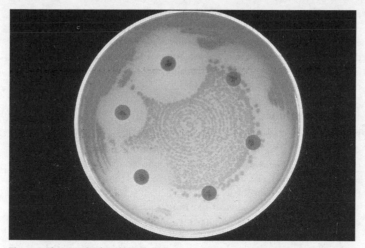

Fig. 17.3 Photograph of a culture plate showing colonies of bacteria growing on the surface of agar. The presence of antibiotics kills the bacteria, leaving clear spaces on the plate.

3. Bacteria may have a change in the structure of their outer membranes so that antibiotics cannot enter them. This is often a problem with the tetracyclines. Some bacteria also produce molecules which interact with tetracycline molecules and pump them out of the cell. The aminoglycosides are normally carried into the cells by an enzyme system, but resistance occurs if bacteria stop producing those enzymes.

4. Some bacteria undergo mutations which change the structure of those molecules which are the targets for antibiotics, such as the enzymes involved in folic acid synthesis (sulphonamides) or protein synthesis (aminoglycosides).

The ability of bacteria to develop resistance to drugs never ceases to astound scientists. The drug vancomycin, described earlier, blocks the formation of bacterial walls by interacting with a pair of unusual amino acids—D-alanyl-D-alanine. The only way that bacteria could develop resistance would be to find an entirely new method of making their cell walls. But that is precisely what has happened. From somewhere—no-one knows where—enterococcal bacteria (which cause some intestinal infections) have obtained genes which allow them to use a different pair of molecules—D-alanine-D-lactate, as a result of which they have become resistant to vancomycin.

The rate of bacterial adaptation, or evolution, is such that scientists are struggling to produce new drugs at a rate which kill resistant strains. Several types of bacteria capable of causing fatal infections are already resistant to all existing drugs. Although there have been many successes in the past, such as the production of new penicillins which are resistant to the β-lactamase enzymes produced by bacteria, the difficulty of identifying bacterial change and then producing new, effective, and safe drugs will keep pharmacologists and other scientists very busy as long as there are both humans and bacteria on the planet.

Fungal infections

Fungi usually cause infections on the surface of the body. They may affect the skin (such as *Tinea pedis*, which causes 'athlete's foot'), hair, and nails. Infections of the nails, or '*onychomycoses*' may need lengthy treatment until the infected portions have grown out. This may take 3–6 months for fingernails and more than 12 months for toenail infections.

Fungi include yeasts and yeast-like fungi such as *Candida albicans*, which causes thrush in the mouth, intestine, and vagina. Occasionally, fungal infections affect the whole body. These 'systemic' infections can be dangerous, but usually occur in patients who are especially susceptible to infections because their immune system is not functioning normally, as in AIDS, or patients receiving anticancer drugs.

Drugs used to treat fungal infections (mycoses) (Table 17.3, p. 277)

Amphotericin and nystatin

Whereas animal cells contain cholesterol in their walls, fungi use a quite different steroid, ergosterol. Amphotericin interacts with molecules of ergosterol in the fungal cell wall to create holes, through which potassium and other important ions and small molecules gradually leak out, causing serious disturbance to the cells and eventually causing their death (Fig. 17.4).

Nystatin is similar and was in fact the first antifungal antibiotic to be discovered. It was isolated from yeasts in 1950 by Elizabeth Hazen and Rachel Brown. At first they called their new substance fungicidin, but when they learnt that another drug had already been given that name, they changed it to nystatin, as they were working in New York State. Nystatin is too toxic to be taken internally. It is reserved for infections of the skin or external membranes such as those in the mouth and vagina.

Imidazoles

The antifungal activity of chemicals with an imidazole structure was discovered in 1944. The Belgian pharmaceutical company founded by Paul Janssen eventually introduced miconazole in the 1960s. At this point, the company decided not to pursue research into fungal diseases and this decision was

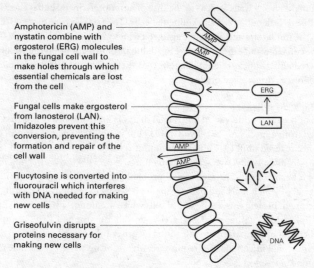

Amphotericin (AMP) and nystatin combine with ergosterol (ERG) molecules in the fungal cell wall to make holes through which essential chemicals are lost from the cell

Fungal cells make ergosterol from lanosterol (LAN). Imidazoles prevent this conversion, preventing the formation and repair of the cell wall

Flucytosine is converted into fluorouracil which interferes with DNA needed for making new cells

Griseofulvin disrupts proteins necessary for making new cells

Fig. 17.4 Drugs used to treat infections caused by fungi.

reversed only because the company received an influx of scientists from Africa when Belgium gave up the Belgian Congo (now Zaire). Many of these scientists had been working to develop anti-fungal drugs and had seen the scale of the health problems caused by fungi in tropical countries. The work subsequently carried out at Janssen led to the discovery of one of the most effective drugs now available—ketoconazole.

Researchers led by Ken Richardson at another company, Pfizer at Sandwich, Kent in England, tried to improve on ketoconazole by replacing the imidazole part of the molecule (which had 3 carbon atoms and 2 nitrogen atoms) with a triazole group (2 carbons and 3 nitrogens). The resulting drug was not destroyed by the body as quickly as the imidazole compound and was, therefore, much more active. Speaking about his discovery of this compound, fluconazole, Richardson has recalled that 'For the first time we could see that we had synthesized a compound that showed a level of anti-fungal activity we had not even dreamed of'.

How do the imidazoles and related drugs work?

The ergosterol which fungi need to produce their cell walls is made from another steroid, lanosterol. The imidazole and triazole drugs prevent the conversion of lanosterol into ergosterol by the fungal cells. The cells cannot then make strong walls and, as in the case of amphotericin, essential chemicals are able to leak out, gradually killing the cells. The triazoles are more effective than the imidazoles and are active against a wider range of fungi.

Tioconazole and amorolfine are available in paints for applying locally to infected nails, but experience suggests that they are not as effective at curing infections as drugs taken orally.

Griseofulvin

One of the most widely used antifungal drugs is griseofulvin. It was first obtained from a species of *Penicillium* in 1939 but its ability to damage fungal cells was not realized until 1946 and it was not introduced into medicine until 1960.

Griseofulvin is effective against many fungi, especially those affecting nails, since it becomes concentrated in and probably incorporated into keratin, the material of which nails and hair are made. It seems to work by disrupting the structure of proteins inside the fungal cells which are important in cell division. Multiplication of the cells is thereby slowed or stopped. The complete eradication of dermatophyte infections by griseofulvin can be a slow process and some nail infections may require treatment for up to two years. The most common side-effect is headaches.

Flucytosine

Fungal cells contain enzymes which take the drug flucytosine into the cells. They also possess an enzyme which converts flucytosine into fluorouracil. This blocks the synthesis of new DNA and, therefore, prevents reproduction. It is also converted into a nucleotide which becomes incorporated into the fungal RNA, so that it cannot be used to synthesize new protein. This combination results in the death of the fungal cells. Fungi can quickly become resistant to flucytosine either by producing less of the enzyme which transports the drug into the cell, or by making less of the enzyme which converts it into fluorouracil.

Terbinafine

This is used to treat fungal infections of the nails, ringworm, and tinea infections. Terbinafine is much more effective than griseofulvin in eliminating fungal infections of the toe-nails.

Thrush

Thrush is the common name given to an infection by the yeast *Candida albicans*. It usually occurs in the mouth or vagina, the first symptoms being a vaginal discharge and soreness. Infection is more likely during pregnancy when the immune defence system is less active. Thrush is best treated with local applications of nystatin, clotrimazole, econazole, or miconazole in the form of pessaries to be inserted into the vagina. Oral thrush is often treated by sucking nystatin lozenges.

Systemic (generalized) fungal infections

Whereas fungal infections are usually localized in part of the body, the whole body can become infected by some types of fungus, especially if the immune system is not functioning correctly. This can happen, for example, in patients with AIDS in whom the immune activity of many of the white blood cells is lost. Drugs such as fluconazole can be used to treat generalized 'systemic' fungal infections, and related drugs are being developed such as voriconazole which are even more effective and have fewer side-effects.

Drugs used to treat viral infections (Table 17.4, p. 278)

Viruses cause a wide range of diseases in humans, including influenza and the common cold as well as more serious ones such as chickenpox, mumps, herpes, rubella (German measles), polio, rabies, and some forms of bronchitis, pneumonia, and meningitis. Even influenza can be life-threatening in the elderly and people with advanced forms of breathing disorder such as asthma and emphysema (see Chapter 2), or heart problems.

The Human Immunodeficiency Virus (HIV) causes AIDS,* in which the immune system is rendered much less able to protect the patient when exposed to attack by all manner of micro-organisms. The immune system normally removes, very efficiently, small numbers of invading bacteria, viruses, and fungi and performs a vital role in checking for the presence of abnormal or foreign cells. The white blood cells, the policemen of the immune system, detect and destroy cells which have been infected with viruses and which have become cancerous. Patients with AIDS have a dramatically increased risk of both infections and cancers.

Whereas bacteria are fully formed cells, viruses may be considered to be only a part of a cell. They are much smaller than cells, and most consist of nothing more than a piece of nucleic acid (RNA or DNA) surrounded usually by a protein 'coat'. While viruses can survive outside the body, they are unable to multiply because they do not possess the necessary enzymes and other molecules. The only way they can reproduce, therefore, is to infect an appropriate host animal or plant, when each virus inserts itself into a cell and takes over that cell's biochemical processes to produce more viruses. When the cell has spawned hundreds or thousands of new viruses, it dies or bursts, releasing the new viruses into the bloodstream (Fig. 17.5). This sequence presents several problems for treatment.

* AIDS is an abbreviation for the Acquired Immune Deficiency Syndrome.

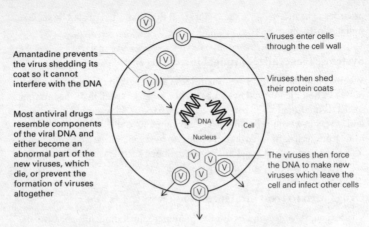

Amantadine prevents the virus shedding its coat so it cannot interfere with the DNA

Most antiviral drugs resemble components of the viral DNA and either become an abnormal part of the new viruses, which die, or prevent the formation of viruses altogether

Viruses enter cells through the cell wall

Viruses then shed their protein coats

The viruses then force the DNA to make new viruses which leave the cell and infect other cells

DNA

Nucleus

Cell

Fig. 17.5 Drugs used to treat serious viral infections.

Firstly, there may be few obvious symptoms at the time when some cells are mass-producing new viruses. By the time that the infected cells release their vast load of new viruses and symptoms start to appear, there may be too many viruses already in the body for drugs to have any effect.

The second problem is that, because the viruses are using the body's own cells to reproduce, it is very difficult to create drugs which can stop the viruses from multiplying without harming the host cells themselves.

Amantadine

For a virus to take over the genetic machinery of a host cell it must first enter the cell and then lose its protein coat. This leaves the nucleic acid at the core of the virus able to attack the cell's nucleus and divert it into producing more viruses. One drug, amantadine, prevents viruses shedding their coats. The viruses are forced to remain inactive inside the cells. Meanwhile, the body's immune system detects the fact that a virus has entered the cell because it leaves tell-tale signs on the outside surface. The cell, along with its trapped virus, is attacked and destroyed. Unfortunately, amantadine is not particularly effective and cannot be used alone to treat most infections. It is given mainly to treat influenza, but even here it acts only on some strains of virus classified as 'type A'.

Inhibitors of nucleic acid synthesis

An alternative approach is to use drugs which interfere with the virus's ability to replicate its nucleic acid within the host cell. Acyclovir is such a drug and is active against the herpes viruses and *Varicella zoster* (which causes chickenpox and shingles). These viruses contain an enzyme which converts acyclovir into another chemical which then inhibits DNA polymerase, an enzyme needed for the replication of viral genes. The host cells in animals contain much less of the converting enzyme and their DNA polymerase is far less sensitive to the chemical produced. Valaciclovir is known as a pro-drug: once inside cells it is converted into acyclovir.

The related drug ganciclovir, as well as vidarabine, didanosine, ribavirin, and tribavirin, are also converted inside cells to compounds which inhibit the enzymes needed to synthesize viral RNA and DNA. Again, the relevant enzymes of the virus and host are sufficiently different that the host cells remain relatively unaffected by these drugs unless high doses need to be given.

Zidovudine (AZT) is the most effective agent currently available for the treatment of HIV* infection (AIDS); it does not cure the disease, but can slow the multiplication of the virus. One of the viral enzymes responsible for producing the viral DNA is not able to discriminate between the molecules it normally uses to make DNA and AZT; the molecules of AZT, therefore, become incorporated into the DNA of the virus, but not of the host.

Foscarnet is an inorganic molecule which can inhibit many of the enzymes involved in nucleic acid metabolism and use.

In view of its toxicity, idoxuridine is now used only for application to the skin. It is incorporated into the nucleic acid of both the virus and the host cells, as a result of which the DNA becomes more fragile and easily damaged.

Protease inhibitors

Two of the genes present in HIV code for proteins which are essential for the virus to be active. These proteins are produced initially as large, complex molecules which need to be split into smaller ones by a protease (protein-splitting) enzyme. Several drugs can inhibit this protease, stopping the formation of the HIV proteins and rendering the virus harmless. They are indinavir, ritonavir, and saquinavir. They are the forerunners of drugs which will be developed from a greater understanding of HIV and which, by affecting targets specific for the virus, should have far fewer side-effects than the drugs used previously.

Parasitic infections

Protozoa are single-celled organisms which can cause a range of diseases in humans and other animals. In general they differ from bacteria in being much more advanced cells, with thinner cell walls resembling those of higher animals,

* HIV is human immunodeficiency virus.

and a nucleus. Most protozoan parasites pass through a series of stages in their life cycle during which they adopt different forms and may need a different host in which to grow.

Amoebiasis (amoebic dysentery)

Dysentery is caused by the protozoan *Entamoeba histolytica*, and causes violent, sometimes bloody diarrhoea. The drugs used most often to treat it are metronidazole, tinidazole, diloxanide, and chloroquine. Metronidazole and the related drug tinidazole have reactive nitrogen groups in the molecule which interact with molecules in the parasitic cells such as proteins and nucleic acids. This interaction seriously disturbs cell function and the parasites are killed. Unfortunately these drugs can also interact with some molecules in the host cells, so that side-effects of nausea, vomiting, and other gastrointestinal disturbances are common.

Diloxanide and the aminoglycoside paromomycin kill parasites in the intestine. Paromomycin has similar effects to those of other aminoglycosides on bacteria, making the walls of the parasite's cells more leaky and inhibiting protein synthesis. Two further drugs, emetine and dehydroemetine also inhibit protein synthesis in the parasites. Chloroquine is able to kill parasitic cells which have passed from the intestine into the body. It will be discussed in more detail when we consider malaria.

Amoebic parasites feed on bacteria in the intestine, so drug treatment often includes the administration of antibiotics to decrease the bacterial content of the gut and 'starve' the parasite.

Toxoplasmosis

The most common protozoan infestation of humans outside the tropics is by *Toxoplasma gondii*. The organism is transmitted in uncooked, infected meat. The most effective treatment is with pyrimethamine, which blocks the use of folic acid by the parasites and leads to their death. Although animals can make their own supply of folate, pyrimethamine may interfere with its use and supplements of folate should be taken together with pyrimethamine. Pyrimethamine is normally taken with a sulphonamide inhibitor of folic acid use, such as sulphadiazine.

Toxocara

The *Toxocara* organism infects the eyes. It is particularly common in the Third World and is a frequent cause of blindness.

Trypanosomiasis

Trypanosomes are protozoan parasites which cause African sleeping sickness and Chagas disease in America. In the early stages of sleeping sickness, the parasites exist mainly in the blood, but in later stages they invade the brain, causing inflammation of the brain and the prolonged sleep that characterizes the disease and which can be fatal.

Melarsoprol is a drug which interacts with sulphur atoms in molecules. It does not distinguish between molecules in the host and parasite cells, but penetrates into the trypanosomal cells more easily than into mammalian cells.

Pentamidine is taken into the cells of trypanosomes where it binds to DNA and other molecules, killing the cells.

Malaria

The most common global example of a protozoan infection is malaria, the life cycle of which is summarized in Fig. 17.6. The word 'malaria' is derived from *mala aria* meaning bad air. Before the realization that mosquitoes transmitted the disease, it was thought to be caused by the foul smells associated with marshes, swamps, and poor sanitation. Malaria still kills huge numbers of people. Around 400 million people contract the disease each year, and between one and two million of them die as a result. So many travellers now visit malaria-affected regions that there are around 3000 cases of malaria each year in the UK and over 10 000 per year in the USA.

The main protozoans causing malaria are *Plasmodium falciparum*, which

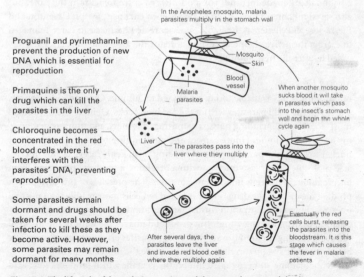

In the Anopheles mosquito, malaria parasites multiply in the stomach wall

Proguanil and pyrimethamine prevent the production of new DNA which is essential for reproduction

Mosquito
Skin
Blood vessel
Malaria parasites

When another mosquito sucks blood it will take in parasites which pass into the insect's stomach wall and begin the whole cycle again

Primaquine is the only drug which can kill the parasites in the liver

Chloroquine becomes concentrated in the red blood cells where it interferes with the parasites' DNA, preventing reproduction

Liver
The parasites pass into the liver where they multiply

Some parasites remain dormant and drugs should be taken for several weeks after infection to kill these as they become active. However, some parasites may remain dormant for many months

After several days, the parasites leave the liver and invade red blood cells where they multiply again

Eventually the red cells burst, releasing the parasites into the bloodstream. It is this stage which causes the fever in malaria patients

Fig. 17.6 The life cycle of the malaria parasite, and drugs used to control the disease.

produces a severe and sometimes rapidly fatal form of the disease, and *P. vivax* and *P. malariae* which cause milder forms. All spend part of their life cycle in the *Anopheles* mosquito, and part in higher animals. When an infected mosquito bites a human, it injects spores of *Plasmodium* (called sporozoites) into the bloodstream. These spores pass through several stages over the next few days, eventually giving rise to gametes (reproductive germ cells) which circulate in the blood. If another mosquito bite is received, some of these gametes pass back into the mosquito, where they fuse and complete the parasite's life cycle.

The symptoms of infection include fever, sweating, headaches, muscle pains, and anaemia. Malaria is characterized particularly by high fever, when the blood cells burst and release parasites. In about 20 per cent of patients, especially those infected with *P. falciparum*, parasites may enter the brain where they cause the serious complication known as cerebral malaria and, not infrequently, death.

Drugs used in the treatment of malaria (Table 17.5, p. 278)

Quinine

The first treatment available for malaria consisted of crude extracts of the bark of a tree in South America, used for centuries by local natives. In 1629 the wife of the Spanish viceroy to South America was cured of malaria in this way. As she was the Countess of Chinchon, the tree was named Cinchona. Imports of cinchona bark made fortunes for a number of entrepreneurs at the time, but also saved millions of lives. In 1817 two French chemists, Joseph Caventou and Pierre-Joseph Pelletier, at the Ecole Supérieure de Pharmacie in Paris, managed to extract the active chemical responsible for the anti-malarial activity. They called it, after the tree, quinine.

Modern Drugs

Many of the drugs available today are related to quinine. Quinine, chloroquine, and mefloquine kill parasites within the red blood cells. Quinine itself produces most side-effects, including nausea, vomiting, dizziness, and tinnitus ('ringing' in the ears). Quinine, chloroquine, and mefloquine block the synthesis of nucleic acids by the parasite cells after being mistakenly inserted into nucleic acid molecules. They also interact with a breakdown product* produced from haemoglobin in red cells infected by parasites. The presence of this breakdown product means that the drugs enter infected red cells more readily than normal ones, reaching a concentration more than one hundred times greater. The combination of drug with haemoglobin product damages the walls of the infected red cells, causing them to burst before the parasites are ready for release. The body's immune system can then kill and remove the immature parasites.

Pyrimethamine and proguanil inhibit the enzyme which produces folic acid

* Ferriprotoporphyrin IX.

and, since folate is needed for DNA and RNA synthesis, the parasites die. Both drugs are more than one thousand times more effective as inhibitors of the parasite enzyme than the human enzyme, so that parasites can be killed at doses that have relatively little effect on their human hosts.

Primaquine kills the form of the parasite (schizonts) which hides in the liver. Primaquine probably works by generating reactive chemicals that oxidize molecules in the parasite. Primaquine is an important drug because some schizonts may remain dormant in the liver for many months or years after infection, producing unexpected and unpredictable relapses. Anyone who develops unexplained fever after travelling in a malaria-infected region may be suffering from a relapse. Primaquine is the only drug capable of killing all the schizonts, including the dormant ones.

Resistance

As with many infections and infestations, resistance is a major problem. Malaria parasites have become resistant to several of the available drugs in some parts of the world, and the particular combination of drugs to be used has to be tailored to the traveller's itinerary. The mosquito carriers have also become resistant to many of the insecticides once used to control them.

Use of anti-malarial drugs

People travelling to malaria-infected areas should take their anti-malarial drugs for about two weeks before travelling. This is partly to ensure that the person does not react badly to the drug, but also allows a sufficient concentration of drug to build up so that any parasites are killed rapidly, even if the traveller is bitten immediately on stepping off the plane. Similarly, the drugs should be continued for at least four weeks after returning from travel to ensure that all the parasites in the blood are killed.

Artemisinin*

As the malaria parasites become resistant to the available drugs, there is an urgent need for new drugs acting in a different way. Rescue may come from an ancient Chinese remedy: the plant *Artemisia*. Extracts of this plant, known as *qinghaosu*, have been used for centuries in China to treat malaria and the active chemical has been isolated and called artemisinin. It is not only quite effective at killing *Plasmodium* parasites but is very safe with few side-effects, and we can expect to see it becoming available in the West in the next few years. It does not seem to be strong enough on its own to eliminate all malaria parasites from infected persons, so it is usually combined with one of the existing drugs such as mefloquine. Artemisinin increases the activity of mefloquine and allows its dosage to be reduced, reducing the risk of side-effects.

---

* Artemisia is a fascinating plant. In addition to the use of artemisinin in malaria, the plant is used in the Middle East to treat diabetes, and research is now trying to determine whether artemisinin or a similar chemical could become a new treatment for diabetes.

Table 17.2 Drugs used in the treatment of bacterial infections

Penicillins	Other β-lactam antibiotics	Tetracyclines
amoxycillin	aztreonam	chlortetracycline
ampicillin		demeclocycline
azlocillin		doxycycline
bacampicillin	**Carbapenems**	lymecycline
benzylpenicillin	imipenem[†]	meclocycline (USA)
carbenicillin	meropenem	minocycline
carindacillin (USA)		oxytetracycline
cloxacillin	**Cephalosporins**	tetracycline
co-amoxiclav	cefaclor	
(amoxycillin	cefadroxil	**Aminoglycosides**
with clavulanic	cefapirin (USA)	amikacin
acid*)	cefixime	framycetin
dicloxacillin (USA)	cefmetazole (USA)	gentamicin
flucloxacillin	cefodizime	kanamycin
mecillinam (USA)	cefonicid (USA)	neomycin
methicillin (USA)	cefoperazine (USA)	netilmicin
mezlocillin (USA)	ceforanide (USA)	paromomycin (USA)
nafcillin (USA)	cefotaxime	spectinomycin
oxacillin (USA)	cefotetam (USA)	streptomycin (USA)
phenoxymethylpenicillin	cefotiam (USA)	tobramycin
piperacillin	cefoxitin	
pivampicillin	cefpiramide (USA)	**Macrolide antibiotics**
procaine penicillin	cefpirome	azithromycin
temocillin	cefpodoxime	clarithromycin
ticarcillin	cefprosil (USA)	erythromycin
	ceftazidime	triacetyloleandomycin (USA)
Penicillinase-resistant	ceftibuten	
penicillins	ceftizoxime	**(4)-quinolones**
flucloxacillin	ceftriaxone	cinoxacin
methicillin (USA)	cefuroxime	ciprofloxacin
temocillin	cephalexin	enoxacin (USA)
	cephalothin (USA)	grepafloxacin
β-lactamase inhibitors	cephamandole	levofloxacin
clavulanic acid	cephazolin	lonefloxacin (USA)
sulbactam	cephradine	nalidixic acid
tazobactam	loracarbef (USA)	norfloxacin
		ofloxacin
		Polymyxin antibiotic
		colistin

Table 17.2 Continued

Sulphonamides	Other antibiotics	Anti-tuberculosis drugs
co-trimoxazole	chloramphenicol	capreomycin
(trimethoprim with	clindamycin	cycloserine
sulphamethoxazole)	fosfomycin	ethambutol
ethionamide (USA)	fusafungine	isoniazid
sulfabenzamide	fusidic acid	pyrazinamide
sulfacytine (USA)	latamoxef (USA)	rifabutin
sulfadoxine	lincomycin (USA)	rifampicin
sulfamerazine (USA)	metronidazole	streptomycin
sulfametopyrazine	nitrofurantoin	
sulphacetamide	novobiocin	**Urinary tract infections**
sulphadiazine	teicoplanin	hexamine
sulphadimidine	tinidazole	nitrofurantoin
sulphafurazole (USA)	vancomycin	
sulphamethiazole (USA)		
sulphamethoxazole		
sulphanilamide (USA)		
sulphathiazole		
trimethoprim‡		

* Clavulanic acid inhibits the bacterial lactamase enzymes that break down the penicillin molecules.
† This drug is often given with cilastatin, a drug which prevents the breakdown of imipenem in the kidney.
‡ Trimethoprim has a similar action to the sulphonamides.

Table 17.3 Drugs used in the treatment of fungal infections

Polyene antifungals	Triazoles
amphotericin	fluconazole
candicidin (USA)	itraconazole
natamycin (USA)	terconazole (USA)
nystatin	voriconazole*

Imidazoles	Other drugs
butoconazole	amorolfine
clotrimazole	ciclopirox (USA)
econazole	flucytosine
fenticonazole	griseofulvin
ketoconazole	terbinafine
miconazole	tolnaftate
oxiconazole	
sulconazole	
tioconazole	

* This drug is in advanced clinical trials and should be available in late 1999.

Table 17.4 Drugs used to treat virus infections

acyclovir	**Reverse transcriptase inhibitor**
amantadine	nevirapine
cidofovir	
didanosine	**Protease inhibitors**
famciclovir	indinavir
ganciclovir	nelfinavir
lamivudine	ritonavir
ribavirin	saquinavir
stavudine	zanamivir
tribavirin	
valaciclovir	
zalcitabine	
zanamivir	
zidovudine	

Table 17.5 Drugs used in malaria

chloroquine
halofantrine
mefloquine
primaquine
proguanil
pyrimethamine
quinine

Summary

- Drugs which kill or stop the growth of bacteria are called antibacterial or antibiotic drugs.
- The penicillins and cephalosporins interfere with the formation of cell walls, stopping reproduction and killing the bacteria.
- Sulphonamide antibiotics are mistaken by bacteria for PABA, one of their own chemicals, leading to disuption of the cells' metabolism.
- Tetracyclines interrupt the synthesis of new RNA in the cells from growing and dividing.
- The macrolide antibiotics block the synthesis of new proteins.
- The 4-quinolones damage bacterial DNA.
- Rifampicin, ethambutol, and pyrazinamide are particularly useful in killing the bacteria which cause tuberculosis. Streptomycin is also effective but bacteria become resistant.
- Bacteria can develop resistance to drugs by producing enzymes to destroy the drug, by pumping the drug out of its cells, or by changing the structure of its molecular targets.
- Fungal infections can be eliminated using drugs to interfere with the formation of cell walls.
- Griseofulvin damages proteins within the fungal cells.
- Flucytosine interferes with the synthesis of new DNA.
- Viruses must invade cells of other organisms in order to produce more RNA or DNA and new viruses.
- Most drugs which are used against viral infections interfere with the synthesis of new DNA or RNA, preventing the production of new viruses.
- Drugs such as saquinavir prevent the splitting of proteins which are needed for viruses to reproduce.
- Aminoglycoside drugs stop protein synthesis in amoeba and are used to treat amoebic dysentery.
- Toxoplasma parasites are killed by pyrimethamine, which prevents the cells from using folic acid for nucleic acid production.
- Quinine and related drugs interfere with nucleic acid synthesis in the malaria parasites. Pyrimethamine and similar drugs prevent the use of folic acid for nucleic acid synthesis. Artemisinin can be used to increase the effects of mefloquine.

CHAPTER 18

Cancer

At the turn of the century, probably less than 10 per cent of people who developed invasive cancers survived or were cured. Now, over 50 per cent of the patients diagnosed with invasive cancers are cured of their disease. In less than a century there has been a remarkable improvement. The most dramatic advances in cancer treatment have come in children and young adults. For example, prior to the National Cancer Act of 1971 [in the USA], the five-year survival rate for acute leukaemia in children was less than 10 per cent. Presently 60–70 per cent of young victims of this disease are alive after five years. Another cancer success story is Hodgkin's disease. In the 1960s, only 10 per cent of patients with this disease survived, but in the 1990s, 90 per cent of patients enjoy long-term survival. This phenomenal improvement has become manifest as a result of new drugs and new approaches to diagnosis.*

Despite the optimism and encouragement offered by this quotation, about one person in three will develop some form of cancer during their lives. Figures for the USA show that in one year, 1994, twice as many people died from cancer as were killed in the Second World War.

The life and death of cells

There are an estimated 100 trillion cells in the human body, all of which are continually renewed, new ones being produced at the same rate as others die. For most of us the rates of cell formation and removal are so closely matched that we see no major change in the size of our organs throughout adulthood. In some cases, however, the total number of cells increases, because the control mechanisms fail and either new cells are produced at a faster rate than cells are dying, or cells are not dying as fast as they should.

This last statement sounds odd, but is very important. In general, cells do not simply get older and die slowly. They seem to be programmed so that after a certain length of time, or a certain number of cell divisions, a series of biochemical reactions causes the cell to die. Many cancers seems to occur

* David Alberts, in *Pharmaceutical News*, 1995, volume 2, p. 24.

because this process of 'cell suicide'* is faulty: cells do not die when they should. As new cells continue to be produced, the total number increases, causing cancer: the affected organs and tissues enlarge into a tumour (from the Greek word *tumor* meaning a swelling). As these grow and press on blood vessels and nerves, they may cause discomfort and pain. The growing tumour may secrete large amounts of chemicals which interfere with other organs such as the heart, brain, and liver. Parts may break away and begin growing in different regions of the body.[†]

Cancer

Types of cancer

Cancer can occur in any tissue. The words 'cancer' and the more usual medical word 'carcinoma' come from the Greek *karkinos* meaning 'crab'. This refers to the crab-like appearance of the roots of some tumours and the appearance of the swollen veins around the tumour. Cancers are often solid, such as those of the breast and lung. Leukaemia is a form of cancer in which the white blood cells multiply far beyond their normal numbers. Some forms of cancer, including some leukaemias and cancer of the testis, can be cured completely by drugs. Others, such as breast (Fig. 18.1), ovarian, and stomach cancer, can often be greatly reduced or controlled by drugs.

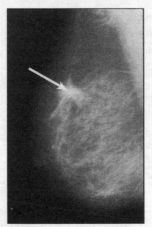 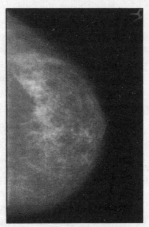

Fig. 18.1 A mammogram, indicating the presence of a breast cancer (showing as a solid area of the picture, indicated by the arrow). The normal breast from the same patient is shown on the right.

---

* This 'cell suicide' is called apoptosis.
[†] This spreading of tumours around the body is called 'metastasis'.

What controls cell division?

The processes which regulate the rate of cell death and match it precisely to the rate of new production are immensely complicated and are only now beginning to be understood. There are, for example, some genes called 'oncogenes' which can make cells divide more rapidly. In normal cells these are suppressed by other genes called 'tumour suppressor genes'.

The balance between these two types of gene is crucial in determining the number of cells in a tissue. If a tumour suppressor gene does not function correctly, then the oncogene which it should suppress is freed from control and may cause cells to grow and multiply beyond their normal numbers. The result is a tumour, in which the tissue cells divide out of control.

Half of all cancers are due to a defect in a tumour suppressor gene called p53. David Lane in Dundee, Scotland and Arnold Levine at Princeton, New Jersey, discovered this gene in 1985. It causes cells to commit suicide if they have been damaged beyond easy repair. If it is defective, cells do not kill themselves, but continue to grow and divide to form a cancer.

Viruses and cancer

Some cancers are caused by viruses. Many cases of cancer of the genitals, cervix, and anus are caused by the papilloma virus. *Helicobacter pylori* (*see* Chapter 4) can cause stomach cancer and some cases of liver cancer are due to the hepatitis B or C virus. Vaccination against hepatitis B has lead to a dramatic fall in the incidence of liver cancer in Taiwan. The viruses seem to damage the delicate control mechanisms of cells, inactivating tumour-suppressor genes or activating oncogenes. The result is a cancer which may be treated by the same range of drugs used in cancers which do not involve viruses.

The use of drugs to treat cancers

Paul Ehrlich's concept of selective toxicity (*see* Chapter 17)—the use of chemicals to kill foreign organisms without harming the infected animal—has been proved feasible when the invading organisms are made of cells very different from those of the host animal. The cells of bacteria and parasites have structures and molecular requirements very different from mammals, and the drugs discussed in Chapter 17 can damage or kill the invaders with much less effect on the human cells. Selective toxicity is far more difficult to achieve when the cells causing illness are derived from the body's own cells, as is the case in cancer. Many of the drugs used to kill cancer cells, therefore, will also damage the body's cells and produce marked and often unpleasant side-effects.

What are the main side-effects of anticancer drugs?

Those drugs which impair the ability of cells to divide will damage not only the cancerous cells, but also those of tissues in which normal cells are dividing rapidly. Cells are always dividing in the bone marrow to replace cells in the blood, so there is a danger that anticancer drugs may upset the formation of red and white blood cells, leading to anaemia, tiredness, bleeding, and an increased susceptibility to infection.

However, if anticancer drugs are used for short periods with a drug-free period in between, the bone marrow recovers much more quickly than most tumours. If drugs are delivered at suitable intervals the tumour cells can be killed with minimal toxicity to the blood cells.

Cells in hair follicles also divide frequently and anticancer drugs may stop this with the result that hair is lost. Hair growth usually resumes when treatment with the drugs is stopped.

Drugs used to treat cancers (Table 18.1, p. 294)

How do drugs work in cancer?

Because the main problem in cancer is that new cells are produced more quickly than old cells die, most anticancer drugs are designed to slow or stop cell growth and division. All cells contain genes made of DNA, very large and complicated molecules which consist of two separate chains of atoms joined at frequent intervals along their length. The individual strands of DNA are made by linking together many thousands of smaller molecules called nucleotides. Before a cell divides into two new cells, the two chains of DNA separate. The cell makes a new copy of each strand, giving two pairs of DNA molecules where there was previously one. The cell then divides so that each new daughter cell has one of the two DNA molecules.

The normal functioning of cells is programmed by their DNA. This is changed (translated) into molecules of messenger RNA (mRNA) by enzymes which line up nucleotides alongside the DNA chain and link them together (Fig. 18.2). The mRNA can then be used by the cell to produce new proteins for use as enzymes, or components of the cell wall. To achieve this the mRNA attaches itself to a large molecule in the cell called a ribosome. Amino acids are brought to the ribosome by molecules of transfer RNA (tRNA) and the ribosome links these amino acids together in the order determined by the mRNA. The result is a protein.

Many of the drugs used to combat cancer interfere with one or more stages in this sequence of reactions (Fig. 18.3).

Cross-linking agents* and cisplatin

Many of these drugs were developed from chemicals produced as agents of chemical warfare. In 1942 two American pharmacologists, Louis Goodman and

* Cross-linking drugs are often called 'alkylating' drugs.

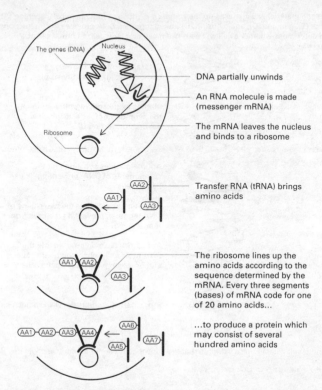

DNA partially unwinds

An RNA molecule is made (messenger mRNA)

The mRNA leaves the nucleus and binds to a ribosome

Transfer RNA (tRNA) brings amino acids

The ribosome lines up the amino acids according to the sequence determined by the mRNA. Every three segments (bases) of mRNA code for one of 20 amino acids...

...to produce a protein which may consist of several hundred amino acids

Fig. 18.2 How proteins are made by the genes.

Al Gilman at Yale University, were asked to test chemicals of possible use in chemical warfare. They showed that these compounds dramatically reduced the number of white cells in the blood, leading them to suggest that the drugs might be useful in treating leukaemias. Gustav Lindskog at Yale University soon showed them to be effective in clinical tests, although their use was limited by their high toxicity.

The first patient, a 48-year-old silversmith was dying from a cancer which virtually covered his chest and face. Two weeks after ten days of treatment with a drug code-named HN3, the tumour had disappeared. Unfortunately, it returned and subsequent treatments were less effective than the first, the patient eventually succumbing to the inexorable progress of the cancer.

Cisplatin was discovered accidentally after a series of experiments by Barnet

DNA is the material which makes up the genes. It is made of four chemicals, adenine (A), thymine (T), guanine (G), and cytosine (C) linked together. DNA provides the instructions which determines whether a cell will be a brain cell or a liver cell, a normal cell or a cancer cell

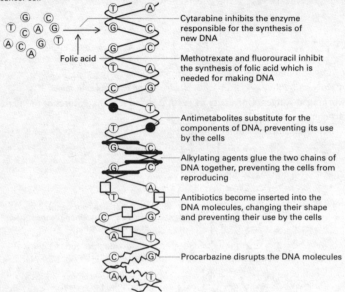

Cytarabine inhibits the enzyme responsible for the synthesis of new DNA

Folic acid — Methotrexate and fluorouracil inhibit the synthesis of folic acid which is needed for making DNA

Antimetabolites substitute for the components of DNA, preventing its use by the cells

Alkylating agents glue the two chains of DNA together, preventing the cells from reproducing

Antibiotics become inserted into the DNA molecules, changing their shape and preventing their use by the cells

Procarbazine disrupts the DNA molecules

The end result with all these drugs is that the cancer cells cannot multiply and will die

Fig. 18.3 How drugs can kill cancer cells.

Rosenberg and colleagues at Michigan State University in 1979. They had been studying the effects of applying an electric current to bacteria and noticed that the cells became longer. They correctly concluded that the current was preventing the cells from dividing, but detailed investigation revealed that the effect was due, not to the electric current itself, but to a chemical produced by interaction of the platinum electrodes and the solution containing the bacteria. Analysis of the effects of other platinum compounds eventually led to cisplatin, a drug widely used today to treat several cancers.

How do these drugs work?
The cross-linking agents and cisplatin stop cell division by binding tightly to the molecules of DNA so that the two strands become distorted and link together. They are bound together so tightly that the cell cannot separate them for reproduction or for the production of new RNA and protein molecules. The cell is unable to divide: cancer growth is stopped.

Two of the drugs in this class are cyclophosphamide and ifosfamide. Inside the body these are changed to another chemical, acrolein, which can damage cells in the urinary tract. They are, therefore, taken together with another drug, mesna, which combines with acrolein and prevents it from producing damage.

Toxic antibiotics

Several antibiotics prevent cells from forming RNA from DNA, so that the cell cannot produce new proteins. Actinomycin was the first of these to be discovered. Selman Waksman and one of his assistants, Boyd Woodruff, working at Rutgers University in 1940, isolated it from cultures of the yeast *Actinomyces*.

Actinomycin, doxorubicin, mitomycin, mithramycin, and bleomycin slide between the different groups of atoms in DNA, altering the shape of the DNA so that it cannot be copied into RNA. Some drugs in this group, such as doxorubicin and daunorubicin also interact with an enzyme in the cell wall* to produce 'oxygen free radicals' (*see* Chapter 22). These are very reactive molecules which damage the delicate structure of the complex nucleic acids and proteins, leading to the death of the cell. Bleomycin has a similar effect, producing reactive free radicals which cause the DNA molecules to split.

The antibiotics also inhibit an important enzyme in cell division called topoisomerase. This controls the shape and structure of the DNA molecules. The antibiotics interact with the enzyme in such a way that it becomes bound permanently to DNA and is no longer active. There are also two drugs, irinotecan and topotecan, which are very powerful and selective inhibitors of the topoisomerase enzyme.

Intercalating agents

The most important drug in this group is amsacrine. It works very like the toxic antibiotics. Amsacrine inserts (intercalates) itself between the components of RNA and DNA molecules, distorting them so that they cannot be copied. This prevents new nucleic acid synthesis and thus cell division.

Procarbazine

Procarbazine seems to have several actions on cancer cells. Like the cross-linking (alkylating) agents described above, it weakens the structure of nucleic acids, causing breakages and serious cell damage. It also leads to the production of free radicals inside cells, as do some of the antibiotics. The highly reactive free radicals interact strongly with nucleic acids and proteins and cause widespread damage to cancer cells.

* Cytochrome P450 reductase.

Folic acid antagonist

The rapid rate of reproduction of cancer cells means that they need a large supply of folic acid in order to make the chemical components (nucleotides) necessary for DNA and RNA synthesis. Methotrexate inhibits the enzyme which produces folic acid. The cells cannot then make the necessary nucleic acids and cell division stops.

Purine antagonists and antimetabolites

Purines are chemicals used by cells to make DNA and RNA. Mercaptopurine and thioguanine are molecules very similar in structure to the natural purines and they can interact with enzymes involved in making them. The cell's supply of purines is diminished, DNA and RNA synthesis cannot occur and cell division stops. These drugs are sometimes known as 'antimetabolites' because they act as antagonists of natural compounds (metabolites) in the cells.

Pentostatin inhibits the enzyme adenosine deaminase, needed for the supply of purine components of RNA and DNA. As the formation of purines is disrupted, cells become unable to divide.

Fluorouracil and cytarabine are converted inside cells to related chemicals which inhibit enzymes needed for the synthesis of new nucleotides and nucleic acids. As in the case of methotrexate, nucleic acid production cannot occur and cell division stops. Cytarabine can also be incorporated into nucleic acid molecules, making them fragile and easily damaged.

Vinca and related drugs

When a cell divides, the two sets of DNA chromosomes are pulled apart by proteins called microtubules. Several chemicals obtained from the periwinkle plant (*Vinca*), including vinblastine and vincristine, damage these proteins so that cell division cannot take place. The vinca alkaloids, as they are known, are components of several drug combinations which have been important in the increasingly successful treatment of childhood leukaemias and Hodgkin's disease.

A different chemical, podophyllotoxin from species of the tree *Podophyllum*, works in much the same way as the vinca compounds. It was discovered because indigenous American Indians used extracts of the plant for centuries to treat some types of wart. The Swiss pharmaceutical company Sandoz* attempted to develop a range of drugs related to podophyllotoxin and produced one which has proved valuable in the treatment of lung cancer. This is etoposide, but we now know that it does not work in the same way as podophyllotoxin. Etoposide inhibits topoisomerase (page 287) which is required for the correct

* Now Novartis.

maintenance and repair of chromosomal DNA. When it is inhibited, the genetic machinery of the cell is damaged irreparably.

Paclitaxel

Paclitaxel (Taxol) was isolated from the yew tree *Taxus brevifolia* after reports that extracts of the bark had beneficial effects in cancer. *Taxus brevifolia* is an endangered species, but the paclitaxel molecule is too complex to allow chemists to make it in the laboratory. The solution to obtaining supplies of paclitaxel has been to use the needles of the related western yew. From these, a very similar chemical can be extracted and then converted into paclitaxel in the laboratory.

Paclitaxel can be used in several types of cancer including lung, breast, and prostate cancers. It works in a manner similar to the *Vinca* alkaloids, interfering with the protein microtubules in the cell which pull apart the chromosomes before cell division. In the presence of paclitaxel, cells can no longer divide into two daughter cells, and the tumour gradually dies.

Hormones and antagonists

Steroids such as prednisolone, which are similar to naturally occurring steroid hormones and are used to treat inflammation (*see* Chapter 19), stop cell division by interfering with DNA synthesis. They can, therefore, also be useful in treating several types of cancer.

Combinations of drugs and other treatments

In many cases, despite increased vigilance on the part of patients and doctors, tumours may become quite large and well-established before they are detected. The cells in the middle of such tumours have a poor blood supply and their rate of multiplication is correspondingly slow. Drugs that stop cell division, nucleic acid, or protein synthesis will not have much effect on such cells. However, if the tumour is partially removed by surgery, or partly killed by radiotherapy (which penetrates throughout the tumour), the remaining cells will start to grow and divide much more rapidly, making them far more sensitive to drugs. A combination of drugs and other treatment is, therefore, often far more effective than either alone.

Thankfully, few patients nowadays have to suffer as did Sigmund Freud.* He was a heavy smoker of cigars and, as a result, developed cancer of the palate, for which he suffered thirty-one operations and a false roof to his mouth. One of the operations was a vasectomy, which was then believed to stimulate the production of rejuvenating hormones of the testis.

* As described by R. Gordon in *Ailments through the ages*.

Breast cancer

Some cancers require hormones for their growth and development. Cancer of the breast in some women, for example, is dependent on a supply of the female sex hormone, oestrogen. Tamoxifen and toremifene block the receptors for oestrogen on the tumour cells, depriving them of the steroid stimulus and causing the tumour to shrink. Drugs with actions similar to the natural hormone progesterone are sometimes used for breast cancer, as their effects tend to oppose those of oestrogen. They include gestronol, megestrol, medroxyprogesterone, and norethisterone.

Androgens are normally converted into oestrogens, and both types of hormone are present in women. Aminoglutethimide, formestane, letrozole, and anastrozole inhibit the enzyme 'aromatase' which brings about this conversion. Consequently they reduce the amounts of oestrogens in the body and reduce tumour growth. These drugs will slow the manufacture of steroids by the adrenal glands and so must be taken with replacement steroids.

Paradoxically, breast cancer in some post-menopausal women can be controlled by drugs which have the same effect as oestrogen. These include stilboestrol and ethinyloestradiol.

GRH analogues

Normally, the amount of sex hormones in the body is controlled by gonado-trophin-releasing hormones (GRH) secreted by the brain. Gonadrotrophin releasing hormones increase the production of sex hormones by the ovaries or testes. As the amount of sex hormone in the blood rises, the secretion of GRH is turned off, so that androgen and oestrogen production slows. Conversely, as the amount of circulating sex hormones falls, GRH is released again to stimulate the sex organs and restore the levels of sex hormones. Several drugs take advantage of this 'negative feed-back' system to control breast or prostate cancer.

The GRH analogues are drugs with molecules which resemble those of GRH so that they mimic its effects. When they are first given to patients, therefore, they activate the same receptors as GRH in the sex organs, increasing the quantities of sex hormones released into the bloodstream. Patients' symptoms may worsen for one or two weeks. As treatment continues, the target cells in the brain adapt by reducing the number of receptors for GRH. The effects of the drugs as well as those of natural GRH decline as a result. The sex organs receive little or no stimulation to secrete sex hormones, and the amounts in the body fall to very low levels. The prostate or breast tumour, no longer supported by sex hormones in the blood, shrinks.

Prostate cancer

In males, cancer of the prostate gland is often dependent on a supply of male sex hormones, the androgens such as testosterone. One successful, if undesirable, treatment is to remove the testes surgically, thus removing the body's source of androgens. An alternative is to use drugs to block the effect of the androgens. Such drugs include stilboestrol. Fosfestrol is a prodrug: it is converted in the body to stilboestrol.

Anti-androgens

Just as some breast cancers thrive on oestrogens in the blood, so some prostate cancers depend on the presence of male sex hormones, the androgens. One method of treatment, therefore, is to use drugs which block the receptors for androgens on the tumour cells. These are known as anti-androgens and include cyproterone, flutamide, and bicalutamide.

GRH analogues are also available for the treatment of prostate cancer, as described above for breast cancer.

Side-effects

The effect of blocking receptors for the male sex hormones inevitably results in a loss of some male characteristics. Impotence is common and patients may experience a loss of libido and enlargement of the breasts.

Drugs of the future

Among the most exciting drugs currently being developed are 'matrix metalloproteinase inhibitors' or MMPIs. As a tumour grows, it secretes enzymes (proteinases) which destroy the proteins which bind together the cells of the nearby tissue. This allows new blood vessels to grow into the tumour to supply it with blood. It also allows the tumour to expand more easily between the surrounding tissue cells, and helps to facilitate the breaking up of the tumour into smaller pieces which can travel around the body and invade other organs and tissues. This may result is tens or hundreds of small tumours (metastases) around the body. Once cancer has spread in this way, it is extremely difficult to trace and kill all the new tumours.

Scientists have been trying to produce drugs which inhibit these proteinase enzymes, slowing the growth and development of the cancer. Several are now being tested in clinical trials, including batimastat, a drug discovered by British Biotech Pharmaceuticals. So far, they have proved very promising in the treatment of a variety of cancers, including ovarian, gastric, and prostate cancers.

Tumours, like all collections of cells, need a supply of blood to bring oxygen and nutrients. Tumours facilitate the growth of blood vessels by secreting a hormone called vascular endothelial growth factor (VEGF). Antibodies to VEGF, or drugs which block its receptors are showing great promise in restricting or stopping the growth of tumours and in some cases limiting the blood supply sufficiently that the tumour cells die. Blood vessels in other areas of the body grow much more slowly than those in a tumour; they do not need VEGF and are little affected by the drugs. Two drugs have now been developed which stop the formation of blood vessels in tumours. These are angiostatin and endostatin and, when given together they have been able to achieve a complete inhibition of tumour growth and cause the death of all cells in the tumour.

Finally, it may be possible to produce drugs which cut off the blood supply to a tumour even when it has become established. The different types of cell in the body possess molecules in their walls which are unique to that cell type—heart muscle, stomach cells, skin cells, and so on. Similarly, tumour cells have their own, unique identifying molecules. Drugs can now be targetted to a specific type of tumour cell by linking them to antibodies or similar large molecules which seek out and attach only to these identifying molecules. If these 'magic bullets' are linked with molecules from the blood which normally trigger clotting, it is possible to encourage clots to form only in the blood vessels used by the tumour cells. Experiments on mice have shown that an approach of this kind can clot the blood inside a breast tumour within minutes, leading to the death of the tumour cells within 24 hours. This is an exciting new method for killing tumours about which we are likely to hear far more in the next few years.

Drug resistance

The problem of resistance to drugs, as discussed in Chapter 17 in connection with bacteria, is encountered with anticancer drugs. Even though most cells in a tumour may be killed by a drug, the proliferation of the surviving cells may include one which is not sensitive to the drug. That single cell can grow and multiply despite the drug, restoring the size and danger presented by the original tumour. This is why doctors try to use the highest possible doses of drugs, in addition to other approaches such as surgery to eradicate the tumour as completely and as quickly as possible, before any cells have a chance to adapt.

The mechanisms by which cancer cells become resistant to drugs are similar to those in bacteria (Chapter 17). The following, for example, are all features which contribute to resistance:

1. The cells stop producing the proteins which carry the drug into the cell. Drugs are normally imported into cells by a protein in the cancer cell wall, and resistance occurs when cells stop producing it.

2. Many cells can produce a protein called the 'P-glycoprotein multi-drug transporter'. As its name suggests, this sits in the wall of cancer cells and forms a pore through which many drugs are pushed out more quickly than they enter. This seem to be an important method by which some cancers become resistant to several different drugs.

3. The cells may produce an altered form of those proteins and enzymes which are the targets of the anticancer drugs.

4. The cells may produce larger amounts of those proteins or enzymes which are disrupted by the drug.

5. The blood supply to the middle of some solid tumours may be so small that drugs cannot penetrate well enough to kill the cancer cells.

6. The cancer cells produce more of the enzymes which repair damage to their molecules, producing repairs just as fast as the anticancer drugs can produce damage.

Table 18.1 Drugs used in the treatment of cancers

Alkylating agents	Vinca and related drugs	Drugs used in breast cancer
busulphan	etoposide	Aromatase inhibitors
carmustine	vinblastine	aminoglutethimide
chlorambucil	vincristine	anastrozole
chlormethine*	vindesine	formestane
cyclophosphamide	vinorelbine	letrozole
dacarbazine		
estramustine	**Taxanes**	**Oestrogen antagonists**
ifosfamide	docetaxel	tamoxifen
lomustine	paclitaxel	toremifene
melphalan		
mitobronitol	**Topoisomerase inhibitors**	**Progestogens**
mustine* (USA)	irinotecan	gestronol
streptozocin (USA)	topotecan	medroxyprogesterone
thiotepa		megestrol
treosulfan	**Other drugs**	norethisterone
	altretamine	
Antibiotics	carboplatin	**Oestrogens for post-menopausal breast cancer**
aclarubicin	cisplatin	ethinyloestradiol
bleomycin	crisantaspase	stilboestrol
dactinomycin	dacarbazine	
daunorubicin	etoposide	**GRH analogues**
doxorubicin	hydroxyurea	buserelin
epirubicin	paclitaxel	goserelin
idarubicin	pentostatin	leuprorelin
mitomycin	procarbazine	triptorelin
mitoxantrone	razoxane	
plicamycin	teniposide (USA)	**Drugs used in prostate cancer:**
	tretinoin	Oestrogens
Intercalating agents		fosfestrol
amsacrine		polyestradiol
		stilboestrol
Antimetabolites		
cladribine		**Anti-androgens**
cytarabine		bicalutamide
floxuridine (USA)		cyproterone
fludarabine		flutamide
fluorouracil		
gemcitabine		**GRH analogues**
mercaptopurine		buserelin
methotrexate		goserelin
raltitrexed		leuprorelin
thioguanine		triptorelin
trimetrexate (USA)		

* These are different names for the same drug

Summary

- *New cells are normally produced at the same rate as others die. Cancers occur when cells are produced too quickly or die too slowly.*
- *Most anticancer drugs exploit the fact that cancer cells grow and reproduce at a faster rate than normal cells. Drugs that interfere with the manufacture of DNA and proteins will, therefore, affect the cancer cells more than normal cells.*
- *Cross-linking drugs and cisplatin bind to the DNA molecules, distorting them so that the cell cannot copy them.*
- *The 'antibiotic' agents slide between the components of DNA, disrupting their structure.*
- *Drugs such as bleomycin produce highly reactive 'free radicals' which damage the DNA molecules. Procarbazine also works by producing very damaging free radicals.*
- *Some drugs interfere with the enzyme topoisomerase which is needed to maintain the normal shape of DNA.*
- *Methotrexate prevents cells from synthesizing folic acid, a compound essential for DNA synthesis.*
- *Purine antagonists and antimetabolites fool the enzymes into reacting with them instead of with natural chemicals and then prevent the enzymes from working.*
- *Vinca drugs and paclitaxel disrupt the cell proteins which move the chromosomes inside the cell and which are essential to cell division.*
- *Breast cancer can be treated with drugs which mimic the body's own female hormones and turn off the secretion of oestrogens which are needed for the survival of some breast cancers.*
- *Prostate cancer can be treated by a similar range of drugs which turn off the production of the male androgen hormones.*
- *Cancers can become resistant to drugs by developing processes to keep the drugs out of the cells or to eject them when they have entered. Cells may also produce more of the enzymes and proteins affected by drugs, so that the drugs become less effective.*

CHAPTER 19

Steroids

Charles Slocomb and Howard Polley injected 100 mg of cortisone into a rheumatoid patient who had proved refractory to many previous therapeutic experiments and who had refused to go home until he had been used as a 'guinea-pig' for yet another trial. The results were spectacular. The pain relief and functional benefits were of a different dimension from those achieved in previous trials. Equally spectacular results were obtained on three other specially selected patients in the same ward. Extraordinary events occurred; thus one of their totally bedridden patients was able to get out of bed and attempt to dance, another took seven baths in one day to compensate for the baths she had missed. Sadly, when the supplies ran out a week later all the patients relapsed completely but Slocomb and Polley were convinced they were on to an important breakthrough.*

That was in September 1948, only just over fifty years ago. The sample of cortisone that was available to Slocomb and Polley at the Mayo Clinic in Minnesota had been produced by the pharmaceutical company Merck and was the result of over a decade's research to isolate and identify hormones produced by the adrenal glands. Interest in the adrenals had in turn been triggered by Philip Hensch, at the Mayo clinic in Rochester, Minnesota, who had observed in 1929 that patients with rheumatoid arthritis improved greatly if they developed jaundice or when they became pregnant. He proposed that this was a result of the stress induced by these conditions and that the adrenal glands, known to be important in the body's response to stress, might be involved. The hunt was on for the body's natural antidote to arthritis.

The early work on the isolation of hormones from the adrenal glands was carried out by the Ukrainian (later Swiss) scientist Tadeusz Reichstein at the Federal Institute in Zurich and Edward Kendall at the Mayo clinic in the USA. They began to isolate a whole new family of hormones—the steroid hormones—from the adrenals. One of these was cortisone, which they identified in 1935. Hensch, Kendall, and Tadeusz shared the Nobel Prize for Medicine in 1950.

* From *The discovery and early use of cortisone* by J. Glyn. *Journal of the Royal Society of Medicine*, vol 91, pp. 513–517 (1998).

The adrenal steroids

The adrenal glands sit on top of the kidneys (hence their name—'ad-renal'). They consist of two parts, an inner medulla and an outer cortex. The medulla secretes the hormones epinephrine and norepinephrine (*see* Chapter 1). The adrenal cortex secretes several hormones which have a common basic molecular structure and are known as steroid hormones. They are also produced from cholesterol (*see* Chapter 15) which is in turn synthesized by the adrenal cells.

The adrenal hormones include aldosterone and cortisol (also called hydro-cortisone) and have two types of action. Firstly, they help to regulate the amounts of minerals, such as sodium and potassium, in the body. Aldosterone mainly affects the mineral balance and is called a mineralocorticoid* (*see* Chapter 5).

Secondly, the adrenal steroids control the levels and use of glucose, and are important in the recovery from inflammation and stress. Cortisol mainly affects glucose metabolism and is known as a glucocorticoid.* The drugs used in medicine are designed to have almost pure mineralocorticoid or pure glucocorticoid activity, thus reducing side-effects as a result of unwanted actions.

What are the effects of glucocorticoid hormones?

The adrenal steroids are secreted in response to stress and one of their main actions is to increase the amount of glucose in the blood so that the body can respond immediately to danger.† They do this by increasing both the release of glucose from the liver and the breakdown of protein in muscles and other tissues. They also suppress the formation of new tissue such as muscle and bone.

Inflammation may occur when a tissue is damaged and invaded by bacteria. White blood cells then leave the blood and enter the affected area, where they kill and destroy the invaders. In the process, however, they also produce chemicals called 'mediators' which were described in Chapter 2, such as prostaglandins, leukotrienes, cytokines, and platelet activating factor. These can cause further damage to the tissue as well as causing reddening and pain. A similar series of events occurs when the white cells attack normal cells in what is called an 'auto-immune' disease. Rheumatoid arthritis (*see* Chapter 20) is one such disease in which the mediators damage the tissues of the joints and bones.

In normal amounts, steroids maintain the body's response to inflammation and normal activity of the immune system. In larger doses—those used by doctors—they have the opposite effect and suppress the inflammatory and immune processes.

---

* The term corticoid is a shortened form of adrenal cortex steroid, or corticosteroid.
† This is also an important role of the adrenal medullary hormone epinephrine (*see* Chapter 1); the adrenal glands have evolved as a whole to provide an integrated response system in times of danger.

How do the steroids work?

In all these conditions, the steroids act on receptors inside cells (*see* Chapter 1) to alter the manner in which the genes produce mediators. They reduce the rate at which the mediators can be produced and secreted by white cells. They also increase the production in cells of a protein, 'lipocortin', which inhibits the production of some of the mediators. Some of the steroids can reduce the rate at which white blood cells are produced so that their overall number in the blood falls and the ability to produce inflammation is correspondingly lowered.

Uses of steroids

The adrenal cortico-steroids are used to suppress the inflammation associated with disorders such as rheumatoid arthritis (*see* Chapter 20), asthma (*see* Chapter 2), and eczema. They are also taken to suppress rejection by the immune system following organ transplantation. Once the immune system recognizes a transplanted organ as foreign, the white cells attack and destroy it. Steroids reduce the activity of the immune system so that this does not occur.

Side-effects

Because the steroids have so many actions, their use for one reason is often accompanied by side-effects resulting from their other actions. For example, when they are used in high doses to control severe inflammation, the increased levels of glucose in the blood may lead to diabetes. Also, the conversion of proteins into glucose causes a loss of muscle strength and destruction of bone, leading to osteoporosis and an increased risk of bone fractures. The depression of the immune system also increases the risk that the patient may be unable to handle infection by bacteria or viruses. If the steroids used have mineralo-corticoid activity, too much sodium may be lost in the urine (*see* Chapter 5) resulting in an increase of blood pressure.

Patients taking steroids for several years are also more likely to develop eye problems such as glaucoma and cataracts and to develop personality changes as a result of effects on the brain. A useful effect of steroids on the brain is to induce euphoria—a 'feel-good' effect which may help patients who are trying to cope with chronic, painful conditions such as arthritis. Taking them in high doses, however, can lead to very abnormal, manic, over-excitable behaviour which is difficult for the patient to control.

Stopping the steroids

In general, if a drug has been taken for longer than a few weeks, it should not be stopped suddenly because the body will have adjusted to the drug's presence. This is particularly important for patients taking steroids.

The amount of natural steroids produced by the adrenal glands is normally controlled by the level in the blood. If the amount of circulating hormone increases, secretion by the adrenal decreases; if blood levels fall, secretion increases. This is a 'feed-back' system which should keep the levels of steroids in the blood constant.* Administration of steroid drugs decreases the production of the natural hormones in the body and the adrenal glands tend to shrink over a few weeks. If a patient ceases to take steroids suddenly, the adrenals will be unable to secrete their natural steroids. He or she may die if then exposed to stresses or simple infections which would not have been a problem if the adrenals had been working normally.

Patients must decrease the dose of steroids slowly; it may take up to a year for the adrenal glands to regain their normal level of activity.

Addison's disease

In Addison's disease, named after the London physician Thomas Addison (1793–1860), the adrenal glands are not producing enough steroids to maintain the patient in normal health, resulting in a greatly increased susceptibility to infection together with marked loss of weight and often a large fall in blood pressure which may lead to shock (*see* Chapter 15). It can be treated by a combination of a glucocorticoid and a mineralocorticoid (usually hydrocortisone plus fludrocortisone) which replace the steroid hormones that are absent in these patients.

Sex steroids

Like so much modern biology, our knowledge of the sex hormones dates back little more than fifty or sixty years. It was only in 1933 that the German scientist Ernst Laqueur isolated the main male hormone, testosterone. He managed to obtain 5 milligrams—about as much as a grain of salt—from one ton of bulls' testicles.

At about the same time several scientists including Alfred Butenandt in Gottingen, Willard Allen in America, and Adolf Wettstein and Max Hartmann in Switzerland obtained a hormone from female ovaries which could prevent abortion and permitted pregnancy. Because it maintained gestation, this hormone was called pro-gesterone.

Male sex hormones

The hormones which determine our sexual characteristics have very similar molecules to the glucocorticoids—they are also steroids. The male sex

---

* This feed-back is mediated by the brain. The steroids in the blood control the production of a peptide hormone called adrenocorticotrophic hormons (ACTH) by the pituitary organ in the brain. It is this which then regulates the secretion of steroids by the adrenal glands.

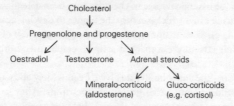

The steroids are inter-related. they are all made in the body from cholesterol

Cholesterol
↓
Pregnenolone and progesterone
↙   ↓   ↘
Oestradiol   Testosterone   Adrenal steroids
↙   ↘
Mineralo-corticoid   Gluco-corticoids
(aldosterone)   (e.g. cortisol)

Fig. 19.1 The relationships between the body's steroid hormones.

hormones are called androgens (from the Greek *andro*, meaning man, and *genes*, to be born). The most important of them is testosterone, produced mainly by cells in the testes, although some is also secreted by the adrenal glands. Like the glucocorticoids, it is made from cholesterol by a series of enzymes (Fig. 19.1). At puberty, changes in the brain result in the secretion of gonadotrophic hormone (GH) which stimulates the testes to produce testosterone. This then produces the changes, such as hair and beard growth, enlargement of the penis and prostate gland, development of the testes and initiation of sperm production, deepening of the pitch of the voice, and the body and muscle development which turn a boy into a man.

Uses of androgens

The most common use of androgens is to replace the natural hormones when the testes are not functioning correctly, or if they have been surgically removed for the treatment of testicular cancer. Androgens can also be used to treat some forms of breast cancer, although we do not fully understand how they work, and they are not very effective. Because they build up muscles, androgens are useful in some diseases in which the muscles waste away because of disuse, such as muscular dystrophy.

Anabolic steroids

The process of building up and developing tissues such as bone and muscle is called 'anabolism' and these effects of the sex steroids are known as 'anabolic' effects.

The idea of using male sex hormones to build up body tissues is usually ascribed to two Austrian scientists, Fritz Pregl and Oskar Zoth. In 1896, they injected themselves with extracts of bulls' testes and measured the effects on the strength of their fingers.

The effects of male hormones on the pitch of the voice and hair growth are known as the masculinizing, or androgenizing effects. By creating molecules very similar to the natural androgens, chemists have been able to separate these actions, producing drugs which can help the tissues to develop again after long and debilitating diseases, major accidents, or surgery. Because of the absence of masculinizing effects, these anabolic steroids can be used both by male or female patients.

In recent years, the anabolic steroids have been widely abused by athletes wishing to build up muscle tissue for competitions. They are, however, sufficiently different from the natural steroids that they can be detected in very small quantities in the blood or urine so that cheating in competitions can be deterred.

Baldness (alopecia)

The use of drugs such as finasteride to reduce enlargement of the prostate gland has been described in Chapter 5.

Testosterone is converted into another chemical, dihydrotestosterone, which is believed to be the chemical partly responsible for male pattern baldness. Finasteride inhibits the enzyme which makes this conversion and has proved successful in treating baldness. It is likely that this drug will be available soon on prescription for the treatment of baldness.

Anti-androgens

The anti-androgens prevent the production of androgens or block their receptors, the overall result in either case being to reduce the activation of androgen receptors throughout the body. Anti-androgens are, therefore, used to treat disorders in which there is an abnormally high level of androgens in the blood, causing excessive hairiness (hirsutism) or baldness in women.

Enlargement and cancer of the prostate gland

Enlargement of the prostate gland and cancer of the prostate are often caused by, or maintained by, testosterone, so anti-androgen drugs may be used to reduce the enlargement and to slow or stop the growth of a cancer. The two most common drugs used are cyproterone and flutamide.

Since the production of testosterone by the testes is promoted by GH secreted by the brain, drugs can also be used to suppress GH production. These include leuprolide, buserelin, and goserelin. They act on the brain to prevent the release of GH and the secretion of testosterone and they can, therefore, be used to treat cancer of the prostate when this is fed by the presence of testosterone.

Finasteride prevents the conversion of testosterone into dihydrotestosterone. The latter is a more potent androgen than testosterone itself and is more important than testosterone for the development of the prostate gland. Finasteride is used to lower the amount of dihydro-testosterone in the prostate and to stop enlargement of the gland and the development of prostatic cancer.

Testosterone as a contraceptive?

One might imagine that, in the search for a male oral contraceptive, drugs which block the effects of testosterone and stop sperm production would be good candidates. Unfortunately such drugs tend to trigger the development of female characteristics (*see next section*) and impotence, which rather defeats the purpose of having a contraceptive in the first place.

Paradoxically, one of the compounds with most promise as a male contraceptive is testosterone itself. Large doses depress the production of GH by the brain so that the testes reduce in size and sperm production stops. The main problem with testosterone treatment is that it does not stop sperm production in all men and sometimes does not stop it completely. It is, therefore, too variable and unreliable to be the sole form of contraception. There are also fears that prolonged use of testosterone at high doses may increase the risk of cancer of the prostate gland.

The use of progestogens as male contraceptives is described at the end of the chapter.

Androgens and sport

Some athletes have misused androgens, taking them to increase muscle mass and strength and to increase the amount of haemoglobin in the blood (which then carries more oxygen, reducing fatigue). The doses used, however, have many long-term effects, causing shrinkage of the testes, and increasing the risk of cancer of the prostate gland. They also decrease the amount of 'good' cholesterol (HDL) (*see* Chapter 15) in the blood, which increases the risk of atherosclerosis and heart attacks.

Side-effects of steroid drugs on the sex organs

Several of the drugs mentioned in this book have side-effects which are a result of their acting on steroid hormone receptors. Cimetidine is an antagonist at H2 receptors for histamine and is used to control stomach and duodenal ulcers (*see* Chapter 4). It can also weakly block the receptors for testosterone. The diuretic drug spironolactone (*see* Chapter 5) and the antifungal drug ketoconazole (*see* Chapter 17) prevent the conversion of the female hormone progesterone into testosterone (Fig. 19.1), increasing the amount of progesterone in the blood.

A decrease in testosterone in the blood also causes the brain to produce more GH, which tries to restore the synthesis of testosterone. In doing so, it increases the production of oestradiol. Together, the increased amounts of progesterone and oestradiol can cause enlargement and tenderness of the breasts in women and some 'feminization' of males, with the development of breasts. Since testosterone is needed to maintain the external male sex organs, these drugs may also cause impotence.

Female sex hormones

The female sex hormones are of two groups. The first are called oestrogens* (from the Greek *oistros*, meaning a frenzy or climax and referring to the fact that most animals show periods of being 'on heat' (oestrus) when they are receptive to male attention). The oestrogens† are steroids made by cells in the ovaries which are activated by hormones produced in the brain at puberty. From that time until the menopause a cycle persists, the menstrual cycle, lasting about 28 days, which is determined by the levels of oestrogens in the blood (Fig. 19.2). The oestrogens are also produced by cells in muscles, liver, and fat.

The second group of female hormones are the progestins, or progestogens. They prepare the uterus to receive a fertilized egg and help to maintain

The level of sex hormones in the blood is controlled by the brain. Two brain hormones, FSH and LH promote the production of sex hormones by the ovaries and testes. As the amount of sex hormone increases, it turns off the production of FSH and LH. In this way the levels in the body are kept roughly constant.

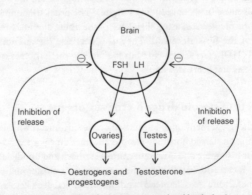

Fig. 19.2 How the levels of steroid sex hormones are regulated by the brain.

* The American spelling of these is 'estrogens', with the individual hormones estradiol, estrogen etc.

† The main estrogens are estradiol, estrone and 17β-estradiol.

pregnancy once it has begun. They also prevent the uterus from contracting before the baby is ready to be born.

The female hormones are responsible for the transformation of a girl into a woman at puberty, causing development of the uterus (the womb), vagina, and external sex organs and initiating the formation of glandular tissue in the breasts. They also cause the deposition of fat in the buttocks, breasts, and thighs, generating the classical female shape, and increase the ratio of 'good' cholesterol (HDL) to 'bad' (LDL) (see Chapter 15). The latter effect partly accounts for the fact that women are less likely than men of the same age to develop atherosclerosis (hardening of the arteries) and to suffer a heart attack.

Uses of oestrogens

The female sex steroids are used as hormone replacement therapy (HRT) either after removal of the ovaries for cancer, or after the menopause. They can reduce some menopausal symptoms, such as hot flushes, and the bone loss which leads to osteoporosis. This subject is dealt with specifically in Chapter 21.

A potentially very important use of oestrogens is in the treatment of Alzheimer's disease. Some doctors noticed that elderly women with Alzheimer's disease, and receiving hormone replacement therapy, showed fewer signs of dementia than before treatment. As a result, oestrogen treatment has been tried with moderate success in a large number of women with dementia. This seems to be a result of oestrogens having several effects on the brain which increase the survival of nerve cells. The adrenal glucocorticoids can damage brain cells if they are present in large amounts for many months, but oestrogens oppose these effects. The oestrogens also increase both blood flow to the brain and the release of the transmitter acetylcholine, which is important for our ability to learn and remember and to think clearly (see Chapter 10). We may eventually see female sex hormones being introduced widely into medicine to slow and perhaps even to reverse some of the signs of Alzheimer's disease and other dementias.

Anti-oestrogens

Drugs such as clomiphene and tamoxifen block the receptors for oestrogens and are used to treat infertility and breast cancer.

Infertility

The production and release of ova (eggs) by the ovary is controlled by hormones known as gonadotrophins. These are secreted by a part of the brain known as the pituitary body. Their secretion is in turn controlled by the amount of oestrogens in the blood: as this increases, gonadotrophin hormone (GH)* production is suppressed. Conversely, as the level of oestrogen falls, gonadotrophin production increases.

This feed-back system can be harnessed to treat women unable to have children because of inadequate stimulation of the ovaries. The drug used is clomiphene. It blocks the effects of oestrogens on the brain, so that the production of gonadotrophins rises and stimulation of the ovaries increases. Many women have benefited from this drug, although the occasional cases in which the ovaries are overstimulated, leading to the birth of three, four, or more babies, tend to hit the news headlines.

Cancer

Some breast cancers depend on the presence of oestrogens for their survival. Anti-oestrogens such as tamoxifen are used to block the receptors for oestrogens and to reduce the growth of the cancer (see Chapter 18).

Contraceptives

The most widespread uses of oestrogens and progestogens are as oral contraceptives—'the contraceptive pill' or often just 'the pill'. Their ability to act as contraceptives is related to the actions of the sex steroids in regulating ovulation—the production and release of an egg.

The discovery of oral contraceptives

In 1950 Gregory Pincus, director of the Institute for Experimental Biology Worcester, Massachusetts, was awarded a small sum of money to try to develop an orally active contraceptive. Since the rise in progesterone levels which maintained pregnancy was believed to prevent further ovulation during this period, Pincus tried giving large doses of progesterone to several rabbits. None of them became pregnant. Several pharmaceutical companies had been producing chemicals related to the natural oestrogens and progestogens in an attempt to develop compounds which could be used to treat disorders ranging from infertility to cancer.

Pincus obtained samples of many of these new chemicals from the companies concerned and soon had several which were more potent and more effective than progesterone itself.

Clinical trials began with one of these, norethynodrel, in Puerto Rico in 1956. By 1958, it was clear that of 221 fertile women on the trial none had become

* The gonadotrophic hormones (GH) are the same in men and women. One is called Luteinizing Hormone (LH). The second is known as Follicle cell Stimulating Hormone (FSH) in women and Interstitial Cell Stimulating Hormone (ICSH) in men to reflect their different actions in promoting development of the ovarian follicles in women and the sperm-producing interstitial cells of the testes in men.

pregnant while taking the drugs. Of several women who had stopped taking the pills, on the other hand, several had become pregnant, indicating that their effects were reversible and that no harm came to the mothers or to their babies. As a result, the American company G. D. Searle launched the first oral contraceptive pill in 1960.

How do the oral contraceptives work?

The menstrual cycle and ovulation

The normal process of ovulation and menstruation is controlled by cyclical changes in the amounts of the female sex hormones in the blood (Fig. 19.2). Normally, the levels of oestrogens and progestogens depress the release of GH (FSH* and LH*) by the brain. Immediately after menstruation the amount of sex hormone is too low to affect the release of GH so that the production of FSH increases and stimulates the development of follicles in the ovary (Fig. 19.3). The follicles are fluid-filled sacs, each of which contains an ovum or egg. As the follicles develop, the largest begin to produce one of the oestrogens—oestradiol. When the amount of oestradiol in the blood is high enough it increases the production of LH which causes the follicle to rupture, releasing its egg into the fallopian tubes on its way to the uterus.

The ruptured follicle becomes the 'corpus luteum' which secretes progestogens to prepare the uterus for receipt and implantation of a fertilized egg. If fertilization does not occur after 14 days, the corpus luteum shrinks, production of progesterone declines, and the thickened lining of the uterus is shed during menstruation. Both oestrogens and progestogens affect amine transmitters such as norepinephrine and 5-hydroxytryptamine (5HT) in the brain. These affect mood and emotional responses (see Chapter 11). The loss of the sex hormones about the time of menstruation probably accounts for the premenstrual behavioural and mood changes experienced by some women (pre-menstrual tension, PMT).

If pregnancy does occur, the placenta begins to secrete another hormone called human chorionic gonadotrophin (HCG), which prevents the corpus luteum from disappearing and maintains the levels of progesterone. This in turn allows the pregnancy to continue.

Oral contraceptives

The 'combined' pill

The contraceptive pill consists of one or more compounds which are similar to the natural sex hormones. It produces a hormonal balance resembling that of early pregnancy. The two drugs together act on the brain to suppress the release of GH and thereby prevent development of the ovarian follicles and ovulation.

* See footnote on p. 306.

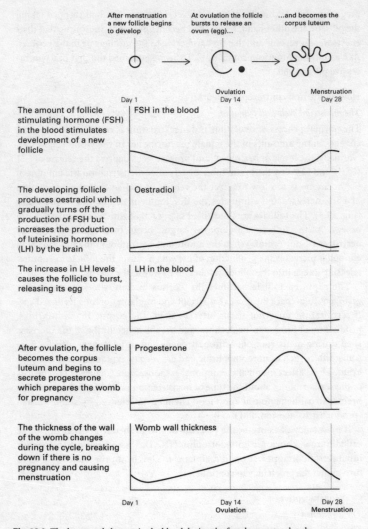

The amount of follicle stimulating hormone (FSH) in the blood stimulates development of a new follicle

The developing follicle produces oestradiol which gradually turns off the production of FSH but increases the production of luteinising hormone (LH) by the brain

The increase in LH levels causes the follicle to burst, releasing its egg

After ovulation, the follicle becomes the corpus luteum and begins to secrete progesterone which prepares the womb for pregnancy

The thickness of the wall of the womb changes during the cycle, breaking down if there is no pregnancy and causing menstruation

Fig. 19.3 The hormonal changes in the blood during the female menstrual cycle.

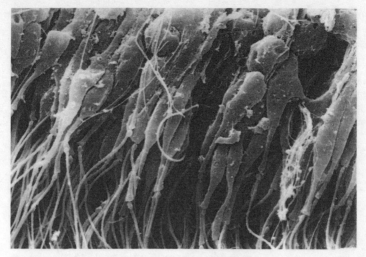

Fig. 19.4 Spermatozoa lining the walls of the testes (magnified approximately 1000 times). (Professor A P Payne)

The pill comes in two varieties. The 'combined' pill contains an oestrogen and a progestogen.

Most packs of contraceptive pills consist of 28 tablets, 21 of which contain the drugs responsible for suppressing ovulation, while the remaining 7 contain an inactive substance. After the first 21 days the levels of drug in the blood falls, causing the uterine lining to be shed as it would during the normal cycle.

Side-effects

Women taking the combined pill may experience weight gain, breast tenderness, reduced libido, headaches, and nausea. The oestrogen content of the pill also increases the risk of thrombosis (blood clotting) (*see* Chapters 14 and 16), while the progestogen content alters the ratio of fats in the blood such that there is a greater risk of atherosclerosis leading to thrombosis and heart disease. However, the overall effects on blood clotting are less than those of pregnancy itself, during which the levels of female hormones are far higher than achieved by the pill. Of every 100 000 women during pregnancy, 60 will develop thrombosis in a vein. Of 100 000 women taking the pill, only about 15 will be affected. This compares with 5 who would be affected when they are neither pregnant nor taking the pill.

Another problem with the pill is its effects on cancer of the breast. The pill increases the chance of developing breast cancer. This risk falls after stopping the pill: ten years after stopping the cancer risk is no greater than in women who have never taken the pill. On the bright side, cancer of the breast which does occur in women who have taken the pill tends to be less advanced and more localized (and therefore easier to treat) than in other women. The pill also seems to decrease the risk of cancer of the ovaries or uterus.

In older women, in whom the risks of thrombosis and cancer are greater, and in women susceptible to blood clotting for other reasons, the progestogen-only pill, sometimes known as the 'mini-pill', is usually preferable.

The 'mini-pill'

The mini-pill contains only a progestogen. This does suppress ovulation in about 25 per cent of women, but its main contraceptive effect is to increase the amount and thickness of the mucus layer which covers the cervix and which acts as a barrier to penetration by sperm. This form of contraception is not as reliable as the combined pill, and there may be irregular bleeding which some women find unacceptable.

The 'morning-after' pill

After unprotected sexual intercourse pregnancy can often still be prevented by taking what has become known as the 'morning after' pill. This is actually a course of two or three tablets containing high doses of oestrogen with or without a progestogen. These must be taken as soon after intercourse as possible and certainly no later than 72 hours afterwards. The effect of this high-dose combination is to stop any imminent ovulation and to alter the state of the uterus so that it cannot accept a fertilized egg. The method is, therefore, one of preventing pregnancy, not of aborting an embryo which has implanted and is growing in the uterus.

The morning-after pill usually causes nausea and vomiting.

The 'abortion' pill

There is also a pill which can induce abortion. This contains the drug mifepristone,* an antagonist at the receptors for progesterone. Progesterone prepares and maintains the uterus for implantation and pregnancy. Mifepristone blocks the effects of progesterone, so causing an early embryo to be rejected by the uterus. A dose of mifepristone is usually followed by a prostaglandin such as misoprostol which causes contractions of the uterus and helps to expel the foetus.

Menstrual disorders

Some women experience heavy and painful periods (called dysmenorrhoea). During the first 21 days of a cycle of contraceptive pills, the degree of thickening

* This drug was formerly known as RU486.

of the uterus wall is much less than during a normal menstrual cycle, so the amount of bleeding is usually quite light. The combined contraceptive pill, therefore, is often prescribed to women who wish to reduce both the amount and the discomfort of their periods.

Contraceptive injections

In addition to the oral contraceptives, some steroids are available for injection, giving protection against pregnancy lasting from a few weeks to several years.

A female hormone as a male contraceptive

The administration of progestogens to men acts on the brain to suppress the release of GH. This leads to loss of testicular function and a cessation of sperm production so these drugs can be used as a male oral contraceptive. They work well and are likely to be available in the near future. Their main drawback is that the lack of testicular function is accompanied by a fall in the production of testosterone. Men wishing to retain their normal physical characteristics and sexual activity will need to take testosterone, probably in the form of injections which last several weeks or months.

Table 19.1 Drugs affecting the steroid hormones: adrenal steroids and sex hormones

Glucocorticoids	GH analogues for infertility and prostate cancer
beclomethasone	buserelin
betamethasone	gonadorelin
cortisone*	gosarelin
deflazacort	leuprorelin
deoxycortone	nafarelin
dexamethasone	triptorelin
fludrocortisone	
hydrocortisone*	**Oral contraceptives**
methylprednisolone	*Combined contraceptives*
prednisolone	*low dose:*
prednisone	ethinylestradiol + norethisterone (Loestrin 20)
triamcinolone	ethinylestradiol + desogestrel (Mercilon)
Female sex hormones	*standard dose:*
dydrogesterone	ethinylestradiol + levonorgestrel (Eugynon®; Logynon®, Microgynon®, Ovran®, Ovranette®, Trinordiol®)
hydroxyprogesterone	
ethinylestradiol	
medroxyprogesterone	ethinylestradiol + norethisterone (BiNovum®, Brevinor®, Loestrin 30®, Norimin®, Ovysmen®, Synphase®, TriNovum®)
norethisterone	
progesterone	
progestogens	
tibolone	ethinylestradiol + norgestimate (Cilest®)
	ethinylestradiol + desogestrel (Marvelon®)
Anti-oestrogens	ethinylestradiol + gestodene (Femodene®, Minulet®, Triadene®, Tri-Minulet®)
clomiphene	
danazol	
gestrinone	*high dose:*
tamoxifen	ethinylestradiol + levonorgestrel (Ovran®, Norinyl-1®, Ortho-Novin®)
Male sex hormones	
danazol	*Progestogen-only ('mini-pills')*
mesterolone	ethynodiol
	levonorgestrel
	norethisterone
Anti-androgens	
cyproterone	
finasteride	**Contraceptive injections**
	levonorgestrel
Anabolic steroids	medroxyprogesterone
nandrolone	norethisterone
stanozolol	

* These steroids also have mineralocorticoid activity.

Summary

- *Steroids are a group of hormones with a similar molecular structure (the steroid nucleus) and are made in the body from cholesterol.*
- *The adrenal glands produce a mineralo-corticoid hormone, aldosterone, which regulates urine formation (see Chapter 5), and gluco-corticoids such as cortisol.*
- *The hormones or drugs derived from them are used to reduce inflammation by suppressing the formation of 'mediators'.*
- *The main side-effects are a suppression of the immune system, increasing susceptibility to infections.*
- *The male sex steroid, testosterone, maintains muscle mass and male characteristics.*
- *Drugs which block the receptors for testosterone are used to slow the growth of prostate cancer.*
- *The female sex hormones control ovulation, menstruation, and pregnancy.*
- *They are used to replace the natural hormones after the menopause (hormone replacement therapy, HRT).*
- *Drugs which block oestrogen receptors reduce the growth of some breast cancers.*
- *Drugs similar to the female hormones are used as oral contraceptives. They work by suppressing ovulation.*

CHAPTER 20

Rheumatic diseases

Rheumatic diseases affect about 10 million people in the UK in one form or another and 50 million in the USA. Only 1 person in 50 will escape some form of rheumatic complaint. 1 child in every 1000 suffers from a juvenile form of the disease. Rheumatic diseases form about 20 per cent of the workload of a general physician. Arthritis is responsible for around 100 million lost working days each year in the UK alone.

What are 'arthritis' and 'rheumatism'?

Rheumatism is a general term, used more by patients than by doctors, to refer to aches and pains arising from the muscles and joints. Arthritis (from the Greek word *arthron* for a joint and *-itis* indicating 'inflammation of') refers to inflammation of a joint from any cause. To many patients, the diagnosis of arthritis suggests a progressive and possibly crippling disease, but this is not necessarily the case; to doctors the word simply means inflammation of a joint.

Rheumatoid arthritis affects about 1 per cent of the population to some degree but only about 1 in 200 women and 1 in 600 men are seriously affected. It can occur at any age and in any part of the world. In severe cases the joints may become progressively damaged, causing serious disability, but many cases are mild and settle completely after a few years.

There are approximately two hundred different types of rheumatic disease (diseases of the joints and associated tissues such as muscles and bone), and these fall into four groups: inflammatory arthritis, osteoarthritis, soft tissue rheumatism, and back pain. Drugs are used in all four groups and, although they cannot *cure* most rheumatic conditions, they can usually control the symptoms. In many cases they can modify the severity of the disease and its progression, allowing patients to live a much more comfortable and normal life than would otherwise have been the case.

The normal joint

At the ends of bones there is a smooth layer of cartilage* which acts as a shock absorber when we move and jump about. Surrounding the joint between two

* Cartilage is the tissue often referred to as 'gristle' in meat.

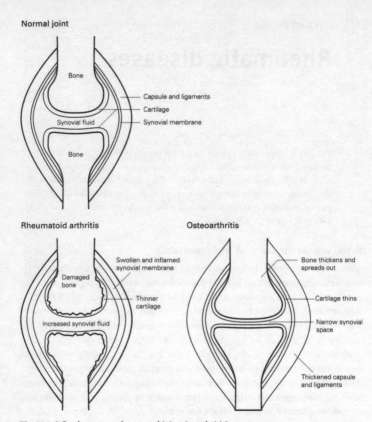

Fig. 20.1 What happens to bones and joints in arthritis?

bones there is a membrane called the synovial membrane which produces a viscous fluid—synovial fluid—to nourish and lubricate the cartilage (Fig. 20.1). Around this is a thicker capsule of ligaments which helps to keep the bones stable and in place relative to each other. Outside the ligaments are tendons which attach the muscles to the bones.

Inflammatory arthritis

Rheumatoid arthritis

Rheumatoid arthritis is an autoimmune disease, which means that the immune system begins to treat the joints as foreign, producing antibodies to some of

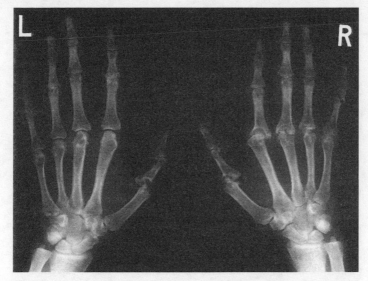

Fig. 20.2 An x-ray picture of the hands of a patient suffering from rheumatoid arthritis. The left hand is much less affected and spaces can easily be seen between the bones at the major joints. In the more severely affected right hand, there is almost no space between the bones of the fingers and the bones have been badly worn away.

the cells in the joint. The reason why this happens is unknown. As cells in the joints are attacked by the antibodies, white cells from the blood begin to enter the joint and secrete chemicals known as cytokines. These can cause the gradual destruction of cartilage and, as this is lost, the bone underneath may also be eaten away and damaged. X-rays may then show damage as pits on the surface of the bones (erosions) (Fig. 20.2).

Since rheumatoid arthritis is primarily a disease of the immune system, there are often other signs of immunological activity. These can include pain and stiffness in and around the joints, tiredness, a general feeling of being unwell (malaise), weight loss, and night sweats. There may also be some swelling of the joint, a reduced ability to move it, muscle weakness, mild fever, and skin rashes. Because immune cells circulate in the blood to all tissues, rheumatoid arthritis sometimes affects many parts of the body in addition to the joints, including muscles, tendons, eyes (dry eyes), nervous system, lungs, and heart. Blood tests often show raised levels of inflammation and of an antibody called rheumatoid factor. This is present in 80 per cent of rheumatoid arthritis patients but is also found in some normal people.

Although some patients may inherit a genetic tendency to develop rheumatoid arthritis, the disease is not transmitted simply from parent to offspring. There are probably other factors needed to trigger the disease in susceptible people. During pregnancy the levels of steroids, such as cortisone (*see* Chapter 19) rise and their anti-inflammatory action often causes a remission of arthritis symptoms. As soon as the baby is born, however, the steroid levels fall immediately and may cause the symptoms to worsen considerably. Even diet can have a major impact on the severity of the symptoms, some patients becoming free of symptoms completely with a suitable change of diet. The changes needed vary enormously from patient to patient and need to be tailored individually.

Drug treatment of rheumatoid arthritis (Table 20.1, p. 333)

Pain

Painkillers are an important part of the treatment of rheumatic diseases, since reducing pain allows patients to remain mobile and improves their overall quality of life. The pain of arthritis can be controlled with analgesics (*see* Chapter 6). Mild pain is controlled by mild analgesics such as paracetamol, moderate pain requires codeine-containing analgesics or dextropropoxyphene, whereas more intense pain may require dihydrocodeine or more powerful drugs in the opioid group, such as buprenorphine.

Non-steroidal anti-inflammatory drugs (NSAIDs)

Inflammation symptoms can usually be controlled by non-steroidal anti-inflammatory drugs, NSAIDs, which were described in detail in Chapter 6. Some 300 million people each year around the world regularly take an NSAID at a cost of US $13 billion in 1998. These drugs, including ibuprofen and diclofenac, can reduce joint swelling and stiffness in addition to relieving pain. They do not modify the disease process itself but they control symptoms, showing benefit after a few days of treatment with a maximum effect in around four weeks. Non-steroidal anti-inflammatory drugs work by inhibiting the COX enzyme and this produces the beneficial anti-inflammatory effect (COX-2 inhibition) (*see* Chapter 6). However, they carry the disadvantage of irritating the stomach, leading to possible ulceration and bleeding (COX-1 inhibition).

Since the NSAIDs are often used at relatively high doses in rheumatoid arthritis, indigestion and gastrointestinal irritation are common side-effects and drugs may be needed to protect against them. Histamine receptor antagonists help to heal gastric and duodenal ulcers as a result of reducing gastric acid output by blocking H2 receptors (*see* Chapter 4). The proton pump inhibitors omeprazole, lansoprazole, and pantoprazole (see Chapter 4) also inhibit gastric acid secretion by blocking the acid-secreting enzyme system (the 'proton pump') of the parietal, acid-producing cells in the stomach. Misoprostol protects against both duodenal and gastric ulcers by stimulating prostaglandin receptors to reduce acid secretion (see Chapter 4) and increase the formation of the protective lining of the stomach. However, it can cause diarrhoea and abdominal pain by increasing movements of the bowel, and it should not be used by women who could become pregnant as it may stimulate contractions of the womb.

Since they inhibit blood clotting, NSAIDs should not be used by people taking anticoagulant drugs because their combined effects may lead to spontaneous bleeding. By interfering with COX, the NSAIDs stop the formation of prostaglandins, hormones which are important for the initiation of labour and childbirth. They can, therefore, delay the onset and increase the duration of labour and should not be used by women in the later stages of pregnancy. The inhibition of COX also results in the increased formation of a group of chemicals called leukotrienes which contract the airways and could trigger, or worsen, an asthma attack in susceptible people.

All these effects of NSAIDs are discussed in more detail in Chapters 6 and 16.

COX-2 inhibitors

Since the anti-inflammatory effects of NSAIDs are produced by inhibition of COX-2, while most of the side-effects are due to inhibition of COX-1 (see Chapters 6 and 16), newer drugs have been produced which affect only COX-2. Such drugs as meloxicam, etodolac, and rofecoxib have good antiinflammatory effects and less effect on the stomach than the traditional NSAIDs.

In the first two weeks after the launch of the COX-2 inhibitor, celecoxib, (Celebrex®) from G. D. Searle and Company in the USA in 1999, almost 100 000 prescriptions were written by doctors, making it the second fastest-selling new drug in history (behind Viagra®, see Chapter 23). More of these preferential COX-2 inhibitors, which should be much safer and yet more effective than the current NSAIDs, are likely to be marketed in the near future.

Slowly acting anti-rheumatic drugs (SAARDs)*

These are more powerful drugs which can suppress the symptoms of arthritis. Some of them suppress the disease process itself, so reducing the amount of joint damage.* For this reason it is often better to take them soon after a diagnosis of arthritis to try to prevent joint damage from developing. SAARDs act rather slowly (hence the name), becoming effective only after treatment for one to six months. They help around 70 per cent of patients.

* These drugs are sometimes known as disease-modifying anti-rheumatic drugs (DMARDs).

SAARDs fall into two categories: the immunosuppressive agents which include azathioprine, methotrexate, cyclophosphamide, and cyclosporin, and a miscellaneous group (gold compounds, d-penicillamine, hydroxychloroquine, and sulphasalazine).

Immunosuppressive drugs

The immunosuppressive drugs are drugs which suppress the activity of the immune system. They are sometimes necessary to control progressive arthritic disease, especially when this is resistant to other treatments, but the blood needs to be monitored carefully for signs of toxicity.

Methotrexate

If NSAIDs are not effective enough to control the arthritis, or if a rapid response is needed, one of the best drugs is methotrexate. A single weekly dose of methotrexate often produces improvement after 4–6 weeks.

Methotrexate inhibits the synthesis of DNA, preventing the division and multiplication of immune cells. It does so by inhibiting activity of the enzyme* which produces tetrahydrofolic acid (see Chapter 18) and folic acid supplements are sometimes needed to avoid folic acid deficiency. NSAIDs can interfere with the effects of methotrexate and should not be taken at the same time (for example, for a headache) unless they have been prescribed by a doctor.

Azathioprine

Azathioprine is useful both for early rheumatoid arthritis and for systemic lupus erythematosus (SLE) (see page 328). It is converted in the body into a chemical called mercaptopurine which then suppresses the immune system by interfering with the synthesis of DNA in the white blood cells, preventing cell division (see Chapter 18). The main side-effects are caused by the drug inhibiting the multiplication of other cells which are dividing rapidly such as those of the bone marrow and liver. It should not be taken during pregnancy, since it may cross the placenta and disturb the rapid cell division in the growing foetus, causing damage and abnormalities.

Cyclophosphamide

Cyclophosphamide also prevents cell division by causing permanent chemical changes (alkylation) in the DNA of the genes (see Chapter 18).

Cyclosporin

Cyclosporin is a fungal metabolite and a powerful immunosuppressant which is used to prevent the rejection of tissues after organ transplantation. In

* Dihydrofolate reductase.

rheumatoid arthritis it suppresses the release of the inflammatory cytokines which cause the destruction of cartilage and bone.

Gold compounds

Towards the end of the 1800s, it had been discovered that metal ions such as arsenic and copper were able to kill some bacteria. The German bacteriologist Robert Koch, at the German Health Office in Berlin, was experimenting with a variety of other metals and their derivatives in order to identify better compounds with antibacterial activity suitable for using in animals and patients. In 1890 he found that compounds of gold and cyanide were among the most effective substances at killing the tuberculosis bacillus. However, perhaps because of its esoteric nature, no-one developed this observation until 1924 when another compound of gold, sodium aurothiosulphate, was tested in Denmark and shown to be suitable for the treatment of tuberculosis in cattle. As a result, a Dr Lande in Germany tested a related chemical, aurothiglucose, in 39 patients who were suffering from fevers he believed were due to bacterial infections. In fact, most of them were experiencing fever associated with arthritis and the most clearcut result of this trial was the discovery that aurothiglucose reduced the joint pain. From this time, tests of gold compounds gradually expanded until a definitive double-blind, placebo-controlled clinical trial was conducted by Sir Thomas Fraser in Glasgow in 1944. The result was clear: 82 per cent of the arthritic patients treated with aurothiomalate obtained relief from their symptoms.

Gold aurothiomalate is now given as an injection into a muscle. A small test dose is injected at first, followed by larger doses until there is improvement. An oral form of gold, auranofin, is a little less powerful than the aurothiomalate injections but also has fewer side-effects and is certainly more pleasant and convenient to take.

As yet, we do not understand how the gold compounds work, although they reduce the multiplication of white blood cells involved in the immune response, and decrease their secretion of free radicals (see Chapter 22) and cytokines which are believed to cause much of the damage to the joints.

d-Penicillamine

Penicillamine was first used for its antirheumatic effect in the 1960s. It is a safe and effective drug in about 70 per cent of rheumatoid arthritis patients, but again we do not know exactly how it works. It seems to combine with metal ions* inside cells, inhibiting those chemical reactions which lead to the formation and release of damaging free radicals. An unusual side-effect of

* A phenomenon known as 'chelation' (from the Latin *chele* meaning a claw).

d-penicillamine is a loss of taste. This is the result of the drug combining with zinc ions, which are needed for the normal sensory activity of the taste buds.

Although it is similar to penicillin, patients with an allergy to penicillin can usually take penicillamine quite safely.

Antimalarial drugs

Although the drugs hydroxychloroquine and chloroquine are usually used to treat malaria (*see* Chapter 17), they are also used for rheumatoid arthritis and systemic lupus erythematosus (SLE) (see page 328). They need to be taken for three to six months before any benefit is felt. They do not cause many side-effects, but they can damage the retina of the eye and any visual symptoms should be reported to a doctor.

The antimalarials work partly by reducing the movement of white blood cells into the area of joint inflammation. Secondly, they reduce the production of free radicals and cytokines by the white cells. Thirdly, they reduce the formation of prostaglandins and related hormones which increase the sensitivity of nerve endings to painful stimuli (*see* Chapter 6). Finally, the molecules of hydroxy-chloroquine and chloroquine can insert themselves (intercalate) (*see* Chapter 18) into the molecules of DNA, suppressing cell division of the immune cells. The overall effect is to suppress many of the symptoms of rheumatoid arthritis and SLE.

Sulphasalazine

Sulphasalazine is broken down by bacteria in the large intestine to produce sulphapyridine and 5-aminosalicylic acid. Sulphapyridine seems to be the more active of these molecules in rheumatoid arthritis, reducing division of the white blood cells. 5-Aminosalicylic acid combines with (scavenges) any damaging free radicals produced by white cells inside the joints. It may damage cells in the bone marrow and kidneys and it causes a fall in sperm count which causes a decrease in male fertility. This usually returns to normal when the drug is stopped.

Corticosteroids

The discovery of the beneficial effects of steroids in arthritis was described in Chapter 19. In 1949, corticosteroids were first shown to reverse the symptoms of rheumatoid arthritis. They suppress inflammation more rapidly than SAARDs and, when given at the same time as SAARD therapy, the symptoms of arthritis are reduced much more quickly. The mechanisms by which steroids work, and some of their side-effects, are described in Chapter 19.

Steroids were once used in high doses for long periods, and patients developed severe side-effects such as a rounded or 'moon' face, easy bruising, obesity, high blood pressure, diabetes mellitus, osteoporosis, thin skin, cataracts, indigestion, stomach ulcers, and an increased tendency to suffer from infections. Some patients, hearing of these problems, may be afraid to take steroids even when they could help to control their inflammatory arthritis safely and effectively, and could perhaps also protect against joint damage. Nowadays, however, steroids are used more carefully and in much smaller doses than previously, so side-effects are far fewer and the overall benefits much greater.

Prednisolone is the steroid most commonly used to treat rheumatoid arthritis and related diseases. It is available as tablets but can be used as an injection into the muscles, veins, or into the joints themselves to obtain the most rapid control of the inflammation. Steroid tablets are usually taken once each day in the morning, with food, to prevent irritation of the stomach. This timing also enables them to fit in with the body's own daily rhythm of steroid production.

Immunizations which involve live viruses, e.g. polio and German measles (*Rubella*) should be avoided by patients taking steroids, because the steroid-induced suppression of the immune system may allow the live viruses to cause illness. Similarly, people taking steroids should avoid contact with anyone suffering from chicken pox or other infections which are very unpleasant and potentially dangerous in adults, as they are more likely to become infected. If they are aware of such contact they should report to their doctor immediately since special protective treatment may be needed.

It is always best not to take any drugs when pregnant but, if steroids are needed and a woman becomes pregnant, steroids are safer than some other anti-rheumatic drugs. Rheumatic disease itself can damage an unborn baby since the activated white blood cells are releasing increased amounts of injurious chemicals such as free radicals, cytokines, and prostaglandins. Uncontrolled rheumatic disease may, therefore, be more damaging to the growing embryo than a low dose of a suitable medication.

Taking steroids should never be stopped suddenly because, as described in Chapter 19, they suppress the body's production of natural steroids. If the natural steroids are suddenly needed to maintain resistance to disease, any exposure to illness or infection can then be much more dangerous.

Biologics

A new group of drugs—the 'biologics' are being developed. These are produced using molecular biology methods and are designed to affect the biochemical pathways which cause inflammation of the joints. Two of the cytokine hormones secreted by white cells, and which cause damage to the joint tissues, are tumour necrosis factor-alpha (TNFα)* and interleukin-1-beta (IL-1β).

* As its name suggests this protein was first discovered as a compound which inhibited tumour growth. It is now known to have a number of other effects which have little to do with tumours.

These are large proteins, and molecules have been isolated or made which interact with them and prevent them from having any effect on the joints. These are 'antitumour necrosis factor alpha' (anti-TNFα) and 'interleukin-1β receptor antagonist' (IL-1βra). It will take time to assess these new treatments in a large enough number of patients, but at present they look interesting and exciting.

Other treatments

Acupuncture has been used to treat pain by trying to stimulate the release of endorphins—the body's own pain-relieving hormones (*see* Chapter 6). Synoviorthesis is a technique in which radioisotopes are injected into joints. This method has been controversial, but some patients who have failed to respond to other treatments seem to improve, particularly when only a limited number of joints is involved. The method has been claimed to produce a prolonged remission of joint inflammation for several years with a slowing of joint destruction. Other forms of therapy are useful in inflammatory arthritis: rest should be used during flares of the disease, with renewed exercise and activity when the flare subsides, to maintain strength and mobility. Physiotherapy and occupational therapy can help to build up muscles and to protect against joint contractures.

Antidepressants

Antidepressants such as amitriptyline and dothiepin (*see* Chapter 11), are frequently used in rheumatoid arthritis, because they have several useful actions. Not only do they help to lift the mood of patients, but they also encourage and improve sleep at night and dull the appreciation of pain by the brain.

Other forms of arthritis

There is a group of rheumatic conditions which tend to occur in families and in which there is inflammation of the spine and joints. They include ankylosing spondylitis, Reiter's syndrome, reactive arthritis, gonococcal arthritis, arthritis associated with inflammatory bowel disease, psoriatic arthritis, and certain forms of juvenile chronic arthritis. Collectively they are known as the 'seronegative spondyloarthritis group' of disorders. There is no rheumatoid factor in the blood but there are often changes in non-joint tissues, including inflammation of the prostate glands (prostatitis), iris (iritis), and conjunctiva (conjunctivitis) and, sometimes, lung and heart problems.

Ankylosing spondylitis (AS)

Ankylosing spondylitis* (AS) is the most important cause of inflammatory back pain, responsible for this in 1–2 per cent of white populations. It is more common in men than in women and usually begins in young adult life with back pain and morning stiffness. There may be inflammation of the joints at the back of the pelvic area† and, in 20 per cent of cases, inflammation of larger joints, such as shoulders and knees. As the disease progresses, movement of the spine and rib cage may be reduced, with stiffness caused first by inflammation and later by deposition of calcium in the ligaments surrounding the spine. As stiffness increases, pain is usually reduced and physiotherapy and exercises are required to help to prevent bending of the spine and to keep the body in the best possible position.

Some patients may be predisposed to AS by inheriting a protein‡ from their parents. This protein, which occurs on white blood cells, is found in 7 per cent of normal European people but 95 per cent of patients with AS. People with this protein may be more susceptible to other factors in the environment which trigger the disease.

Mild forms of AS are common and may cause very little disability. Juvenile spondarthropathy affects teenage boys and often causes arthritis of hips, knees, or ankles. It may persist into adulthood, when it becomes ankylosing spondylitis.

Treatment of AS

The most useful drugs for AS are the NSAIDs (see Chapter 6). One of these, phenylbutazone, was once used frequently but an annual blood test is now needed to detect any developing bone marrow toxicity. Sulphasalazine can suppress AS in more severe cases and azathioprine can suppress joint but not spinal inflammation. Radiotherapy was once used in severe cases but is rarely used nowadays because of the small risk of leukaemia. Surgery is sometimes needed, particularly for hip replacement.

Reiter's syndrome

Hans Reiter (1881–1969) was a German medical officer on the Balkan Front with the 1st Hungarian Army. In 1916 he described the case of a young lieutenant who had diarrhoea and developed arthritis together with inflammation of the urethra (urethritis), and conjunctivitis. Although this combination of symptoms is still known as Reiter's syndrome the condition had first been reported a century earlier by Sir Benjamin Brodie (1783–1862)

---

* The name derives from Greek words meaning stiffening (ankylosing) and inflammation of the spine (spondylitis).

† The sacroiliac joints.

‡ Known as human leukocyte antigen—B27. (HLA-B27)

in a textbook entitled *Diseases of the bones and joints* (1818). Reiter's syndrome follows an infection from the intestine (for example, with *Salmonella, Shigella, Campylobacter,* or *Yersinia* bacteria), or urethra. Most cases occur in young adults, men being twenty times more likely to have the condition as women.

Treatment

NSAIDs can be taken or steroids injected into the affected joints but, in some cases, sulphasalazine or azathioprine are needed. The antibiotic tetracycline reduces the urethritis, and eye symptoms can be treated with anti-inflammatory eye drops. Although the acute arthritis usually settles within a few months, about half of patients have long-term joint, spine, or eye inflammation.

Other forms of arthritis

Gonococcal arthritis consists of arthritis of a few large joints following infection with gonorrhoea. Gonococcal organisms are found in the genitourinary tract in most cases and the arthritis is treated with antibiotics, to clear the infection, and with NSAIDs and analgesics to suppress the inflammation and pain. *Reactive arthritis* is the commonest form of arthritis in young men and is the result of infection but without micro-organisms being found in the joints.

Psoriasis is a common, scaly skin rash which often affects the elbows and knees. One in ten patients may also inherit the tendency to develop an inflammatory arthritis—*psoriatic arthritis*—which usually affects the small joints of the hands. The treatment of psoriatic arthritis is with analgesics, NSAIDs and, in progressive cases, with sulphasalazine, methotrexate, or azathioprine.

Lyme disease is caused by the micro-organism *Borrelia burgdorferi* and is spread by tick bites. The symptoms include various forms of arthritis. Most patients with Lyme disease are cured by antibiotics.

Septic arthritis is inflammation of a joint caused by the presence of live micro-organisms inside the joint. It usually affects just one joint, with redness, swelling, severe pain, and signs of generalized illness such as fever and malaise. Septic arthritis tends to occur in the very young and the elderly and in those whose immune system is not working correctly (such as people taking immunosuppressive drugs, patients with rheumatoid arthritis, and those with AIDS). This form of arthritis is best treated with the correct antimicrobial drugs (*see* Chapter 17).

Osteoarthritis

Osteoarthritis is the commonest type of arthritis, occurring in about 20 per cent of the population as a whole and in 50 per cent of people over sixty years of age. It usually begins after the age of 50, though it can appear as early as age

30. It is twice as common in women as in men and is much more common in white than in black populations.

In osteoarthritis (which is also known as osteoarthrosis, arthrosis, and degenerative joint disease), the surface of the joint is damaged and there is an abnormal reaction in the underlying bone. It is probably caused by biochemical abnormalities of the cartilage, made worse by mechanical problems such as trauma or previous inflammatory joint disease. The cartilage, which normally acts as a 'shock-absorber', then becomes worn and thin, so that the bone underneath is less protected and becomes thicker. The disease progresses slowly over the years and occurs most in the weight-bearing joints such as the knees. As the bone thickens, spikes of bone (osteophytes) grow out from the joint edges, and the joint membranes usually becomes inflamed with extra synovial fluid production making the joint swell slightly.

A certain amount of osteoarthritis is common, especially as people grow older, with about five million people affected in the UK and 30 million in the USA. It may cause very little trouble, but severe osteoarthritis is a major problem for many people which may seriously threaten mobility and quality of life. It is characterized by joint pain and stiffness, often with reduced movement, a creaking noise on movement and, sometimes, by joint deformities. Losing weight will help by reducing the load on the affected joints, and physiotherapy will build up the muscles around them.

Treatment

At present there is no specific drug treatment to control the disease process but analgesics (*see* Chapter 6) help to control pain, as do NSAIDs, particularly when osteoarthritis is accompanied by a degree of joint inflammation. Injections of steroid into the joint itself may also be valuable.

Hylans

A new concept in the treatment of osteoarthritis is the use of hylans. These are lubricating substances injected directly into the knee joint—a process called 'visco-supplementation'. The idea is that the injected substance will lubricate, protect, and absorb shocks, while reducing sensitivity to pain and restoring knee mobility in a way similar to the natural synovial fluid in the knees of healthy young people. These substances have great potential but their value in osteoarthritis is still being assessed by doctors.

Soft tissue rheumatism

Soft tissue rheumatism applies to several related conditions in which musculo-skeletal pain arises not from bones or joints but from the soft tissues around them, such as the tendons. They include conditions such as 'tennis elbow' and 'housemaid's knee'. These are not threatening conditions and they usually settle with time. Most can be treated with local injections of steroids rather than by anti-inflammatory drugs.

Fibromyalgia is associated with widespread pains in muscles and their connections onto the tendons. There may be a psychological component to the condition, which is accompanied by sleep disturbance and soft tissue tenderness at painful trigger points. Local steroid injections at these trigger points often helps, together with drugs such as amitriptyline to improve sleep.

Polymyalgia rheumatica (PMR), which means many (poly-) muscle pains (-my-algia), often strikes suddenly and almost always in people over fifty years of age. It is characterized by pain and stiffness of the shoulders and hips and the muscles of the thighs and upper arms, usually with high levels of inflammation detectable on testing the blood. The cause is not known.

Fortunately, corticosteroid therapy (*see* Chapter 19) using moderate doses of prednisolone will usually make the symptoms disappear very quickly. PMR normally burns itself out after a few years and the steroids can then be withdrawn at a rate which keeps the symptoms well controlled, but with minimal side-effects.

Connective tissue diseases

This group includes three diseases: systemic lupus erythematosus (SLE), systemic sclerosis, and polymyositis with dermatomyositis. The cause of these conditions is unknown but they all have abnormalities of immunological function, with arthritis and inflammation of blood vessels (vasculitis) in many different parts of the body.

Systemic lupus erythematosus (SLE)

This is the commonest of the connective tissue diseases and affects around one person in every thousand. The female to male ratio is about 9 to 1 and SLE is much more frequently found in black women in the USA. The cause is unknown, but the symptoms include arthritis. Other tissues may also be affected, mainly as a result of the inflamed blood vessels which supply them. Skin rashes are common and are often made worse by exposure to light, while the tissues lining the heart and lungs can become inflamed, causing chest pains and discomfort or difficulty with breathing.

Mild cases can be treated with NSAIDs to reduce the inflammation and analgesics (*see* Chapter 6) to control the pain. For moderately severe disease the antimalarial drug hydroxychloroquine (see above) is useful if NSAIDs and analgesics do not work sufficiently well on their own. For more severe disease, corticosteroid therapy may be needed, usually in small doses for short courses, to suppress the disease with as few side-effects as possible. In the most severe cases, immunosuppressive drugs such as azathioprine, chlorambucil, and cyclophosphamide are used, particularly to treat kidney disease and usually in combination with corticosteroids. They may also allow the doses of steroids to be kept to a minimum, reducing the problems of side-effects.

Polymyositis with dermatomyositis

Polymyositis is a muscle disease with damage, inflammation, and degeneration of muscles. In patients who also have a skin rash the condition is known as dermatomyositis. Those afflicted exhibit muscle weakness and wasting, with muscle pain and tenderness, and joint pains or arthritis are present in about half of the cases. The cause of these diseases is not known. Steroids are normally used for treatment; a high dose of prednisolone at first, slowly reduced to a level that can be maintained for several months or years.

Back pain

Back pain is extremely common and varies greatly in severity. In most countries of the world 1 in every 100 people lose some time from work each year because of back pain. Drug treatments for back pain vary according to the cause of the pain; antibiotics are used to treat spinal infections (*see* Chapter 17), chemotherapy, or radiotherapy for malignant diseases of the spine (*see* Chapter 18), NSAIDs and occasional steroid injections for inflammatory conditions (*see above* and Chapter 6), and analgesics to relieve the pain of mechanical back problems (*see* Chapter 6). All are usually used in conjunction with rest, corsets, physiotherapy, and occasionally, surgery.

Gout

Gout has been known for thousands of years and can be one of the most painful forms of inflammatory arthritis (Fig. 20.3). It can run in families and occurs in six out of every thousand men and one in every thousand women, primarily those who are post-menopausal. It is rarely found in children or premenopausal women and does not occur in eunuchs. This suggests that male hormones are associated with gout while female hormones protect against it.

Gout is a disorder frequently associated with rich living and above average intelligence: Julius Caesar and Alexander the Great are both believed to have suffered from it. It can, however, be found in teetotallers and people who are certainly not rich. The belief that too much red meat and alcohol can cause gout has been disproved, but the idea of an association with decadent living

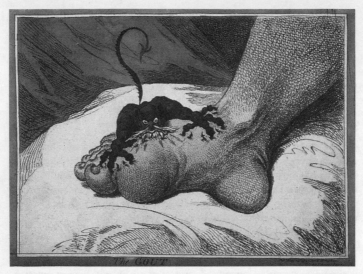

Fig. 20.3 An eighteenth-century etching conveying the devilish 'exquisite agony' of a sufferer with gout of the foot.

probably arose from the fact that a diet rich in protein and alcohol and a tendency to obesity will make attacks of gout more likely. This is because the chemical responsible for gout—uric acid—is produced by the destruction of proteins. The more protein consumed, the more uric acid will be produced and the greater the chance of gout. The incidence of gout in the UK was at its lowest level during World War I and II, when food was often in short supply.

What causes gout?

Gout is usually characterized by severe, inflammatory arthritis in one joint, often the big toe. It is usually associated with raised levels of uric acid in the blood. The level in blood is a balance between the quantity we produce and the quantity we excrete. Uric acid is the breakdown product of protein and is carried in the blood in quite large quantities until the blood becomes saturated and tiny crystals of uric acid or its salt, monosodium urate, are precipitated out of the blood and deposited in joints and tendons. Wherever they are deposited these crystals set up an inflammatory reaction because white blood cells invade the tissues to try to engulf the uric acid crystals and digest them as alien particles. In doing so, they release inflammatory chemicals (such as prostaglandins and cytokines) which produce the classical, severe, inflammatory reaction of acute gout. The condition is very painful—indeed it is often described as 'exquisitely' painful. Acute gout frequently occurs in joints which have been traumatized, so most cases of gout appear first in the bunion joint of the foot since, when walking, human beings push on that joint in order to push forward as they walk.

Gout can occur as a result of treatment with diuretic drugs (see Chapter 5), some of which raise the levels of uric acid in the blood, or kidney damage because the uric acid cannot be excreted in the urine.

Drug treatment of acute gout

Non-steroidal anti-inflammatory drugs (NSAIDs)

Acute attacks of gout are usually treated by NSAIDs, (see earlier and Chapter 6) which reduce pain and suppress inflammation. Medicines which contain aspirin should be avoided since, at the doses usually taken for aches and pains (one or two 500 milligram tablets), it can raise uric acid levels by competing with uric acid for excretion by the kidney. As a result, aspirin may encourage attacks of gout.

Colchicine

Although there is clear evidence that the meadow saffron plant (or autumn crocus, *Colchicum autumnale*) has been used medicinally for over 2000 years, it was not until 1552 that the German botanist Hieronymus Tragus first officially documented its use by Arabian physicians for the treatment of gout. From then it was used increasingly for this purpose, often in a concoction known as *Eau Medicinale*, despite its rather poisonous nature. Eventually, in 1820, the French chemists Pierre-Joseph Pelletier and Joseph Caventou at the Ecole de Pharmacie in Paris, managed to isolate the chemical responsible for the antirheumatic activity, calling it colchicine. Although colchicine can be quite poisonous if taken in doses larger than those prescribed by doctors, most of the poisonous property of the meadow saffron is due to another chemical, veratrine, which stimulates nerve fibres, causing excitement, convulsions, and death.

Colchicine in medicinal doses, however, has proved to be a safe and valuable drug which can help in both the diagnosis and treatment of gout at the same time. If a patient has an attack of inflammatory arthritis, which may or may not be gout, they may be asked to take one colchicine tablet every two hours for one day. If the arthritis is improved by the colchicine it is usually gout—a very useful test for a patient which simultaneously cures his or her symptoms. Colchicine is remarkably effective in abating an acute attack of gout. 'A patient who is in helpless agony with a tumefied, red, hot joint is sufficiently relieved so that he can walk about in a few hours'.*

* From *The pharmacological basis of therapeutics* by A. G. Goodman, 1985, p. 709.

Colchicine works by suppressing the activity of the white cells that engulf the uric acid crystals, preventing the release of inflammatory hormones and the development of the full-blown attack of gout. It inhibits the white cells by disrupting complex molecules within the cells known as microtubules. These form part of the 'cytoskeleton'—a system of interconnecting large molecules which act rather like muscles and give the white cells their ability to move around the body. When the cytoskeleton is damaged the white cells cannot move into the joints. Equally, microtubules are needed by those white cells already in the joint to move the inflammatory cytokine and other molecules to the cell surface from where they can be released into the joint. Disruption of the microtubules prevents this release.

Steroids

Occasionally, steroids such as prednisolone (*see* Chapter 19) can be taken by patients whose gout is slow to respond to treatment with NSAIDs, or a severely painful joint may need to be injected directly with steroids. Steroids should be taken as early as possible and as soon as a patient begins to feel the symptoms, since this may prevent the development of the very painful full attack.

Preventative therapy of gout

Preventative therapy for gout is completely different. The pills which help to prevent gouty attacks are of *no value at all* in treating an acute attack, and can sometimes make it *worse*. The main aim of preventative treatment is to control the levels of uric acid in the blood so that uric acid will remain in solution in the blood and not crystallize out in the tissues to provoke an acute attack of gout. There are several drugs which will do this, the best known being allopurinol, probenecid, and sulphinpyrazone. These all lower uric acid levels in a few weeks. On stopping these drugs, uric acid levels begin to rise again and gouty attacks may occur once more.

Allopurinol

Allopurinol is the drug used most commonly to lower uric acid levels in the blood. The final stage in the breakdown of proteins into uric acid is brought about by the enzyme xanthine oxidase. Allopurinol inhibits this enzyme, causing less protein breakdown and the formation of less uric acid. It is used in people who are producing urate at an abnormally high rate, leading to high blood levels and the deposition of crystals in tissues, crystallization in the bladder or kidney to form kidney stones,* and frequent, acute attacks of gout.

It is an effective, safe drug with few side-effects but it may take weeks or months to become fully effective. During this time it should be taken together

* Kidney stones can be formed as crystals of uric acid or of calcium (*see* Chapter 5).

with an NSAID to avoid triggering an attack of acute gout. After a while, when the risk of producing acute attacks of gout has passed, the NSAID may be stopped and the allopurinol continued alone.

Probenecid and sulphinpyrazone

As urine is being produced in the kidney (*see* Chapter 5), some of the uric acid in it is re-absorbed back into the bloodstream by a transporter enzyme. Probenecid and sulphinpyrazone inhibit the transporter, preventing reabsorption of uric acid and increasing the rate at which it is excreted in the urine. If the levels of uric acid are high enough, crystals of uric acid may precipitate in the urine, potentially causing damage to the kidneys. The best way to prevent this is to drink plenty of water when taking these drugs to ensure that uric acid remains in solution and is excreted.

Table 20.1 Drugs used in rheumatic diseases

NSAIDs	NSAIDs *continued*	Miscellaneous
acemetacin	salsalate (USA)	penicillamine
aloxiprin	sulindac	sulphasalazine
aspirin	tenidap	
azapropazone	tenoxicam	**Corticosteroids**
benorylate	tiaprofenic acid	dexamethasone
diclofenac	tolfenamic acid	hydrocortisone
diflunisal	tolmetin	methylprednisolone
etodolac		prednisolone
felbinac	**SAARDs:**	triamcinolone
fenbufen	**Gold compounds**	
fenoprofen	auranofin	**Drugs used in gout:**
flurbiprofen	aurothioglucose (USA)	*for acute attacks*
ibuprofen	aurothiomalate sodium	colchicine
indomethacin		NSAIDs (see list)
ketoprofen	**Immunosuppressants**	
ketorolac	azathioprine	*for prevention*
meclofenamate (USA)	cyclophosphamide	allopurinol
mefenamic acid	cyclosporin	probenecid
meloxicam	methotrexate	sulphinpyrazone
nabumetone		
naproxen	**Antimalarials**	
oxaprozin (USA)	chloroquine	
phenylbutazone	hydroxychloroquine	
piroxicam		
salicylate sodium		

Summary

- Rheumatoid arthritis involves inflammation of the synovial membranes surrounding a joint and is a result of immune cells producing antibodies to molecules in the joint.
- The pain associated with the disease can be controlled using analgesic drugs.
- The inflammation can be controlled by non-steroidal anti-inflammatory drugs (NSAIDs).
- The disease itself can be controlled to some extent by drugs (SAARDs) which reduce the number or activity of the white blood cells, such as gold compounds (auranofin and aurothiomalate), penicillamine, and the antimalarial drugs such as chloroquine.
- Steroids injected into affected joints also depress immune cell activity and relieve the symptoms.
- Gout is a form of arthritis which results from the precipitation of crystals of uric acid in the joints.
- Gout can be treated by drugs such as colchicine and NSAIDs, and attacks may be prevented by lowering the amount of uric acid in the blood with allopurinol, probenecid, or sulphinpyrazone.
- Osteoarthritis involves thinning of the cartilage 'shock-absorbers' at the ends of the bones, leading to damage to the bones.
- This and many other forms of rheumatic disease are treated with analgesics, NSAIDs, or steroids.

CHAPTER 21

Osteomalacia and osteoporosis

Our bones are strongest at about age 30, after which they gradually become weaker. Osteoporosis is, therefore, largely a disorder of ageing, with women at particular risk because the loss of bone increases after the menopause. One hundred million people in the world either have, or are at risk from osteoporosis.

Without bones the human body would be shapeless and unsupported. Bones provide a framework to which muscles are attached and which can then act as levers to support and move the various parts of the body. They must be strong and not break easily. Bone is continually being made by specialized cells called osteoblasts and broken down by others called osteoclasts (Fig. 21.1). It is made of fibrous proteins known as collagen upon which minerals, mainly calcium salts, are laid down.

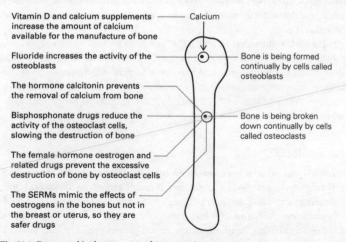

Vitamin D and calcium supplements increase the amount of calcium available for the manufacture of bone

Calcium

Fluoride increases the activity of the osteoblasts

Bone is being formed continually by cells called osteoblasts

The hormone calcitonin prevents the removal of calcium from bone

Bisphosphonate drugs reduce the activity of the osteoclast cells, slowing the destruction of bone

Bone is being broken down continually by cells called osteoclasts

The female hormone oestrogen and related drugs prevent the excessive destruction of bone by osteoclast cells

The SERMs mimic the effects of oestrogens in the bones but not in the breast or uterus, so they are safer drugs

Fig. 21.1 Drugs used in the treatment of osteoporosis.

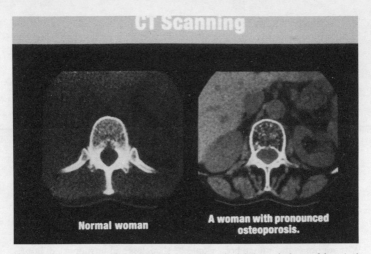

Fig. 21.2 CT scans through the spine. The picture on the *left* shows the bone of the spinal column (white), which surrounds and protects the spinal cord. In the picture on the *right*, from a woman with severe osteoporosis, the bone is very much thinner and more fragile.

If a bone is to be strong it must contain enough calcium salts. Two thirds of the weight of bone is in these mineral salts, which are responsible for the hardness of the structure. Bone exists in both a dense form (compact bone) and a less dense form with a spongy appearance under the microscope (cancellous bone).

There are two disorders in which the bones can become weakened, brittle, and easily broken. People with osteomalacia lack minerals in their bones, which become 'softer' than normal and may result in pain and deformation of the skeleton. In osteoporosis there is a generalized deficiency in the whole bony structure, collagen fibres, and calcium salts, causing the bone to become fragile and easily broken (Fig 21.2).

Osteomalacia

Vitamin D and calcium are essential for the normal development of bone and both substances are required, not just through growth in childhood and adolescence but throughout life (*see* Chapter 22, Table 22.4). Vitamin D is found in fish oils, egg yolk, and liver but is also made in the body by the action of ultraviolet light, from sunshine, on the skin. A growing child lacking vitamin D may develop soft bones which bend easily—a condition known as 'rickets'.

The bones of the legs are particularly susceptible to bending under the weight of the body.

In an adult a lack of vitamin D produces weak bones which break easily, possibly with bone pain and weakness, a condition known as osteomalacia. Healthier diets nowadays have made osteomalacia less common in Britain than in the past but it can still occur in the elderly and in some ethnic groups whose diet may not contain enough Vitamin D and who may not often have sunshine on a large enough area of their skin. Middle Eastern women, who traditionally have clothing covering all of their body, may fall into this category. Treatment is usually easy, with vitamin D given as tablets or by injection and the condition usually responds well to treatment.

Osteoporosis

As we grow and develop, our skeletons become stronger until they reach a peak strength around 30 years of age. After that, the bones begin to lose calcium salts so that, as we grow older, they become thinner, lighter, and more fragile. If the bones are very fragile the condition is known as osteoporosis. Old people may break a bone very easily and some shrink in height and develop a stooped appearance because the bones in their spines (vertebrae) become squashed under the weight of the body. Sometimes this even produces fractures visible on X-ray examination. These are known as 'vertebral crush fractures' and can be extremely painful. Indigestion and bladder or bowel problems may occur since the loss of height squashes these organs in the abdomen.

Both men and women lose calcium salts from their bones as they grow older. The rate of loss is greater in women than in men because, as the levels of female hormone (oestrogen) begin to fall after the menopause, women lose calcium salts more quickly than before. Osteoporosis affects over 20 per cent of white women in the UK over the age of 50. By the age of 70 to 80 years women may have lost as much as 30 per cent of their bone mass and up to two thirds of them have some vertebral fractures. Some may develop a fracture of the hip which may seriously reduce the ability to walk and presents a significant threat to independence.

Osteoporosis in men is often the result of factors such as steroid therapy (*see* Chapter 19), excessive consumption of alcohol, or poor absorption of calcium.

Risk factors, prevention, and treatment

Osteoporosis is a very good example of prevention being better than cure. Once bones have become weakened and fragile it is difficult to strengthen them again. The most important aim is to prevent osteoporosis from occurring in the first place.

Since bone loss increases in women around the menopause, women who have an early menopause have an increased risk, particularly if the early menopause is the result of surgical removal of their ovaries. Small amounts of the female sex hormones (*see* Chapter 19) can be made by fat cells in women even after the menopause and this hormone may help to protect the skeleton. Women who lose fat cells in the course of losing weight will reduce this production of oestrogens and may increase their risk of osteoporosis.

Exercise and diet

A good calcium intake throughout life is important to provide the mineral content of bone, and a poor diet increases the risk of both osteoporosis and fractures. Children and adolescents need to have a healthy diet rich in calcium and to take plenty of exercise in order to produce healthy bones which will remain strong throughout life.

Lack of exercise allows calcium to be lost from bone, weakening the skeleton and increasing the risk of fracture. These effects are seen particularly in people who have illnesses such as rheumatoid arthritis, multiple sclerosis, or strokes in which mobility is reduced. The best forms of exercise are against gravity, for example, walking, tennis, and badminton. Swimming is excellent for keeping fit but, because it is not against gravity, owing to the buoyant effect of the water, it is less good for protection of bones. Even in more elderly patients, physical exercise may reduce bone loss. Walking for a few hours each week may be sufficient but exercise with a risk of injury should be avoided. Active exercise in the elderly improves balance, strength, and flexibility and makes falls less likely.

Drugs

Cigarette smoking and excessive alcohol intake increase the risk of osteoporosis. Cigarette smoking should always be avoided and an alcohol intake of three units of alcohol per day in a man or two units in a woman is the maximum intake believed to be safe for the liver, bones, and brain, (where one unit of alcohol is one glass of wine, one single measure of spirits, or one half pint of beer). Drugs such as steroids may, if used for several years, increase the risk of osteoporosis. This is one reason why doctors try to prescribe steroids, such as prednisolone (*see* Chapter 19) in the lowest possible dose for as short a time as possible.

Hormone replacement therapy (HRT)

The female hormone, oestrogen, protects against bone loss. In most women replacing oestrogen restores the protection they had before the menopause. Oestrogen cannot be used alone because it can increase the chances of cancer of the womb (uterus). It is combined, therefore, with a related hormone, progesterone, which greatly reduces this risk. In women who have had their uterus removed (an operation known as a hysterectomy), oestrogen alone can then be used since there is no longer any risk of uterine cancer.

The effect of taking hormone replacement therapy (HRT) is to protect the whole body and not just the bones. Bone protection is believed to last at least until age 75, but beyond that age the bones may again be at risk. The amounts of hormone used in HRT are very small and simply aim to return the woman to a 'pre-menopausal' state. Risks of heart disease and strokes are reduced and overall death rate is lower than in women not taking HRT.

There are sometimes minor side-effects such as breast tenderness, ankle swelling, headaches, feelings of bloating, and weight gain but, with care, a form of HRT can usually be chosen to suit each woman. Many women do not wish to return to having a monthly period and they can be given a form of HRT which is continuous so that they do not have a withdrawal bleed each month as do women taking oral contraceptives.

The biggest worry for many women, however, is that of breast cancer. After five and ten years of HRT treatment there is a small increased risk to the breasts. To put this risk in perspective, it is less than the risk of heart disease and strokes which may occur in women not taking HRT. It is also less than the risks produced by taking the oral contraceptive pill. Nevertheless, the risk is real in spite of being very small and, with breast cancer risks in women generally now running at around one woman in twelve, or even more in some areas, it is understandable that some women should be anxious. In general, however, if a woman does not have a family history of breast cancer, and if she takes HRT in a low oestrogen form for not more than five years, any increased risk of breast cancer is probably very small indeed.

The risk of thromboses (blood clots) is increased in women taking HRT (from 1 in 10 000 woman-years in untreated women to 3 in 10 000 woman-years on HRT) but the risk is again obviously small, appears to be related to the dose of oestrogen (being lower in women using transdermal patches from which the hormone is absorbed through the skin), and the risk falls with continuing use.

Steroids used for HRT (see Chapter 19)

The two most common oestrogenic steroids used are oestradiol and mestranol (Table 21.1) and these are combined with a progestogenic hormone such as dydrogesterone, medroxyprogesterone, or norethisterone. Progestogens alone are not suitable for the majority of people with osteoporosis.

Tibolone

Tibolone is a synthetic steroid drug with weak effects like those of the female hormones, oestrogen, and progesterone, and of the male hormones (androgens). It does not stimulate the lining of the womb, so cancer of the womb should not be a risk on this drug, and it does not cause significant withdrawal bleeding. In post-menopausal patients, with or without established osteoporosis, it prevents rapid bone loss and it increases bone mass in the spine and hip.

Selective oestrogen receptor modulators (SERMs)*

One aim of medical research has been to produce a drug with the advantages of HRT without the side-effects. A breakthrough came from the use of tamoxifen, which is used in the treatment of breast cancer (*see* Chapter 18). Some breast cancers are dependent on a supply of oestrogen, and tamoxifen was found to interrupt this dependency by blocking the oestrogen receptors, stopping their stimulation of the cancer. Tamoxifen was introduced on prescription in 1971 and rapidly became, and still is, a valuable drug in the control of breast cancer, but over several years of clinical use it was realized that it had complex effects on the oestrogen receptors.

In the breast, tamoxifen does indeed block the oestrogen receptors but in other tissues it stimulates them. For example, tamoxifen slows the loss of bone and reduces the levels of damaging LDL-cholesterol in the blood (*see* Chapter 15). It was the ability of drugs like tamoxifen to modulate the activity of oestrogen receptors differently in different tissues that led to their being called 'selective oestrogen receptor modulators' or SERMs.

Unfortunately, tamoxifen can stimulate oestrogen receptors in the uterus, and this can increase the risk of cancer here. Nevertheless, the realization that compounds could be produced with such a remarkable range of effects stimulated research to find an ideal oestrogenic drug. Many compounds similar to tamoxifen were produced, and in 1998 one of them, raloxifene, was finally introduced by the Eli Lilly company.

The main effect of raloxifene is to stimulate the oestrogen receptors in bone, slowing the loss of calcium and proteins which lead to bone softening after the menopause. At the same time, raloxifene blocks the receptors in breast tissue so that the risks of breast cancer are no greater than in women not taking the drug and may even be lower. Raloxifene also has a very important advantage over tamoxifen: it does not stimulate oestrogen receptors in the uterus. This means that the risk of uterine cancer is no greater than in women not taking the drug. It also means that the uterine lining does not grow and break down as it does in women before the menopause. There should, therefore, be no bleeding from the uterus, a problem which many women find inconvenient when using tamoxifen and which causes many to stop taking the drug.

There is a small increased risk of thrombosis but, overall, raloxifene appears

* The abbreviation SERMs is based on the American spelling of 'estrogen'.

to be one of the most promising drugs for the treatment of osteoporosis and is likely to be the first of many such drugs with even greater efficacy and selectivity.

Calcium and Vitamin D

If there is not enough calcium in the diet, for example in people following diets low in dairy products, then calcium supplements may be useful. Elderly people absorb less calcium from the intestine and most elderly women have a small calcium deficiency. Other groups at particular risk are people who cannot absorb food normally through the stomach and intestine, those with milk intolerance, and those who have had surgical operations on the stomach, all of whom may be unable to absorb adequate amounts of calcium.

Not all 'calcium tablets' bought over the counter contain sufficiently useful quantities of calcium. Calcium gluconate and calcium lactate tablets contain too little calcium to be really effective. Calcichew (calcium carbonate), Sandocal (calcium lactate, gluconate, and carbonate), and Cacit (calcium citrate) are calcium supplements which can be obtained on prescription or bought over the counter from a pharmacy.

Calcium alone, however, does not prevent bone loss, because calcium and vitamin D are needed together. In women whose skin is not exposed to sunlight, this combination reduces the risk of hip fracture, especially in women aged 70 years or above. To be of benefit these supplements need to provide a total intake of about 1 gram per day for pre-menopausal, and 1.5 grams per day for post-menopausal women.

Calcitriol

Calcitriol is the active form of vitamin D (namely 1,25-dihydroxyvitamin D). It is used to treat post-menopausal osteoporosis and increases the absorption of calcium from the intestine. It is necessary to check that this increased absorption does not result in blood calcium levels which are too high because this may cause the formation of kidney stones and may damage the kidney. Blood calcium level and kidney function should be measured one, three, and six months after beginning treatment and then at six-monthly intervals.

Calcitonin

Calcitonin is one of the body's natural hormones for controlling calcium levels in the blood and bone. It is normally produced by cells in the thyroid glands and its main action is to prevent the loss of calcium from bone. However, it is not often used for treatment because it is expensive, it needs to be injected, and its effects on the bone only last a short time. It is sometimes used in the early stages of an osteoporotic bone fracture to reduce pain and help the patient to become mobile again as quickly as possible.

Bisphosphonates

The bisphosphonates are used to treat osteoporosis when it has already developed and include cyclic etidronate, alendronate, and pamidronate. They suppress the activity of the osteoclast cells, reducing the breakdown of bone. All the bisphosphonates reduce the risk of bone fractures by about half.

Bisphosphonates produce a 6–10 per cent increase in bone density over two years of treatment and this benefit persists for several years. Cyclic etidronate, in the form of Didronel PMO, is a cyclical programme of 14 days of etidronate and 76 days of calcium citrate supplement.

Alendronate reduces the number of vertebral and hip fractures at a dosage of only 10 μg per day. It is very important for a person to take alendronate on an empty stomach and with at least 200 ml of water, after which he or she should remain upright for half an hour and not have anything else to eat or drink. These precautions prevent the indigestion which has been the worst problem for people taking alendronate. Treatment with cyclic etidronate may be continued for five to seven years.

A third bisphosphonate is pamidronate, which is very successful in treating severe osteoporosis and can be valuable when pain is a significant problem. It has to be given by injection into a vein daily for seven days, but it is particularly useful for patients who cannot absorb medicine taken by mouth.

Etidronate, alendronate, and pamidronate are, therefore. valuable in the treatment of osteoporosis when it has already occurred. HRT is of particular use in preventing the development of osteoporosis in the first place.

Anabolic steroids

The role of anabolic steroids, such as androlone decanoate, in osteoporosis is controversial. They are synthetic steroids related to the male sex hormone, testosterone, and they have a limited role in men who lack adequate quantities of this hormone.

Fluoride

Fluoride has probably been the most controversial chemical suggested for the treatment of osteoporosis. People with mild forms of osteoporosis are most likely to benefit from fluoride. It facilitates the formation of bone by increasing the activity of the osteoblast cells which make bone tissue. A combination of calcium and fluoride increases the bone density in most subjects by around 20 per cent. The problem with fluoride is that, despite the increased formation of bone, the strength of the bones is not increased to the same extent, so that the risk of fractures is only slightly reduced. The reason for this is that the structure of bone formed under the influence of fluoride is slightly different from normal. Drug companies are now trying to produce a 'slow release' preparation so that a single tablet will produce a gradual delivery of fluoride into the bloodstream over 24 hours. The presence of fluoride in the body at low levels over a long period seems to improve the quality of the bone made by the osteoblasts and reduces the chance of side-effects.

Monitoring of treatment with anti-osteoporotic drugs

Bone density is usually measured either with a densitometric (DEXA) scanner —a simple process not in any way unpleasant—or by ultrasonic assessment of the bone density of the heel of the foot. Results may help to decide whether osteoporosis is present in the first place and whether treatment is effective. Rescanning with a DEXA scan about two years after starting treatment can often encourage doubting patients to persevere with treatment as they see the improvement in the scan reading as a result of therapy.

Drugs of the future

Although a range of drugs is available to treat or control osteoporosis, none is perfect. The ideal drug would increase the formation of bone by stimulating the natural activity of the osteoblasts and reducing the activity of osteoclasts. Together these effects should build up new bone with a completely natural, strong microarchitecture and density, restoring their strength towards that of a 30-year-old person.

In fact, substances exist which do all these things. They are the natural hormone parathyroid hormone and proteins called fibroblast growth factors (FGF). These are responsible for the natural formation of bone in our child-hood and youth. Unfortunately, being proteins, they would not be effective if taken by mouth, as they would be digested in the stomach, and they would have to be given by frequent injections. Researchers are trying to develop drugs which reproduce the effects of these hormones and which can be taken easily.

Many other new drugs are being assessed to treat osteoporosis including oestrogens with specific effects on the bone, integrin antagonists, proton pump inhibitors, amylin (a protein produced by the pancreas and which seems to affect the formation and structure of bone), new drugs related to vitamin D, zeolite A (a relative of silicon), and strontium salts. All of these need more testing before they can be used routinely.

Osteoporosis in people taking steroid therapy

About a quarter of a million people in the UK are treated continuously with steroids, mainly for conditions such as asthma or arthritis, and this may increase the risk of developing osteoporosis and fractures. Bone is lost most rapidly in the first six to twelve months of treatment with steroids, post-menopausal women being particularly at risk. The lowest risk is in pre-menopausal women, who are still protected by oestrogen. The lowest possible dose of steroid should be used, to prevent the development of osteoporosis. If steroids are being taken for three months or more, drugs may be needed to protect against osteoporosis, although regular exercise, care to prevent falling, the avoidance of excessive alcohol and smoking all help to increase bone density and reduce the need for drugs.

In men, testosterone supplements may be used if necessary. It is sometimes possible to change the steroid given to deflazacol, a steroid with fewer damaging effects on bone.

Treatment summary for osteoporosis

- Every woman at the menopause should be assessed and her personal hereditary and lifestyle risk factors should be considered to see whether she needs to be protected against osteoporosis.
- Hormone replacement therapy (HRT) is often the best treatment, in that it prevents osteoporosis and also protects against disease of the heart and blood vessels. However, it also carries the possibility of a slightly increased risk of breast cancer.
- If a woman is not willing to take HRT, there are several drugs which can be used to prevent bone loss, such as cyclic etidronate or alendronate.
- Elderly people sometimes do not have an adequate intake of vitamin D. All postmenopausal women should ensure that they have an adequate intake of calcium which, in practice, may mean they should take a calcium supplement.
- Calcitriol is usually prescribed only by doctors with specialist knowledge of this treatment, and even then in relatively few cases. Other drugs such as calcitonin, tibolone, anabolic steroids, and progestogens should also only be used under medical supervision.
- Exercise, a healthy lifestyle, and prevention of falls in the elderly are also very important.
- Steroid therapy causes weakening of the bones. Most of the bone loss occurs early in the course of treatment, so the doses should be adjusted to minimize the problem.
- In men, if there is a lack of the male hormone, testosterone, this can be replaced. Treatment is otherwise similar to that for post-menopausal women.

Table 21.1 Drugs used for osteoporosis and osteomalacia

Calcium-increasing agents	Anabolic steroid
alfacalcidol	nandrolone
calcitonin	
calcitriol	**Other agents**
cholecalciferol	fluoride
dihydrotachysterol	
ergocalciferol	**HRT**
salcatonin	mestranol
	oestradiol
Bisphosphonates	
alendronic acid	
clodronate	
etidronate	
pamidronate	
risedronate	
tiludronic acid	

Summary

• *Strong bones require calcium. A deficiency of vitamin D leads to poor absorption and use of calcium, resulting in weak bones.*

• *As we age, calcium is lost from bones, making them weaker. The loss is increased by smoking, alcohol, and steroids. Calcium loss can be reduced by exercise. Increased intake of calcium or drugs such as calcitriol can improve bone strength.*

• *The female hormones, the oestrogens, protect against the weakening of bones. As the levels of oestrogen fall at the menopause, the risk of bone loss— osteoporosis—increases.*

• *Osteoporosis can be reduced by hormone replacement therapy (HRT) using oestrogens, but this may slightly increase the risks of breast cancer, uterine cancer, and thrombosis.*

• *The selective oestrogen receptor modulators (SERMs), such as raloxifene, stimulate oestrogen receptors in bone and maintain bone quality but do not stimulate receptors in the breast and uterus. They do not increase the risks of cancer but carry a small increased risk of thrombosis.*

• *Fluoride increases the rate at which bone is produced and strengthened. Bisphosphonate drugs reduce the rate at which bone is broken down.*

CHAPTER 22

Vitamins

The word 'vitamin' was coined by a Polish scientist, Casimir Funk, in 1910. He had extracted from rice a chemical which prevented and cured the symptoms of a disease called 'beri-beri', in which patients suffered loss of weight, lack of appetite, vomiting, and constipation, and led to generalized weakness and eventually paralysis. Funk called his new chemical 'vitamin', as it seemed to be an amine which was vital to prevent the disease. Since Funk's discovery, the word vitamin has come to refer to a variety of organic nutrients which the body needs in small quantities for a range of activities.

Why do we need vitamins?

Vitamins perform several vital roles. One of these is as 'cofactors' for enzymes. Enzymes are the protein molecules which carry out many of the chemical reactions in cells, but to do so most enzymes need to enlist the help of smaller molecules called cofactors. These may be simple atoms of elements such as iron or selenium, or more complex molecules such as vitamins. Cofactors are usually needed by the body in very small quantities—micrograms (μg) or milligrams (mg) per day.

A second important function of some vitamins is to destroy, or scavenge, molecules known as 'free radicals'. These can severely damage cells and tissues and are responsible for several major disorders such as rheumatoid arthritis, some cancers, brain damage after strokes, and damage to the heart after a coronary thrombosis. Antioxidant vitamins and other chemicals can reduce that damage.

What are free radicals?

Each atom is made partly of charged particles called electrons which exist in layers, called orbitals. There are normally two electrons in the outermost orbital and if an atom loses one electron it becomes a free radical.

Free radicals are unstable and within a fraction of a second one radical will snatch a replacement electron from another atom, sometimes combining with it in the process. That creates another atom with only one electron which steals a further electron, and so on. In this way one single free radical can start a chain reaction involving thousands of other atoms. When those atoms are part of molecules such as proteins, RNA, DNA, or the fatty molecules which make up cell membranes, those molecules may be severely damaged.

Antioxidants

The chain reaction initiated by a free radical can be stopped only when one of the radicals in the chain meets a molecule which can rearrange itself so that a single electron is shared by other atoms. Such molecules are called antioxidants, and they include vitamins C and E. Cells also contain enzymes* whose main function is to interact with free radicals, stopping them in their tracks and limiting the amount of damage they can inflict.

The vitamins

Most of the vitamins we need must be supplied by the diet. A lack of vitamins in the diet can lead to diseases such as scurvy (vitamin C deficiency) and anaemia (vitamin B_{12} deficiency). Vitamins are divided into two main groups, depending on whether they dissolve in water or in fat. Water-soluble vitamins are the B vitamins and vitamin C, while the fat soluble vitamins are A, D, E, and K.

Water-soluble vitamins

The B vitamins which are essential for human health are thiamine (vitamin B_1), riboflavin (vitamin B_2), niacin (also called nicotinic acid or nicotinamide; vitamin B_3), pantothenic acid (vitamin B_5), pyridoxine (also called pyridoxal or pyridoxamine; vitamin B_6), biotin, cobalamin (vitamin B_{12}), and folic acid (pteroylglutamic acid). Because all of these dissolve in water, any excess can be excreted in the urine, and it is rare for them to be found in toxic amounts in the body. On the other hand, because they are only stored in small quantities, except for cobalamin, they must be supplied regularly in the diet.

The B vitamins (Table 22.1, p. 349)

Thiamine (vitamin B_1)

The first B vitamin to be purified and identified was thiamine. Although employed as the chemical director of the Bell Telephone Laboratories in the USA, Robert Williams studied vitamins in his leisure time. Working in the

---

* These include superoxide dismutase (SOD), catalase, and glutathione peroxidase.

Table 22.1 The B Vitamins

Vitamin	Daily requirement*	Food Sources	Deficiency symptoms
B₁ Thiamine	1.0-1.5mg/day (levels reduced by prolonged cooking)	Many foods, pork, beef, beans, wholegrain cereals, peas, lentils	Beri beri: exhaustion, poor appetite, abnormal functioning of heart, nerves, and muscles, fluid retention. Common in alcoholics who eat little food.
B₂ Riboflavin	1.3 mg levels reduced by prolonged cooking	Milk, milk products, meat, cereal grains, yeast, some green leafy vegetables	Sores on tongue and corners of mouth; dislike of light. Deficiency may occur in newborn with high blood bilirubin: treated with light—phototherapy.
B₃ (Also called B7, nicotinic acid, niacin, niacinamide, nicotinamide)	6.6 mg/1000 Kcal except maize. Can also be made from	Meat, fish, milk, yeast, wholegrain cereals tryptophan, an amino acid found in protein foods	Pellagra: weight loss, diarrhoea, dermatitis, depression, and dementia. Deficiency results from diet lacking both niacin and tryptophan e.g. populations eating maize (corn) as the staple food.
B₅ Pantothenic acid, pantothenate	4-7 mg	Many foods, meat, eggs, nuts, seeds, cereals, legumes	Burning feet.
B₆ pyridoxine	15 μg/g protein (levels reduced by cooking and if food is kept hot after cooking)	meat, fish, egg yolks, wholegrain cereals, potatoes, bananas, red peppers, watercress, avocados, nuts, seeds, green vegetables	Lack of B₆ alone is rare. May occur in alcoholics, nursing infants of mothers deficient in vitamin B₆. Use of isoniazid in tuberculosis may cause deficiency.
B₁₂ Cobalamin or cyanocobalamin	1.5 μg per day Easily destroyed by cooking	Meat, especially liver, fish, milk, yeast	Pernicious anaemia, confusion, depression, numb or tingling hands or feet, unsteadiness. May be deficient in vegetarian or vegan diets.
Folic acid (folate, folacin)	200 μg per day. Lost by cooking and if food is kept hot. Tinned vegetables lose much of this vitamin	Eggs, nuts, yeast, wholegrain cereals, green vegetables, liver	Anaemia. May occur on drug treatment, e.g. on methotrexate. Spina bifida in babies—reduced by giving folic acid to pregnant women.
Biotin	30-300 μg	Meats, milk products, wholegrain cereals. Made by bacteria in the intestine	Depression, hallucinations, muscle pain, hair loss, dermatitis. Deficiency may result from eating raw eggs.

* Reference nutrient intake, (RNI).

basement of his own home in New Jersey, he isolated thiamine from huge quantities of rice in 1936. Severe thiamine deficiency causes *beri-beri*, with mental confusion, muscle thinning (dry beri-beri), fluid accumulation in the body (wet beri-beri), high blood pressure, difficulty in walking, and disturbances of the heart. It used to be common in sailors as well as the people of Japan and China living on polished white rice. The frequency of the disease dropped, however, when they were given additional meat, vegetables, and whole rice. Beri-beri is still found in parts of Asia where white rice still supplies up to eighty per cent of dietary calories in some areas.

Thiamine is destroyed when in contact with alcohol, coffee, tea, or sulphites. In people who drink too much alcohol, the combination of thiamine deficiency and alcohol toxicity may produce the Wernicke–Korsakoff syndrome—a serious brain disorder which causes problems with memory, walking, and vision. Treatment with thiamine has been claimed to have beneficial effects in Alzheimer's disease and age-related senility. No toxicity from thiamine has been reported.

Riboflavin (Vitamin B_2)

Riboflavin, or vitamin B_2, was first recognized as a yellow green pigment in milk in 1879. It is found in liver, kidney, and heart, whole grain cereals, green leafy vegetables, and mushrooms and is destroyed by light but not by cooking. Riboflavin is important in energy production and in regenerating the compound glutathione, which protects cells against free radical damage. Mild deficiency of riboflavin is quite common in the elderly. Severe deficiency produces cracking of the lips and the corners of the mouth, an inflamed tongue, disturbed vision, and anaemia. No toxic effects seem to occur from consuming too much riboflavin.

Niacin (Vitamin B_3)

The amino acid tryptophan is present in the diet and is converted in the body to niacin (vitamin B_3), so that niacin is not itself essential, provided that tryptophan intake is adequate. Niacin is involved in many chemical reactions in the body including those responsible for energy production, the metabolism of fats and carbohydrates, and the production of adrenal and sex hormones. It also helps to regulate blood sugar and antioxidant processes. It is found in liver, eggs, fish, peanuts, whole grains, milk, and avocados.

A deficiency of niacin produces pellagra, a condition characterized by the '3D's' of dermatitis, dementia, and diarrhoea. The disease was first described by a Spanish physician Gaspar Casal, in 1735, although the name pellagra was coined later from the Italian words *pelle* meaning 'skin', and *agra* meaning 'rough'. Too much niacin can be toxic, with flushing of the skin, irritation of the stomach, and liver damage. Supplements should not be taken by diabetics, unless supervised, since niacin can reduce their tolerance of glucose, or by patients with liver disease, gout, and peptic ulcers.

A deficiency of niacin, and the pellagra which would have resulted, could have been the origin of vampire legends in the eighteenth and nineteenth centuries. Pellagra was first described in 1735, following the widespread introduction of corn (maize) into European agriculture. Corn farming greatly increased the calorific value per acre of farmland, but the niacin and tryptophan content of corn is tightly bound to other molecules and cannot be readily absorbed after eating. Jeffrey and William Hampl have suggested that the symptoms of pellagra closely resemble the features attributed to 'vampires', and that the legends of vampires such as Dracula arose from the existence of severely ill pellagra-sufferers (pellagrins). For example, pellagrins avoid sunlight, because this causes the skin to become sensitive and painful, as well as red, thickened, and scaly; they become irritable, sometimes violent, and suffer insomnia, just as vampires seek victims for their violent attacks at night.

Pyridoxine (vitamin B_6)

Pyridoxine is important in maintaining a normal hormonal balance and immune system. It is also involved in the production of proteins, transmitters in the nervous system, and red blood cells. Pyridoxine occurs in whole grain cereals, bananas, seeds, nuts, potatoes, Brussels sprouts, and cauliflower. Deficiency produces depression, convulsions, impaired nerve function, skin diseases, intolerance of glucose, anaemia, and cracked lips and tongue.

Taking too much pyridoxine can cause tingling in the feet, loss of muscle co-ordination, and damage to nerves. Some substances, including food colourings, oral contraceptives, and alcohol, can interfere with the effects of vitamin B_6.

An unusual syndrome produced at least in part by pyridoxine deficiency is the 'Chinese Restaurant Syndrome'. With the growth in the number of Chinese restaurants in the 1970s, it was realized that some customers were suffering tingling and weakness of the face and upper body, with feelings of warmth and flushing of the skin, associated with palpitations, anxiety, thirst, and nausea. The symptoms were produced in people who reacted to monosodium glutamate, a chemical used as a flavour enhancer in food. Pyridoxine is needed by the body to metabolize and remove glutamate. Those people lacking pyridoxine were unable to destroy the glutamate and so suffered from the toxic effects of glutamate.

Cobalamin (vitamin B_{12})

Vitamin B_{12}, or cobalamin, was isolated from liver in 1948 and found to be the nutritional factor that prevented 'pernicious anaemia', a severe anaemia associated with large, immature red blood cells and damage to the nervous system. Vitamin B_{12} is found only in foods obtained from animals, especially liver, kidney, eggs, fish, cheese, and meat. Pernicious anaemia is unlikely to occur in people taking a healthy diet, including vegetarians who consume milk products and eggs. A deficiency may develop in the elderly and people with medical conditions, such as Crohn's disease, which impair the absorption of vitamin B_{12} from the intestine.

Vegans are at much greater risk and, if intake of vitamin B_{12} is inadequate, may develop an anaemia. This may not be obvious immediately if the diet is rich in leafy vegetables containing folic acid (another B vitamin which protects temporarily against the anaemia of vitamin B_{12} deficiency). However, folic acid cannot replace vitamin B_{12} in its role in the nervous system and, even if the anaemia is prevented by folic acid, nerves may be damaged irreversibly before the deficiency of vitamin B_{12} is diagnosed.

Early signs of nerve damage are confusion, depression, numbness or tingling in the hands or feet, and unsteadiness when walking, as a result of the loss of sensation in the feet and legs. People on macrobiotic or strict Rastaferian diets are also at risk of vitamin B_{12} deficiency as are the breastfed babies of vegan mothers. Vegans are often told that fermented foods such as tempeh are good sources of vitamin B_{12} but this form of B_{12} is not the type which the human body needs. Strict vegetarians and vegans are advised to supplement their diets with vitamin B_{12}.

Folic acid

Folic acid received its name from the Latin word *folium* meaning foliage, since it is found in high concentrations in green, leafy vegetables. Folic acid is essential for the division of cells to produce new ones, because it is necessary for the production of the large molecules in DNA which make up the genes of the cell. A deficiency of folic acid can, therefore, cause anaemia, diarrhoea, and poor growth. Folic acid is essential for the development of the nervous system before birth, and its deficiency during pregnancy is linked to birth defects.

Much of the benefit from supplements of folic acid is from a reduction in the amounts of the amino acid homocysteine in the body. This promotes atherosclerosis ('hardening of the arteries') probably by damaging the artery walls. It can also contribute to the development of osteoporosis (*see* Chapter 21) since it interferes with collagen formation, leading to a weak bone structure. Folic acid reduces homocysteine levels, and thereby protects against both these disorders.

Folic acid can mask many of the symptoms of vitamin B12 deficiency, and if not recognized by doctors, B_{12} deficiency can seriously damage the nervous system. If there is any possibility of B_{12} deficiency, folic acid should not be given without vitamin B_{12} since it may encourage damage to the nervous system. High doses of folate may cause nausea and loss of appetite, while epileptics may suffer an increase in the frequency of fits.

Vitamin B complex

Members of the B family of vitamins affect each others' absorption from the intestine. Taking a supplement of one B vitamin alone can, therefore, cause more problems than it solves. As a result, B vitamins are usually taken as supplements of the whole group as a 'Vitamin B complex' tablet.

Vitamin C (Ascorbic acid) (Table 22.2)

An important function of vitamin C is in the manufacture of collagen proteins, which provide the supporting structure for the organs of the body. Since collagen is such an important structural protein, vitamin C is vital for wound repair, healthy gums, and protection from bruising. It is also essential for immune function and for the manufacture of neurotransmitters and hormones, such as epinephrine. In addition, vitamin C helps the absorption of iron from the intestine and, as an antioxidant, may be protective against cancer and other diseases. It occurs in citrus fruits, vegetables, and salad foods but is destroyed by exposure to air and by cooking.

Table 22.2 Vitamin C

Reference nutrient intake (RNI)
60 mg per day.
Good sources
Most fruits, particularly blackcurrant, strawberries, oranges, grapefruit, kiwi fruit, avocado pears, fresh parsley, watercress, green or sweet peppers, raw cabbage, and potato.
Effects of cooking
Destroyed by heat; cooking should be as light and for as short a time as possible. Also destroyed by oxygen, metal cans, an alkaline environment, and light.
People at risk of deficiency
Those living on canteen or 'convenience' foods and the elderly, demented, alcoholics, and food faddists. More needed after surgery or trauma.
Signs and symptoms of deficiency
Scurvy: tendency to bruising and bleeding. Swollen, bleeding gums, loose teeth, dry, scaly skin, muscle weakness, and poor wound repair.
Results of excessive intake
Diarrhoea, kidney stones, and scurvy may occur if a high intake is suddenly stopped.

Vitamin C has been used in an enormous range of conditions from asthma to atherosclerosis, from the common cold and cataracts to cancer, from hepatitis to high blood pressure and from peptic ulcers to Parkinson's disease. However, much more work is required to assess its true role, if any, in treating these conditions.

The late Nobel prize winner Linus Pauling recommended an intake of 2–9 grams per day during health. These high doses often lead to diarrhoea and probably no more than 500 milligrams to 1 gram per day should be taken. Because vitamin C is an acid, chewable tablets may damage tooth enamel. A disorder known as 'rebound scurvy' may occur when people taking high doses of vitamin C stop taking the supplement suddenly.

Vitamin C deficiency produces scurvy, characterized by bleeding gums, poor wound healing, and extensive bruising. Scurvy has been known for centuries since food given to soldiers and sailors on long journeys rarely contained adequate amounts of vitamin C. Some explorers realized that eating certain foods on long journeys protected against, or helped to cure, scurvy. Some ate spruce tree needles, others limes, berries, oranges, and lemons, the last two being first recommended by the Dutchman Balduinus Ronsseus in 1564 after his observation that sailors returning to land ate large numbers of oranges and lemons to cure themselves of scurvy.

In 1742 the British physician James Lind wrote the first real scientific discussion suggesting that scurvy was a form of dietary deficiency and showed in a classic experiment that patients given lemon juice recovered from scurvy. By providing fresh fruit, Captain Cook avoided scurvy altogether in three long voyages between 1768 and 1779, but the British Navy did not adopt lime juice rations for its crews until 1804.

Fat soluble vitamins

The body cannot make these vitamins which must, therefore, be supplied in the diet. They can be absorbed efficiently only when there is normal absorption of fats from the intestine. The fat soluble vitamins are vitamins A, D, E, and K. Because the body stores fat soluble vitamins in fatty tissues, any excess taken in the diet and not used immediately will tend to accumulate in the body fat. As a result, fat-soluble vitamins can reach levels which may be high enough to cause toxic effects.

Vitamin A (Table 22.3)
Vitamin A (retinol) was the first fat-soluble vitamin to be recognized. The initial discovery was made almost at the same time by researchers at the University of Wisconsin and at Yale University. Vitamin A is taken in the diet, but the body

Table 22.3 Vitamin A (retinol)

Daily requirements **Reference nutrient intake (RNI)**
4–5000 IU per day.
Good sources
Milk, butter, eggs, kidney, liver, margarine. Made in the body from beta-carotene (found in carrots, red peppers, mangoes, and dark green leafy vegetables.
People at risk of deficiency
Those who cannot absorb food properly i.e. pancreatic or small bowel disease and people with zinc deficiency. Those with poor diets and lack of fruit and vegetables, e.g. alcoholics.
Signs and symptoms of deficiency
Poor vision in dim light, dry eyes and, in extreme cases, blindness.
Results of excessive intake
Accumulates since fat-soluble. Vitamin A and beta-carotene excess in pregnancy may cause defects in the baby. Otherwise headache, vomiting, and visual disturbance. Excess of beta-carotene causes a yellow appearance.

can also make it from carotenoids. Foods containing the greatest quantities are liver, kidney, butter, and milk. The best sources of carotenes are dark green, leafy vegetables (broccoli and spinach), and yellow or orange vegetables (carrots and squash).

Carotenoids

There are more than 600 different chemicals called carotenoids, of which 30 to 50 behave like vitamin A. Carotenoids make up a large group of naturally occurring pigments in nature with intense colours (red and yellow). Photosynthesis, the process by which plants and some other organisms produce chemical energy in the presence of sunlight, requires carotenoids, not only to assist in the process itself but also to protect the plant against free radicals produced during photosynthesis.

Vitamin A is called retinol since it is involved in the function of the retina of the eye. The retina has four light-sensitive pigments made from vitamin A and which are linked to proteins. When light strikes the retina, the pigment is split from the protein. This splitting excites 'rod' and 'cone' cells in the retina which send impulses to the brain and cause us to 'see' the outside world.

Vitamin A is believed to be important in growth and development since it is necessary for the synthesis of molecules called glycoproteins, some of which control the development of cells and the expression of genes. Vitamin A and carotenes are essential for the health of epithelial tissue which lines the airways and reproductive tracts and which makes up the skin and the cornea of the eye. Vitamin A is also important in fertility and reproduction, for good immune function, and as an antioxidant.

The antioxidant effect of carotenes is probably the factor responsible for the anticancer effect which has been reported and, since ageing is also associated with damage produced by oxidizing free radicals, carotenes are believed to offer some protection against ageing.

Vitamin A deficiency causes poor immune function, with reduced ability to combat infectious diseases, night-blindness, severe eye diseases (xerophthalmia), skin disorders, and cataracts in the elderly. However, women must *avoid* vitamin A supplements during pregnancy since they may produce defects in the baby. Since vitamin A is a fat-soluble vitamin, it can accumulate in fat cells to levels which cause toxic effects such as dry skin, brittle nails, hair loss, loss of appetite, nausea, fatigue, and irritability.

Vitamin D (Table 22.4)

Vitamin D is both a vitamin and a prohormone: it is broken down by the body to give a hormone, known as calcitriol, which plays a central role in the use of calcium and phosphate. Vitamin D is found in cod-liver oil, fish, butter, and egg yolks, with some in dark green leafy vegetables.

Table 22.4 VItamin D

Daily requirements
No dietary intake required if exposed to sunlight. If living indoors, or covered from head to foot with clothing as in some ethnic groups, 10 μg per day.
Good sources
Oily fish, egg yolk, liver.
People at risk of deficiency
Those not exposed to sunlight or with inadequate vitamin D in the diet, especially the elderly.
Signs and symptoms of deficiency
Adults: osteomalacia; children: rickets; weak bones and muscles with pain from poor calcification.
Toxicity
Malaise, drowsiness, nausea, abdominal pain, constipation, and thirst. Excessive amounts produce high blood calcium levels and abnormal calcification of tissues.
Drug interactions
Thiazide diuretics increase blood calcium. Cabamazepine, phenytoin, and phenobarbitone may increase need for supplement.

There are two main forms of vitamin D: ergocalciferol (vitamin D_2) and cholecalciferol (vitamin D_3). Ergosterol occurs in plants and a very similar chemical, 7-dehydrocholesterol, occurs in animals. Ultraviolet rays from sunlight break up both ergosterol and 7-dehydrocholesterol to give ergocalciferol (vitamin D_2) and cholecalciferol (vitamin D_3) in plants and animals respectively. Both of these vitamins can also be absorbed from the diet.

Vitamin D is involved in cell development and immune function. It has a range of anticancer properties, especially against cancer of the breast and colon—the incidence of both is higher in areas where people are exposed to the least amount of light. Vitamin D is also involved in making bone. Bones are made of two important parts—a complex network of collagen fibres and other proteins which form a strong framework and crystals of calcium phosphate salts laid down on the framework to make the collagen rigid. Vitamin D is responsible for controlling the absorption of calcium and phosphate in the intestine and for preventing their loss in the urine. It also helps with the deposition of calcium on the collagen framework of the bone.

Vitamin D deficiency results in rickets in children and osteomalacia (see Chapter 21) in adults. Rickets is a condition characterized by poorly calcified, soft bones which tend to give bowed legs, spinal curvature, and bone pain, with delayed eruption of teeth. It used to be common in childhood but is now extremely rare. In adults osteomalacia often causes muscle weakness and tenderness, or pain in the spine, shoulders, ribs, or pelvis. Elderly people who do not get sunlight are particularly at risk.

Vitamin D supplements should not be taken, however, unless prescribed by a doctor because it can produce too high a level of calcium in the blood, causing muscle weakness or paralysis. If the calcium crystallizes out of solution there is also a danger that kidney stones may form, with possible damage to the kidneys.

Vitamin E

Vitamin E, also known as tocopherol, is available in many different forms, both natural and synthetic. The word tocopherol comes from the Greek *tokos* meaning 'offspring' and *phero* meaning 'to bear' so tocopherol means to bear children. This name arose from the discovery in 1922 that when rats were fed a diet without vitamin E they could not reproduce but, when vitamin E was added to their diet, they became fertile again. Vitamin E became known as the 'antisterility vitamin'.

The richest natural sources are sunflower seeds, sunflower oil, safflower oil, margarine, wheatgerm, and sweet potatoes. There are smaller amounts in eggs, milk products, peanuts, and avocados and many vegetables, especially lettuce, celery, chick peas, and beans. Vitamin E is destroyed by cooking, food processing, and by deep-freezing.

There are several naturally occurring forms of vitamin E (tocopherols). The two main types have molecules which are mirror images of each other, just as the right hand is a mirror image of the left hand. They are indicated by the letters d- and l-. Natural forms of vitamin E are d-, as in d-alpha-tocopherol, which is the type most widely distributed in nature and has the greatest biological activity. Most of the vitamin E in humans is in this form. The human body can use only the d- or natural form.

Synthetic forms are a mixture of the d- and l- types (such as dl-alpha-tocopherol) but the l-form stops the d-form from entering cells and being used. It is, therefore, far safer to take supplements of the natural vitamin E (d-alpha-tocopherol) than the synthetic dl- form.

Supplements of natural vitamin E, which contains mixed tocopherols and the related tocotrienols offer the greatest benefit to health, particularly when the *d*-alpha-tocopherol is present as its acetate or succinate forms, since these are more stable.

Although the official daily requirements of vitamin E are only 10 milligrams (or 15 international units) the amount required depends on the intake of polyunsaturated fatty acids (PUFAs) in the diet as well as alcohol intake, smoking, exposure to air pollution, and time spent in the sun, since sunshine produces free radicals in the skin. Vitamin E is an important antioxidant which is believed to protect the body from the damaging effects of free radicals produced by sunlight and which could damage cell membranes.

Foods containing large quantities of PUFAs but little vitamin E, such as oily fish, create an increased need for vitamin E. Other foods, such as some cooking oils, seeds, and nuts use up vitamin E as they are broken down during digestion. Supplements of vitamin E are then needed to maintain the body's stores. The currently recommended daily intake of vitamin E is 0.4 mg vitamin E per gram of PUFA. The average intake of PUFAs in western diets is about 18 g per day so 7 mg per day of natural alpha-tocopherol are needed as a daily minimum. Vitamin E has an excellent safety record. Doses up to 1000 units per day appear to be quite safe.

Tocopherols are absorbed during the digestion of fat. Vitamin E deficiency is found in conditions where there is abnormal absorption of fat, such as after surgery in which part of the intestine is removed, and in liver disease. It is also seen in premature infants, in hereditary disorders of red blood cells (such as sickle cell disease and thalassaemia), and in patients with kidney failure receiving haemodialysis. People with low levels of vitamin E and other antioxidants such as selenium may be more likely to develop certain types of cancer, particularly of the gastrointestinal tract and lungs.

Vitamin E and heart disease

Vitamin E may offer protection against heart disease and strokes. It is believed to reduce the amounts of harmful low density lipoprotein (LDL) (*see* Chapter 15) and increase the levels of protective high density lipoproteins (HDL) in the blood. It also makes platelets less sticky (*see* Chapter 14) and assists in the breakdown of clots. It has also been suggested that the explanation for the 'French Paradox'—i.e. why the French have a lower rate of heart disease and strokes than the Americans in spite of a higher cholesterol and fat intake—may not only be the greater consumption of red wine by the French, with its content of antioxidants, but may also be because the French have higher vitamin E levels.

Diabetes mellitus

Vitamin E is believed to improve the action of insulin and to prevent the long-term complications of diabetes (*see* Chapter 3). Its main effect is probably as an antioxidant to counteract oxidative stress.

Fibrocystic breast disease and menopausal symptoms

Fibrocystic breast disease (FBD) consists of painful, benign cystic breast swelling, most noticeable before menstruation, and may be a risk factor for breast cancer. FBD is relieved by vitamin E although the mechanism is not yet fully understood.

Immune function

Vitamin E improves the functioning of the immune system, with increased protection of the body against stress and infection.

Sexual activity

Vitamin E supplements have been considered to improve general well-being and sexual performance but scientific studies are required to confirm or reject the suggestions.

Vitamin K (Table 22.5)

Vitamin K, or phytomenadione, has been mentioned in Chapter 14. It is essential for the manufacture of factors needed for normal blood clotting. Several of the anticoagulant drugs work by interfering with the role of vitamin K in this process.

Table 22.5 Vitamin K

Daily requirements

1 µg per kg (2.2 lb) of body weight. This would be about 0.07mg per day for an 'average' 70kg person.

Natural sources

Parsley, cabbage, broccoli and other 'greens'—the greener the leaves the more vitamin K they contain. Liver, margarine, vegetable oils, milk. Bacteria in intestine produce vitamin K.

Deficiency problems

Abnormal blood clotting especially in the newborn. Osteoporosis.

People at risk of deficiency

Anyone not eating green vegetables or taking courses of antibiotics which kill intestinal bacteria (which manufacture Vitamin K). Anyone with poor absorption of fat or taking anticoagulants. High doses of vitamin E make vitamin K deficiency worse.

Summary

- The vitamins are chemicals required by the body in small but regular quantities to maintain the activity of enzymes within the cells.
- The B vitamins have a wide range of functions. A lack of vitamin B_{12} can result from the inadequate formation of a chemical, 'intrinsic factor', in the stomach which is needed for B_{12} absorption. This can lead to pernicious anaemia.
- Vitamin C is needed for wound repair and as an antioxidant to destroy the very damaging free radicals which are produced in cells.
- Vitamin A is important for healthy vision. The related carotenoid chemicals are powerful antioxidants, protecting cells against free radicals.
- Vitamin D is needed for the proper absorption and use of calcium.
- Vitamin E is one of the most important antioxidants. Supplements of vitamin E improve general health and the immune system, and slow some aspects of ageing.
- Vitamin K is needed for the manufacture of 'clotting factors' needed for coagulation of the blood.

CHAPTER 23

Love potions and aphrodisiacs

Calsonia, wife of Caligula, gave the mad Roman Emperor a love potion which is said to have made:
> 'the blood run hissing through his veins, 'til the mad vapour mounted to his brains'.

Love and sex are extremely important to most of us and we feel the need to be successful in both. The fact that a belief in aphrodisiacs is so widespread in cultures all over the world is proof of the importance of potency to human beings to an extent far greater than is required to perpetuate the human species.

There is a large cultural and traditional literature, extending over many centuries, on techniques to increase sexual desire. The earliest recipes for love potions were written on Egyptian medical papyri from the Middle Kingdom between 2200 and 1700BC. The *Anunga runga* manuscript by Kullian Mull, in the fifteenth century, and the *Kama sutra* of Vatsyayana, written between the first and fourth centuries, have become well known for advice on love and social conduct. The Arab text *The perfumed garden* has become extremely well known for advice on sexual techniques and recipes for improving sexual performance, and modern scientific literature includes factual books on technique for the use of those who are sexually inexperienced or wish to improve their performance. In the process of reading such literature a degree of sexual arousal will frequently occur in the reader, so these books may themselves be considered to have aphrodisiac properties.

What is an aphrodisiac?

An aphrodisiac has been defined as 'a drug or other substance capable of inducing venereal desire or lust', and science has usually concluded that aphrodisiacs defined in this way do not exist. However, if the definition includes substances which enhance the pleasure of sexual activity, then a whole range of drugs, foods, and other substances may be considered to be aphrodisiacs.

Aphrodisiacs may increase desire, improve performance, or increase sexual pleasure or, indeed, may have a combination of all three actions.

To be loved, potent, and fertile are basic needs for most people, and enormous numbers of pills and potions are consumed in the often mistaken belief that sexual success will be achieved. If we try to measure the effects of any aphrodisiac we run the risk of equating sexual success with quantitative measures of sexual performance and of ignoring qualitative performance, which to most intelligent people is much more important. How can we compare the lovemaking between two people who are deeply in love and are both giving and receiving pleasure, with the mindless gymnastics of someone selfishly trying to better their own sexual record?

Lovemaking is a serious matter and its success or failure can ruin lives and relationships. There is no 'correct' level of sexual activity: two people with a low sex drive can live together as happily as a couple with a high sex drive. A mismatch of libido (sexual drive), however, may cause enormous tensions in relationships and provides a rich market for those who claim to sell aphrodisiacs. The effortless physical relationship which may be taken for granted by one couple is not always easy to achieve by another couple, and an aphrodisiac may be seen by a person who is sexually dysfunctional as a way to retrieve their self-esteem.

Successful lovemaking is a dream which, at least until recently, science has largely failed to help. Not only is there no such thing as an effective aphrodisiac, but many drugs have been produced which, when taken for other reasons, have impaired desire, potency, and fertility.

It is difficult to measure the increase in sexual desire produced by an 'aphrodisiac' since libido varies with many factors, such as tiredness, anxiety, hormonal cycles, and the conditioning effects of earlier unpleasant encounters which may have long-lasting effects on later sexual responsiveness. Desire in women is believed to increase to a peak after a menstrual period, (which may sometimes reflect abstinence during menstruation), with a peak in the rate of intercourse and orgasm in mid-cycle, i.e. at ovulation, and again three days before the next period.

For men the effect of tiredness, disease, anxiety, alcohol, and ageing may reduce libido and sexual potency and may encourage faith in aphrodisiacs. In the Kinsey report on human sexuality, impotence or inability to create an erection sufficient for intercourse was found in 1.3 per cent of men up to 35 years of age, 6.7 per cent at 50 and 18.4 per cent at 60.

The placebo effect

A 'placebo' (a Latin word meaning 'I shall please') was originally a mourner employed to sing at funerals for a fee to protect the bereaved from having to do so. In medicine at the end of the eighteenth century, a placebo became an inactive drug used as a way of pleasing a patient by making him believe he was being treated when in truth there was no real remedy. By the end of the nineteenth century a placebo was widely known as a dummy medicine, a 'sugar' or 'chalk' pill.

The power of placebos is enormous, particularly when people are desperate, and the field of sexual desire and performance is perfect for placebos to play a successful role, thus increasing the reputation of so-called aphrodisiacs. Whatever the mechanism of success, the power of placebo aphrodisiacs can be harnessed to increase human confidence and happiness and, with few side-effects, their global value is difficult to deny.

Sex hormones and sexual activity

Sex hormones are crucial to the normal sexual and reproductive health of human beings (*see* Chapter 19). Oestrogens and progesterone are the main female hormones required for health and reproduction, while testosterone, made in the testes, is the main male hormone necessary for normal libido and potency. The production and release of sex hormones is under the control of the pituitary gland at the base of the brain.

Testosterone

Testosterone is required for normal sexual performance in the male and, if testosterone levels are abnormally low, the administration of additional testosterone can often restore potency. There is, however, a considerable range in the levels of testosterone circulating in the blood of men with normal sexual desire and performance which suggests that the level of testosterone has little influence on these. There is no evidence that giving extra testosterone can increase sexual desire or performance if a man's own testosterone level is within the normal range for his age. This is because hormone feedback controls act on testosterone synthesis (*see* Chapter 19) and giving extra testosterone simply causes the body to reduce its own production.

In fact, testosterone levels are known to be lower when men are not sexually active than when they are, at which stage levels rise again. This is probably because testosterone is necessary for the production of mature sperm and is relatively unimportant when mature sperm are not needed. Libido and sexual activity, therefore, regulate testosterone levels rather than the reverse.

These facts, unfortunately were not known at the time when testicular transplants of 'monkey glands' were popular therapy for sexual dysfunction. Such transplants were the understandable but ineffective result of the work of people like the French doctor Charles-Edouard Brown-Séquard. In May 1889, at the age of 72 years, he prepared an extract of guinea-pig testes in water, filtered it, and injected it into himself (an action which many of his colleagues felt certainly indicated the need for some form of therapy!). Brown-Séquard claimed to experience a 'rejuvenating' effect of this preparation and triggered untold numbers of senior citizens around the world to seek similar treatment. However, since testosterone does not dissolve easily in water, and the German scientist Ernst Laqueur in 1933 needed more than a ton of bulls' testicles to extract enough testosterone to treat the effects of castration in one patient, Brown-Sequard was demonstrating a placebo effect, rather than a hormonal one.

Other people described experiments in animals in which extracts of testicles were injected to reverse the effects of castration. All this culminated in Paris around 1900 with a Franco-Russian surgeon, Serge Voronoff, who was the first to transplant testicles from monkeys into human subjects and claimed that the recipients (more than 500) were amazingly improved in youthful vigour. He became very famous, his treatments being euphemistically referred to as 'monkey gland therapy'. Unfortunately for his patients, the transplanted tissue would probably have been rejected by the body and any transplanted hormone would only have been active for a short time. One can only hope for their sake that the placebo effect was powerful enough in these patients to compensate for the trauma and potential disappointment of the process they had undergone.

A little later, in 1911, an American doctor, Victor Lespinasse, used the testicles from a recently dead youth and transplanted them into a 38-year-old man who had lost both his own in an accident. The operation was reported to be successful, though we do not know for how long. Nevertheless, the story prompted a Dr Stanley in San Quentin to set up business transplanting, into those who needed them, the testicles from criminals executed in the local prison. Fortunately the later isolation of testosterone by Laqueur meant that it could be used as a pure hormone, and the use of 'monkey glands' and other dubious sources of testicular tissue was abandoned.

Oestrogens

Frigidity is defined as a lack of interest in sex or an inability to achieve orgasm. In women, sex drive and desire are mainly the result of psychological and social factors which usually outweigh any hormonal effects. However, in the absence of psychological causes of frigidity, hormonal therapy may help many women. Sexual pleasure in women is based on the clitoris and clitoral sensitivity is maintained by androgenic hormones (see Chapter 19) produced by the ovaries. The levels of these androgens vary during the menstrual cycle and may account for the variation in libido experienced during the cycle. Chemotherapy for cancer, radiotherapy, or long-term use of oral contraceptives can suppress the ovaries, leading to reduced clitoral sensitivity and making orgasm more difficult to achieve.

In 1943, Dr U. J. Salmon used androgens to treat frigidity in women, but later research suggested that only auto-erotic behaviour was increased. The side-effects of male hormones, such as deepening of the voice, an increase in facial hair, and deterioration of relationships between partners, also prevented their becoming more widely used.

Female hormones, or oestrogens, are mainly produced from the ovaries (see Chapter 19). A deficiency of oestrogens following the menopause can reduce libido, but it can be restored readily by oestrogen replacement.

Prolactin

Prolactin is a protein hormone which exists in both men and women. In women, it initiates and maintains milk production after childbirth, but it also acts on the brain to affect libido. An increase in the levels of prolactin in the blood is associated with reduced libido and sexual activity. This is sometimes seen in patients, men or women, on haemodialysis treatment for kidney failure, in whom prolactin levels are raised.

Bromocriptine, a drug used in Parkinson's disease (see Chapter 8), blocks the release of prolactin from the pituitary gland and has been used successfully to treat sexual problems in dialysis patients. Unfortunately it has too many side-effects to be widely acceptable as an aphrodisiac, but drugs with similar actions against prolactin could be developed in the future. Bromocriptine has no effect, however, on the libido of normal males and lowering prolactin levels in the blood does not have any aphrodisiac effect in men.

Oral contraceptives

Oral contraceptive pills may either increase or decrease libido: libido may be increased by removing the fear of unwanted pregnancy, but a proportion of women seem to find sex less exciting without the possibility of pregnancy, and sex drive is reduced as a result. Oral contraceptive pills, rich in oestrogen, can increase libido but progesterone in the pill can suppress the secretion of ovarian androgens and so reduce sex drive. This is a problem which can be prevented by using a progestogen which has some androgenic activity.

Anti-androgens

Anti-androgens, such as oestrogens and progestogens, can be used as anaphro-disiacs (i.e. drugs which suppress sexual desire and performance) by preventing the body's own testosterone from acting normally. They can be used to treat male hypersexuality, habitual sex offenders, and excessive hairiness in women (hirsutism) in addition to prostatic cancer (*see* Chapter 18).

Erectile dysfunction

Erectile dysfunction, or impotence, is the inability to produce and maintain an effective erection. It is experienced by about 7 per cent of men at age 50 and nearly 20 per cent of men aged 60. There are several methods and drugs available to treat the problem, though some of these are inconvenient and clumsy. (The methods of assessment of erection can be equally crude. One of the most widely used is the Buckling Test, which assesses the ability of the erect penis to withstand a weight of 1 kilogram). Sildenafil (Viagra®) was introduced recently specifically for the treatment of erectile dysfunction.

Erection

The penis contains spongy tissue, the corpora cavernosa, which swell up when filled with blood. In the resting state, most of the cavernous blood vessels contain very little blood and the penis is relaxed. During sexual arousal these vessels dilate, allowing more blood in to fill and swell the tissue, causing erection (Fig. 23.1). Dilation of the vessels is brought about by the sympathetic and parasympathetic nerves (*see* Chapter 1) which release norepinephrine to act on beta-receptors and acetylcholine to act on muscarinic receptors, respectively.

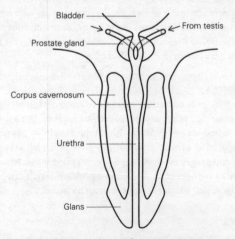

Fig. 23.1 Internal structure of the penis, showing the spongy corpus cavernosum which swells with blood to produce an erection. Injections of some drugs can be made into this tissue to induce an erection in patients suffering from impotence.

Acetylcholine in turn promotes the formation of nitric oxide which further relaxes the vessels. Factors that reduce erection include thickening of the arteries (atherosclerosis, *see* Chapter 15) since this prevents the blood vessels from dilating normally, beta-blockers, which prevent the activation of beta-receptors (*see* Chapter 15), and diseases which cause damage to nerves, such as diabetes (*see* Chapter 3).

Drugs for injection

Before the arrival of Viagra®, the most effective drug treatment involved the patient making an injection directly into the corpus cavernosum through the side of the penis. This is not as unpleasant as it sounds (apparently) and, provided that patients adhere to the instructions not to inject more than three times a week, most find it a very acceptable method. Indeed, it has the advantage over Viagra® that erection can be achieved less than ten minutes after injection.

The drug used is alprostadil, another name for prostaglandin E1. One of its most prominent effects is to relax and dilate blood vessels. By injecting it directly into the penis a local increase of blood flow is produced which causes an erection lasting up to an hour. Alprostadil can also be given as a small pellet inserted into the urethra* at the tip of the penis.

Other drugs used by injection into the penis include thymoxamine and phentolamine. These drugs block the alpha-receptors for norepinephrine (*see* Chapter 1) which maintain contraction of the blood vessels. Once these receptors are blocked the vessels relax, allowing more blood into the penis and producing an erection.

Sildenafil (Viagra®)

We saw in Chapter 15 how Robert Furchgott came to realize that the relaxation of blood vessels by acetylcholine was caused by an intermediary chemical which was later identified as nitric oxide. We now know that nitric oxide is important in the transmission of information between nerves and between nerves and muscle (*see* Chapter 16).

Both acetylcholine and nitric oxide cause blood vessels to relax by stimulating an enzyme, guanylate cyclase, which increases the amount of cyclic GMP† inside the cells. This lowers the amount of calcium in the cells and produces the relaxation. The cyclic GMP is then destroyed by another enzyme called phosphodiesterase.‡ Sildenafil (Viagra®) inhibits this latter enzyme, allowing the levels of cyclic GMP to rise and producing greater relaxation of the vessels.

---

* The tube bringing urine from the bladder to the exterior.
† Cyclic guanosine 3′,5′-monophosphate.
‡ Type 5 guanosine-cyclic-3′,5′-monophosphate phosphodiesterase (PDE5).

When Pfizer Pharmaceuticals began to develop sildenafil, they did not envisage its being used for the treatment of impotence. The drug was developed for the treatment of angina (*see* Chapter 16), because its ability to relax the coronary vessels was expected to increase blood flow to the heart, relieving the pain of angina and lowering the risk of a heart attack. When its was being tested on patients, however, during clinical trials, several patients who had been having difficulty obtaining a full erection during sexual activity reported that the problem disappeared when taking the drug. This alerted the company to the possibility that sildenafil might be an appropriate treatment for impotence and this has indeed proved to be the case. In the first two weeks after Viagra® was launched, over 20 000 prescriptions were written for it in the treatment of erectile dysfunction.

By inhibiting phosphodiesterase, sildenafil allows a larger increase of blood flow to the penis and a more effective erection. It works, therefore, by enhancing the body's own natural mechanisms to restore normal erectile function. It is extremely successful and easy to use since it is only necessary to take one tablet about an hour before sexual activity is anticipated. Because it works only on blood vessels which are being relaxed by the nervous system, it acts only during sexual stimulation and does not produce erections at inappropriate and possibly inconvenient times. Its effects last for about three to five hours. An effective erection can be induced and allowed to subside several times during that time, though ejaculation may not be possible every time. It also appears to be safe: side-effects are generally mild and include headache and dyspepsia.

Sexual activity itself, like any other physical activity, is associated with a degree of cardiac risk and sildenafil should only be taken after consultation with a doctor. The deaths which have occurred so far in men taking sildenafil have nearly all occurred in those with cardiovascular risk factors. Since it can dilate blood vessels throughout the body, not just in the penis, it should not be used by men taking nitrates or nitrites or by those with low blood pressure, a recent stroke, or coronary thrombosis. In these people, the drug may cause a large and dangerous fall of blood pressure or cause blood to be diverted away from parts of the heart and brain where it is needed.

If appropriately prescribed, however, sildenafil is a highly effective drug giving a more natural experience than other methods of treating erectile dysfunction, such as injections, insertion of drugs in the urethra at the end of the penis, or mechanical hydraulic devices. In spite of discussions about cost, it is still cheaper per person than certain alternative drugs freely prescribed for treating erectile dysfunction and, according to information available so far, is an extremely effective way of bringing inadequate erectile performance back to normal—an enormous relief to many men and to their partners.

Other treatments

A variety of mechanical treatments are available for erectile dysfunction. They include devices in which a cylinder is placed around the penis and a vacuum pump used to reduce pressure around the organ, encouraging (sucking) blood into it and producing an erection. The erection is maintained for sexual intercourse by placing a ring around the base of the penis to prevent blood leaking out. An alternative method is to implant a flexible tube into the penis which can be inflated as required.

Alcohol

Alcohol (*see* Chapter 24) has been used, and abused, by men and women for thousands of years and rules to regulate its sale are described in the laws of Hammurabi of Babylon around 1700BC. It is certainly the most widely used substance with aphrodisiac properties of our time, and in a sexual relationship the disinhibiting effects of alcohol and the associated feelings of relaxation and confidence make it a social lubricant and assist in encouraging sexual activity.

Alcohol plays an important part in legend and in religious rites; its aphrodisiac properties are described in the story of the Arabian prince, Jemshed, who stored fermented grape juice in the cellar of his palace in bags labelled 'poison'. One of his wives, whom the prince no longer loved, decided to kill herself by drinking this 'poison' but, instead of dying, she became decidedly happier and very loving, sufficiently so to regain the prince's affection.

In ancient Greece, wine was used in the orgiastic rites of the god Dionysius while the Romans, who called this god Bacchus, used to honour him at mixed baths by leaping naked into pools of wine, particularly champagne.

There is, however, a problem in using wine as an aphrodisiac, a problem described by Shakespeare's porter in Macbeth who reminds Macduff that of alcohol: 'Lechery, sir, it provokes and unprovokes; it provokes the desire, but it takes away the performance'.* Furthermore, when alcohol is drunk in large quantities for a long time, it produces more permanent damage which threatens sexual function. Alcohol-induced liver disease, for example, may produce atrophy of the testes. Even a single dose of six pints of beer can produce a significant reduction in the amount of testosterone in the blood which can last 10–20 hours after drinking it.

Alcohol, therefore, has certain aphrodisiac properties: by reducing inhibition it can encourage sexual desire and activity and, in women, may encourage intercourse by its muscle relaxing and anaesthetic properties, although it may delay the achievement of orgasm. There is no evidence that it increases sexual satisfaction directly, however, and quantities should be limited since an excess will produce a definitely anaphrodisiac effect.

* Act 2, Scene 1.

Other abused drugs

In addition to alcohol, other drugs which are abused have been thought to increase sexual ability. In 1979, Barnes and his colleagues described the preferences of men and women in certain sexual groups for drugs which they claimed increased their sexual performance (Table 23.1). The properties of these drugs are listed in Table 23.2. The nitrites are more popular with male homosexuals because they relax the anal sphincter; they do not increase the ability to have an erection. Any increase in sexual desire or activity obtained from abused drugs is unpredictable and is bought at the price of a significant risk to health, to normal relationships, and to society as a whole, and, cannot be recommended or felt to be safe.

In contrast to the drugs listed in Table 23.2, opium and narcotic drugs induce sleep: so morphine, heroin, and methadone all reduce libido, may cause sexual dysfunction and reduce or abolish potency, i.e. they are anaphrodisiacs.

There is no evidence that nicotine has any aphrodisiac properties.

Table 23.1 Drugs believed to improve sexual performance, in order of preference by different groups of users

Males	Preferred drugs
Heterosexual	cocaine, cannabis, alcohol, LSD, MDA
Bisexual	cannabis, nitrites, LSD, cocaine, MDA
Homosexual	cannabis, nitrites, MDA, LSD, amphetamine

Females	Preferred drugs
Heterosexual	cannabis, alcohol, methaqualone, cocaine
Bisexual	nitrites, MDA, cannabis, LSD, methaqualone, cocaine
Homosexual	MDA, nitrites, cannabis, methaqualone, cocaine, LSD

Drugs and libido

Any condition which brings with it mental or physical discomfort is likely to reduce libido. As health improves, enthusiasm for sex increases but the drugs used in treatment cannot really be described as aphrodisiacs since they are actually treating the underlying medical conditions. The antidepressants, for example, have been associated with increased libido, but this may simply be due to the improvement in mood.

After its introduction into medicine in the mid-1960s, the antiParkinsonian drug L-dopa (*see* Chapter 8) was said by some patients to increase their sex drive. The news spread rapidly and soon led to the drug being hailed in the press as an aphrodisiac and sold widely for this purpose. However, it does not seem to have any effect on sex drive, desire, or performance in normal people. The

Table 23.2 'Aphrodisiac' effects of abused drugs

DRUG	Potential aphrodisiac effect	Problems, side-effects, and dangers
Cocaine	1. genital anaesthetic effect prolongs pleasure. 2. stimulant effect on the brain increases feeling of power.	No evidence of genuine aphrodisiac effect and side-effects include tolerance, slurred speech, tremor, chest pains, hallucinations, and paranoia. Excess causes impotence in men and sterility in women.
Cannabis	Relaxation. May increase desire in men.	Reduces testosterone levels in blood and reduces sperm count, with some impotence.
Alcohol	Reduces inhibitions, delays orgasm. Produces relaxation and has some anaesthetic effect on the skin.	Reduces testosterone levels. Disinhibition may cause inappropriate behaviour. In excess it reduces performance.
LSD	In some people can induce a gentle mood which may be helpful in a sexual context.	Visual hallucinations and altered mental state. Delusions, e.g. of ability to fly, which may be dangerous.
MDA*	Produces relaxation and increased empathy between individuals.	Psychedelic effects. Decreased desire for orgasm. Dangerously addictive.
Nitrites	Relaxes blood vessels, facilitating erection, and relaxes the anal sphincter.	Many side-effects, e.g. nausea and muscle weakness. May be dangerous if user has high blood pressure, anaemia or heart disease.
Amphetamine	In males, delays ejaculation and in women, delays orgasm, thus potentially prolonging pleasure.	Delays in achieving orgasm may be frustrating. May unmask paranoia, aggression, and perversion and there is frequent dependence on the drug with withdrawal symptoms on cessation.
Methaqualone (Mandrax)	May increase desire and said to intensify orgasm.	Many side-effects and may be fatal if taken with alcohol.

* 3 methoxy-4,5 methylene dioxy amphetamine (Chapter 24).

improved sexual function in patients is simply the result of the drug's increasing the ability of patients to move normally.

Far more drugs reduce libido, potency, and sexual function than improve them (Table 23.3, p. 372). Those which induce it include antihypertensives such as hydralazine, prazosin, and beta-blockers (*see* Chapters 15 and 16), antipsychotic drugs (*see* Chapter 9) and some diuretics (*see* Chapter 5). Although the percentage of patients with sexual side-effects from these drugs is small, the effects are often not reported by patients to their doctor, and indeed may not even be recognized by patients as a side-effect of drug treatment at all. The associated unhappiness may be considerable. Any patient who feels a

Table 23.3 Drug effects on sexual activity

MALES

Type of drug	Example	Biological mechanism	Effect on sexual activity
Alpha-receptor block	Prazosin; some drugs lowering blood pressure	Reduced contractions of muscle in the vasa deferentia (sperm ducts)	Diminished erection and ejaculation
Androgen antagonists	Drugs used for prostate cancer	Block receptors for testosterone in the brain	Diminished libido
Beta-receptor blockers	Propranolol	Reduce blood flow to the penis	Diminished erection and ejaculation
Dopamine receptor block	Anti-schizophrenic drugs	Increased secretion of prolactin	Diminished libido
Increased sympathetic nervous activity	Amphetamines	Reduced blood flow to the penis	Diminished erection

FEMALES

Type of drug	Example	Biological mechanism	Effect on sexual activity
Acetylcholine antagonists	Atropine	Reduced blood flow to the sex organs	Reduced vaginal secretions; delayed or inhibited orgasm
Beta-receptor blockers	Propranolol	Reduced blood flow to the sex organs	Reduced vaginal secretions; delayed or inhibited orgasm
Increased sympathetic nervous activity	Amphetamines	Reduced blood flow to the sex organs	Reduced vaginal secretions
Dopamine receptor block	Anti-schizophrenic drugs	Increased secretion of prolactin	Diminished libido
Oestrogen and progestogens	Oral contraceptives	Reduced secretion of FSH/LH	Diminished libido

reduction in libido or sexual function while taking a new drug treatment should report it to their doctor since it might be possible to use a lower dose or find an alternative drug which does not have this side-effect. Even if this is not possible, it is at least reassuring to know that the problem will disappear when the drug is eventually stopped.

Pheromones

Pheromones are hormones acting outside the body which allow animals to communicate with each other. They include the sex pheromones, which could be classed as aphrodisiacs since, in non-human animals, they alter sexual behaviour. These are among the most powerful of biological chemicals. The males of some species of moths are said to detect the pheromones produced by a female of the species up to four miles away. The scents deposited by some animals contain chemicals which appear to have a strong sex attractant and stimulant effect. They include civetone from the civet cat, and muskone from the musk deer.

Are there human pheromones?

The vaginal secretions of women contain several simple chemicals such as butyric acid, iso-butyric acid, and isovaleric acid. Similar mixtures of these induce sexual activity in some monkeys, but there is no evidence that they do so in humans. Perhaps the behaviour of men was once determined by these secretions, but modern man has lost the ability to respond to such primitive stimuli.

Many perfumes now have a base which includes chemicals related to the pheromones of other animals, including muskone, civetone, and exaltolide. The assumption is that these will have some effect as sexual stimulants in people and will enhance sexual attraction.

There are several hormones present in the sweat secreted by glands in the groin and axilla (armpit), including steroids related to testosterone, such as androstenol and androstenedione. There is a wealth of anecdotal reports of women sitting close to chairs or other object sprayed with these hormones, but careful scientific trials have failed to produce any convincing evidence that they do act as sexual attractant or stimulant molecules.

Yohimbine

Yohimbine is a chemical isolated from the bark of the African yohimbéhé tree. It is one of the few drugs to have any real scientific justification for an aphrodisiac action. It works by blocking the receptors for amines such as norepinephrine (see Chapter 1) and 5-hydroxytryptamine (5HT). The amount of sexual activity and desire of animals is determined, like all aspects of our behaviour, by the brain. In particular, a small part of the brain called the hypothalamus near the base of the brain and roughly in the middle of the head, controls many 'unconscious' aspects of our daily lives. These include control of our body temperature, our appetite for food and water, and our level of sexual activity. These various functions are performed by nerve cells releasing norepinephrine or 5HT as their neurotransmitters (see Chapter 1). This is why drugs such as amphetamine, by stimulating the release of norepinephrine and 5HT, decrease appetite. Yohimbine also increases the release of norepinephrine but blocks the receptors for 5HT and this change of amine balance in the brain increases sexual drive. Unfortunately, yohimbine can also block receptors for norepinephrine on some of the muscles involved in ejaculation, such as those of the vas deferens (the tube carrying sperm from the testes and which is cut during a vasectomy operation). The net effect—stimulating libido but preventing ejaculation—is, therefore, not unlike that of alcohol.

'Aphrodisiac' foods

Over the centuries, the search for aphrodisiacs has taken men and women into the worlds of food, plants, and animals. Many of the substances used may well contain chemicals we could call drugs, but since the historical, botanical, and anthropological descriptions of all the substances used as aphrodisiacs would easily fill a book on its own, we have limited ourselves in this chapter to a few examples from each group. In most cases scientific support for an aphrodisiac effect from any of these substances is lacking:

- **Chocolate**, sometimes mixed with vanilla
  Favoured in seventeenth-century Europe, young women were forbidden to drink it in case they were tempted by 'the sins of the flesh'.
- **Honey and sweetmeats**
  Popular as sources of energy needed for sexual performance.
- **Nuts**
  Popular as aphrodisiacs since Victorian times, but with no justification.
- **Seafood**, especially oysters
  The association between oysters and libido arose from the myth that Aphrodite, the goddess of desire was born from the sea when Cronus castrated his father and threw his genitals into the sea.
- **Fruits and vegetables**
  Over the centuries several fruits and vegetables have been claimed to be useful, including apples, oranges, peaches, figs, truffles, asparagus, and tomatoes.

'Aphrodisiac' plants

In addition to these, aphrodisiac (or anaphrodisiac) properties have been ascribed to a range of other plants, herbs, and flavourings:

- **Coriander**
  Men gave this herb to their women before seducing them in the Middle Ages since it has a mildly narcoleptic (sedative) effect—hence its name of 'Dizzy Corn'.
- **Damiana**
  Another herb claimed to have aphrodisiac properties.
- **Dill**
  This has been used to treat impotence in men.
- **Fenugreek**
  Used in the harems of the Middle East and North Africa, supposedly to stimulate conception.
- **Feverfew**
  Said to have a specific aphrodisiac effect on women.

- **Flowers**

  Many heavily scented and brightly coloured flowers such as cyclamen, fuschia, and roses have been claimed to stimulate desire, as have tropical plants such as bamboo, sago, kava-kava root, marijuana, ginseng, and even the stinkhorn.

- **Ginseng**

  Among many other properties, this herb has often been claimed to treat impotence.

- **Guarana**

  This is a South American herb which has been described as a potent 'energizer', increasing sexual drive.

- **Hot spices** such as chillies and peppers.

  These have been applied directly to the sexual organs to encourage blood flow and potency. They were feared by the English Puritans because of their supposed ability to provoke unseemly passions.

- **Mandrake**

  The mandrake plant has been prominent in the legends of Greek, Roman, Indian, Arabic, and Chinese literature. There are two types of mandrake: the real mandrake plant with a long, forked root and with hypnotic and sedating properties from the alkaloids it contains, and the magical mandrake which has never existed but which has always been described as growing at the foot of a gibbet and glowing in the dark. When pulled from the ground it was supposed to give a shriek which was instantly and agonizingly fatal to anyone who heard it, and a dog was therefore used to uproot such plants. When the drug methaqualone (Mandrax®) was launched in 1965 the name was probably chosen to reflect the sleep-inducing properties of the mandrake plant. However, since it also produced euphoria (an elevation in mood) it was soon being abused. By 1973, it was the most popular street drug of abuse. It was claimed to intensify orgasm and to improve sexual performance, but it could be fatal if used with alcohol and had many side-effects. It is no longer available.

- **Nettles**

  Pliny in ancient Greece recommended that the sexual organs be rubbed with nettles. There is no doubt that this would produce considerable local irritation because of the presence of acetylcholine and histamine in the stings, driving a man to seek stimulation. Both substances would also increase local blood flow in the penis, thus helping an erection.

- **Orchids**

  The roots of some orchids, especially *Cynos orchis* were also recommended on the basis that they resembled dogs' testicles. (In fact the word orchid comes from the Greek *orkhis* meaning a testicle.)

- **Peppermint**
  Named after Persephone, Queen of Hades, whose husband loved the nymph, Menthe.
- **Rocket** (*Brassica eruca*)
  This was sown around the shrine of the phallic god, Priapus. It was also described by Pliny as inducing 'a great provocation of lust'.
- **Saffron**
  Modern Chinese and American research describes stimulation of the uterus (womb) which may be a result of the presence of chemicals such as veratrine. An aphrodisiac effect is unproven.
- **Satureia**
  Used by the sex-hungry satyrs of mythology for its lust-provoking power.
- **Saw Palmetto**
  Said to stimulate and strengthen the male reproductive system.
- **Springwort**
  To be rubbed on the limbs to give superhuman sexual strength.
- **Thyme**
  This was worn on the head as wreaths which were believed to stimulate desire.
- **Verrain**
  Virgil and Horace described its 'lust-provoking powers'.

'Aphrodisiac' animals

There are also many animal products that have been claimed to have aphrodisiac properties, primarily for the commercial benefit of the marketeers and with a reputation deriving largely from their esoteric and mysterious nature:

- **Elephant tusks**
  These have no known aphrodisiac effect but a mistaken reputation for sexual power.
  Hippomanes
  A fleshy substance from the forehead of a newly-born foal.
- **Rhinoceros horn**
  There is no evidence of any aphrodisiac effect but rhinoceros hunting poses a major threat of extinction of the species. The word 'horny' is a legacy of the mistaken belief in its power.
- **Reindeer antlers**
  Once crushed to a powder, these were taken by Csars and Emperors for their supposedly extraordinary effects on male potency.
- **Spanish flies** or cantharides
  These are actually beetles (blister beetles, usually *Cantharis* species) which contain a chemical called cantharidin. Because of its ability to induce

blistering of the skin, it has been used to remove warts, but if taken by mouth it is a dangerous poison with a toxic dose as low as 3 milligrams and a fatal dose of only 32 milligrams (about one thousandth of an ounce). The damage it causes to the lining of the stomach and intestines produces severe stomach cramps, with vomiting of blood. When it reaches the bladder and urethra it causes swelling of their linings, making the passing of urine very difficult and extremely painful. Death is caused by kidney damage. Livia, mother of the Roman Emperor Tiberius was said to have used it as a poison in the imperial family. In more recent times, Dr M A Lecutier described in 1954 the case of a fisherman who pricked his finger while putting some Spanish fly on his fish-hook. He died within six hours.

The reputation of Spanish fly as an aphrodisiac comes from the use of very low doses which, while still causing cramps and painful urination, also cause sufficient irritation of the urethra that an erection may occur and be sustained for several hours. This was the case with a group of French soldiers described by Dr J Meynier in 1893. They had eaten frogs which had in turn fed upon *Cantharis* beetles and their spontaneous erections, reported to the camp doctor, were maintained for several hours. Madame de Pompadour is said to have used Spanish fly to keep the love of King Louis XV of France.

Miscellaneous

Finally, there is a group of miscellaneous 'aphrodisiacs':

- **Arsenic**
  Believed in the eighteenth century to be a sexual stimulant. Arsenic was popular among prostitutes to produce rosy cheeks. We now know this is caused by damage to blood vessels in the skin. It is a dangerous poison (*see* Chapter 25).
- **Gold and silver**
  These were used in medicinal mixtures up to the 1970s.
- **Gerovital** and **Aslavital**
  In the 1950s, Dr Ana Aslan in Bucharest claimed to have discovered revitalizing injections which included the local anaesthetic procaine and which were said to affect libido. Clinical trials failed to find any real effect.
- **Hot pitch**
  This was popular among Arabs because of the stimulating effect when rubbed on to the penis.

Preparations available today of some of the ingredients listed above as aphrodisiacs tend to be in the forms of creams or pills, often in 'hot colours' of red, orange, yellow, or gold—the colours of the hot spices they may contain and which are believed to have aphrodisiac effects. Some preparations are of single components while others, such as Potensan Forte® are a mixture of several drugs or herbs. New, equally esoteric preparations are coming onto the market all the time, such as a preparation from fertilized, partly incubated chicken eggs (Libid®, Erosom®, Ardorare®) which is claimed to increase male sexual desire.

Final thoughts

We may smile at the gullibility of people buying these commercial 'aphrodisiacs' but at least most of those available nowadays are safe, and anticipation of benefit can produce a very useful placebo effect on potency. Care must be taken with some, however, such as Spanish flies and arsenic which may be toxic or even fatal.

Finally, however, it should be remembered that, happily for most of us, love potions are not required for love to grow, and the reasons why one person loves and desires another are far more complicated than can be explained by the action of drugs on receptor organs. Love, thank heavens, remains more powerful and more gloriously unpredictable than either chemistry or pharmacology.

Summary

- *An aphrodisiac has been defined as 'a drug or other substance capable of inducing venereal desire or lust'.*
- *In men, testosterone has little influence on sexual activity. Rather, libido and sexual activity probably affect the production of testosterone.*
- *Prolactin reduces libido and drugs which prevent its formation increase libido.*
- *Erectile dysfunction (impotence) in men can be treated with drugs such as alprostadil, thymoxamine, and phentolamine injected directly into the spongy erectile tissue of the penis.*
- *Sildenafil (Viagra®) inhibits the destruction of a chemical, cyclic GMP, which is involved in erection.*
- *A range of other drugs has been claimed to have aphrodisiac properties but for most of them these effects have never been proved scientifically. Some of these drugs are quite dangerous.*

CHAPTER 24

Drugs of recreation and misuse

Darker than opium, sweeter than hashish, it consoles the dejected, seduces the shy, refreshes the weary. It is humanity's most popular, most delectable drug—an object of mild pancultural addiction—and yet it can be sold without a prescription. At least for now.*

On the kitchen shelf of most homes sits a tin of the most potent drug, innocent and unknown, a drug sold in every grocery store, used by every cook and ignored by the sleuths of the narcotics division of the justice department. This strange exotic drug from the Orient is a household byword and yet within its innocent spiciness lurks a chemical capable of drugging one completely out of the world of reality and sending him into a hypnotic trance where a world of golden dreams and euphoric bliss wraps itself around him.†

Cannabis? LSD? Amphetamine? No, the first quotation applies to chocolate and the second to nutmeg and we shall see later the possible reasons for their popularity. Most of the drugs we shall describe in this chapter are often misused. Some, such as caffeine, are not appreciated as drugs at all. Some can produce dependence (addiction).

What is dependence?

Dependence has been defined as 'a state characterized by (1) a compulsion to take a drug, (2) a loss of self-control in limiting the intake of the drug, and (3) withdrawal signs which may include a psychological craving for the drug and physical signs such as headaches, sweating, hallucinations, and convulsions'.

Why are some drugs addictive?

In the 1950s, a group of American psychologists including Olds, Milner, and Skinner were exploring the functions of different parts of the brain by placing electrodes into the brains of rats during anaesthesia and, after allowing the

---

* Christine Chianese writing in *The Sciences*, March/April 1997.
† From *The hallucinogens* by A Hoffer and H Osmond, 1967, Academic Press, p.53.

animals to recover from the anaesthetic, delivering tiny electric shocks through the electrodes. The electrical stimuli did not seem to disturb the animals in the least. In fact, the researchers discovered that when the electrodes were placed into a small region of brain called the ventral tegmental area (VTA), the rats actually seemed to enjoy the stimuli. If the animals were allowed to press a lever which triggered a stimulus through the electrodes, most animals would soon spend most of their time pressing it. Some animals did so at the expense of sleeping, eating, and drinking and had to be taken away from the lever if they were not to die from exhaustion and starvation. Animals in which the electrodes were not connected to the lever pressed it a few times, accidentally or out of curiosity, but soon became bored and went back to their normal routine of eating, drinking, and sleeping.

Olds and Milner proposed that the rats' behaviour could best be explained if they experienced the VTA stimuli as some kind of 'reward' for pressing the lever. The VTA and the brain pathways associated with it have become known as 'reward' centres.* In humans, similar behaviour might be explained by saying that the subjects found the stimuli 'pleasant'. We do not, of course, have any way of knowing whether rats feel pleasure, as humans understand the word. We can only infer something akin to pleasure reflected in the animals' devotion to pressing the lever.

This experiment has turned out to be far more important than anyone could have imagined. Scientists soon discovered that the main nervous pathway from the VTA uses dopamine as its neurotransmitter. If drugs which block the effects of dopamine are given to rats with electrodes in the VTA, they no longer bother to press the lever for their stimulus reward: the activity of dopamine is essential for the reward experience.

We now know that many of the drugs which produce dependence (addiction) in humans, including amphetamine, morphine, and cocaine, can promote the release of dopamine from these nerve cells. Moreover, their tendency to cause dependence can be prevented by giving antagonist drugs which block dopamine receptors. Addiction to these drugs in humans seems to be an attempt to stimulate the reward pathways of the brain, except that in humans this is achieved using chemicals rather than electrical stimuli.

Does this mechanism apply to *all* drugs producing dependence? As more scientific evidence is obtained, it does look as though most drugs can affect the activity of the dopamine-releasing nerve cells of the VTA pathway. Drugs such as amphetamine act directly on these neurons to induce a release of dopamine from the nerve endings in the brain. Cocaine stops the nerve cells retrieving dopamine after they have released it naturally, so that more dopamine remains

* The reward pathway includes those areas of brain connected with the VTA, especially areas called the nucleus accumbens and the ventral pallidum.

outside the cells to act on receptors. Morphine acts on its own receptors (*see* Chapter 6) which in turn activate dopamine receptors indirectly.

Drugs as different as nicotine, cannabis, and benzodiazepines may also produce dependence in this way. In the presence of nicotine or cannabis, cells in the VTA can release dopamine more easily than usual. Benzodiazepines act by a rather complicated sequence of events, increasing the effects of the transmitter GABA on cells which control the VTA. The result is that activity of the VTA cells increases, releasing more dopamine onto its receptors.

Tolerance

If some drugs, such as morphine, are given to patients for more than a few days, the dose must be increased to produce the same degree of pain relief (*see* Chapter 6). This requirement for more drug is known as tolerance. Dependence and tolerance often go together.

What is the basis of withdrawal signs?

There are probably different mechanisms of dependence and withdrawal for each drug of misuse, but several common features can be identified. Many drugs, as we have seen already in this book, act as agonists, activating the receptors for a natural hormone or neurotransmitter. When an agonist is used repeatedly, cells try to compensate by lowering the number of receptors for it, a process called down-regulation. If the subject stops taking an agonist suddenly, the cells are 'caught napping', with too few receptors for the normal transmitter or hormone. The cells do not respond efficiently to the natural substance and the subject will experience withdrawal symptoms.

Similarly, if a drug acts as an antagonist at a receptor, blocking the actions of a natural transmitter or hormone, cells try to increase the number of receptors so that they can regain their natural sensitivity. The sudden cessation of the drug will now leave the cells too sensitive to their normal chemical, and withdrawal symptoms will again occur. This aspect of dependence at the cellular level has been discussed in Chapter 6.

Alcohol

The substance we refer to in everyday speech as 'alcohol' is only one of a large group of alcohols.* Scientifically it is known as ethanol or ethyl alcohol.

Alcohol has been used for medicinal purposes since antiquity, often as a means of dissolving preparations of plants or animal tissues. Large doses, either alone or in combination with opium, also seem to have been used, long before

---

* An alcohol is a chemical with an oxygen and a hydrogen atom forming a 'hydroxyl' grouping (-OH).

the discovery of anaesthetics, to reduce sensitivity to pain during the crude forms of surgery used in ancient times. It also had its recreational uses, as reflected in ancient Sumerian references to fermented barley drinks and its later use as wine in ancient Greece and Rome.

Alcohol's effects at different concentrations in the blood were summarized by the 'D signs' listed by the British pharmacologist Sir John Gaddum:

- dizzy and delightful (at 1mg per ml of blood)
- drunk and disorderly (at 2 mg per ml of blood)
- dead drunk (at 3 mg per ml of blood)
- danger of death (at 4 mg per ml of blood).

How does alcohol work?

Alcohol readily dissolves in fatty tissues and cell walls. As it does so, it squashes those walls so that the receptors and other molecules present are distorted and cannot work properly. Because the brain is so intricate and depends on the precise interactions of millions of cells, it is more susceptible to this disruption than other organs. The effects of alcohol are, therefore, largely the result of a generalized confusion of the nerve cells.

Alcohol also depresses the activity of nerve cells in the brain. It does so by two main methods. Firstly, it acts on the receptors and channels responding to the transmitter GABA (see Chapter 13). This is an inhibitory transmitter, which opens channels for chloride ions. This in turn makes nerve cells less likely to set up the electrical impulses (action potentials) by which they interact with other cells in the brain. Alcohol acts on these channels so that, when they are activated by GABA, they are 'wedged' open and cannot easily close again. The effect of GABA is thereby greatly prolonged and activity of the nerve cells is suppressed.

The second action of alcohol is to block receptors for glutamate, an excitatory transmitter which is responsible for most of the interactions between nerve cells in the brain. By blocking excitation, alcohol is again interfering with the ability of the nerve cells to 'talk' to each other, so that the brain cannot work normally.

Together, these two actions of alcohol produce a depression of the brain which is seen first in the areas which contain most connections between the cells. These include the cortex, responsible for thinking, reasoning, and judgement, and the cerebellum, responsible for some aspects of movement. Thus the first signs of taking alcohol are a decline in the clarity of thinking, impaired judgement of situations and distances, and a decreased performance of movement tasks which are the result of training (playing an instrument, balancing, typing). Tests can easily show that performance declines in all these cases even when alcohol has been consumed in quite small quantities, less than those at which we become aware that we have been drinking.

After slightly larger amounts of alcohol, similar to those which do begin to make us aware that we have taken alcohol, we start to lose concentration and our memory processes become affected.

In many people, alcohol may stimulate their social interactions and overall behaviour, because the cortex is normally responsible for restraining our behaviour and social interactions. As the cortex is depressed by alcohol, these restraints are lost. Some people become more talkative, some become less inhibited sexually, some become aggressive, and some even violent.

As people consume more alcohol, the brain is depressed more and more, until the individual becomes drowsy and falls asleep. In the highest doses, equivalent to about 10 pints of beer or most of a bottle of spirits drunk over a couple of hours, the person may fall into a coma, those parts of the brain which control breathing become depressed, and death may ensue.*

Regular consumption of large amounts of alcohol can lead to serious health problems, gradually destroying the liver (cirrhosis) and damaging several parts of the brain. Eventually, areas of brain involved in learning and memory are destroyed almost entirely, so that chronic alcoholics lose the ability to retain information for more than a few seconds. It may sometimes be quite difficult to distinguish between patients with this advanced form of alcoholic brain damage and those with early Alzheimer's disease.

Alcohol and sleep

Alcohol is sometimes taken as a 'nightcap', as the initial calming, relaxing effect has a sedative action and can help us to get to sleep. However, it also disturbs the pattern of sleeping (see Chapter 13) so that less time is spent in the important REM phases, and individuals usually waken early. The overall quality of sleep is, therefore, reduced, and the use of regular alcoholic nightcaps may result in people being more likely to lose concentration or fall asleep during the day.

Alcohol and blood pressure

Alcohol relaxes blood vessels. This is the reason for feeling warm after taking moderate amounts. It is also the reason why alcohol should never be given to people suffering from haemorrhage, or being treated for shock at the scene of accidents, as the blood pressure will be low in such people and alcohol will depress this further to a level which might be very dangerous.

If alcohol is taken in moderate to large amounts regularly over several years, it seems to produce a gradual increase in blood pressure, probably by an effect on the brain, with an increased risk of stroke. Conversely, the regular consumption of small amounts of alcohol, equivalent to about one glass of wine or a measure

* In 1999, the legal limit for driving in the UK is a blood alcohol level of 80 mg per 100 ml. In the USA it is less than this, but varies in different States. The lethal level is around 400 mg per 100 ml.

of spirits per day, seems to lower the risk of a heart attack. This is probably because alcohol produces a rise in the amount of 'good' high-density lipoprotein (HDL) (see Chapter 15) in the blood, and a decrease in the amount of 'bad' low-density lipoprotein (LDL), although scientists do not yet understand how alcohol produces these changes.

Alcohol and the stomach

Alcohol also dilates blood vessels in the stomach wall. It should not, therefore, be taken with drugs such as aspirin which can cause irritation, bleeding, and the formation of ulcers. For the same reason, alcohol should not be taken by anyone with an ulcer, partly because the dilatation of blood vessels may cause the ulcer to burst and bleed, and partly because it increases the secretion of acid by the stomach (see Chapter 4).

Alcohol and the liver

Alcohol increases the storage of fats in the liver and, over a period of several years, these gradually reduce the effectiveness of the liver. The condition is known as cirrhosis of the liver and causes very serious health problems. Until it is very advanced, however, liver function can be restored by stopping or greatly reducing the intake of alcohol.

Alcohol and the kidney

It is well known that alcohol increases the frequency and volume of urination. Normally the amount of urine produced in the kidney is controlled by a hormone, antidiuretic hormone (ADH), secreted by the hypothalamus in the brain. ADH acts on the kidney to reduce urine formation and is secreted by the brain when there is a need to retain water. Alcohol reduces the secretion of ADH so that more urine is produced. One of the causes of hangovers after taking large amounts of alcohol is the degree of dehydration produced by this loss of water. That is why people are advised whenever possible to drink the same volume of pure water as of an alcoholic beverage.

Red wine and antioxidants

No discussion of alcohol would be complete without a mention of what has become known as the 'French paradox'. Despite the consumption of large amounts of meat, saturated fats, and alcohol in France, the incidence of heart attacks is much lower than in other European countries. One view is that the reason lies in the very high consumption of red wines.

The use of wine as a medicinal preparation is not new, as described in the book by Salvatore P. Lucia *A history of wine as therapy*. Red wines in particular contain over twenty chemicals which are antioxidants* (see Chapter 22) and are, therefore able to remove or stop the formation of free radicals which can damage or kill cells. One of these is a chemical called resveratrol, which is now available as a separate drug. Some scientists believe that the cell damage caused by free radicals can lead to cancer. If true, this might explain the evidence that a small, regular intake of alcohol can reduce the incidence of some cancers.

In fact, red wine has an intriguing pharmacology of its own. Several compounds find their way into red wine from grape pips, including proanthocyanidin. This counteracts the ability of alcohol to produce the signs of drunkenness and helps remove free radicals (see Chapter 22) produced by alcohol. Similar chemicals are present in Japanese green tea and may also help to explain the lower incidence of cancers in people consuming red wine or green tea in moderation on a regular basis.

Memory

There are many jokes made by and about people who have spent an evening drinking heavily only to find the next day that they cannot remember clearly where they were or what they were doing. In fact, even quite small quantities of alcohol can make us more forgetful. Memories seem to be formed as a result of nerve cell interactions in a region of the brain called the hippocampus (because it is shaped rather like the sea-horse *Hippocampus*). One of the most important neurotransmitters in memory formation is the amino acid glutamate, which acts on receptors called NMDA receptors.[†] Alcohol can block these receptors, thereby impeding the formation of new memories.

The NMDA receptors are also believed to be important in the formation of correct nerve cell connections and one of the dangers of consuming alcohol during pregnancy is that the development of the baby's brain may be damaged.

On the other hand, repeated drinking can cause cells in the brain to increase the number of NMDA receptors in their walls. This overstimulates the cells and can kill them. Chronic drinking of alcohol, therefore, increases the possibility of brain damage and dementia in old age.

Balance

The middle part of the ear contains several tubes, or canals, some of which contain nerve cells which respond to the position of the head. Alcohol changes the density of the fluid in these canals and that in turn changes the activity of the sensory nerve cells, causing the brain to believe that the body's position in space is not the same as that being signalled by the eyes. The result is a tendency to stumble and fall.

* Red wine antioxidants include resveratrol and quercetin.
[†] NMDA is an abbreviation for N-methyl-D-aspartate.

Tolerance and dependence

Alcohol is destroyed in the liver by an enzyme called alcohol dehydrogenase. If alcohol is taken regularly, the liver produces more of this enzyme, so that more alcohol has to be drunk to achieve the same degree of pleasurable intoxication and relaxation. The need for larger amounts of alcohol is called 'tolerance'.

Although a large proportion of people regularly consume alcohol in small to moderate amounts, most can abstain from alcohol for several days or longer with no ill effects. A few, however, become dependent. They come to depend on alcohol psychologically to control the stresses and strains of a difficult job or domestic problems. As they become tolerant, they increase their daily intake to several times the safe limits and may be in danger of liver cirrhosis. It is usually obvious to friends and colleagues that someone is under the influence of alcohol, either from their behaviour or the smell of alcohol on the breath, even though the individual concerned may be fooled by their own intoxication into believing their problem is undetected.

Such people are unable to stop taking alcohol. Abstaining for 24 hours or so induces an intense craving, as well as physical symptoms such as headaches, trembling, anxiety, restlessness, and inability to sleep. After very long-term abuse of alcohol the trembling can be a long-lasting or even permanent result of cessation, associated with vivid dreams or hallucinations. This withdrawal condition is known as 'delirium tremens'.

What causes dependence on alcohol?

The answer to this question is not known with certainty, although there are many theories. The most popular among pharmacologists at present is that alcohol activates those brain cells which produce the transmitter dopamine. It is not clear how alcohol achieves this, but one idea is based on the discovery that alcohol can interact with other chemicals in the brain, including dopamine and 5HT, to produce chemicals whose molecules closely resemble morphine. Possibly, therefore, addiction to alcohol is related to addiction to morphine and the related drug heroin.

There is good evidence that alcoholism can run in families as a result of a defect in the genes for the dopamine receptors in the brain. Kenneth Blum at the University of Texas and Ernest Noble in California found that alcoholics had more dopamine receptors in their brains than normal people. The activation of dopamine receptors appears to be important in the reinforcing, addictive properties of drugs such as cocaine (*see later*), so this explanation may apply also to the excessive consumption of alcohol.

Scientists have also found that the amount of alcohol consumed by rats depends on the levels of a transmitter in the brain called neuropeptide Y. If the levels are high, the animals drink less alcohol; if the peptide levels are low, the animals drink more. If this relationship is also found in humans, it may be possible to understand alcoholism as a disorder of neuropeptide Y production in the brain and to develop drugs which increase the amounts of peptide or stimulate its receptors on brain cells.

Treatment of alcohol dependence

Diazepam

Dependence can be treated by placing alcoholics on diazepam for about seven days. This produces a sufficient sedative and relaxant effect to remove the immediate need for alcohol. After seven days, the worst of the physical withdrawal signs will have passed, so that the main hindrance to permanent cure is the psychological craving, or need, for alcohol. If effective counselling is started immediately to find ways of circumventing or dealing with the patient's problems at work and home, and to give them emotional support, long-term abstinence can often be achieved fairly readily.

Disulfiram

An alternative method to treat alcoholism is to use disulfiram. We have seen that alcohol is destroyed by alcohol dehydrogenase, but this produces another chemical called acetaldehyde. This is in turn destroyed by another enzyme, aldehyde dehydrogenase.

Disulfiram is a chemical once used in the manufacture of rubber products. Many years ago it was noticed that two workers in the industry became extremely sensitive to drinking alcohol after working with disulfiram. Similar reports were made by two scientists involved in the development of drugs to kill intestinal parasites. Jens Hald and Erik Jacobsen in Denmark had discovered a compound which killed the parasites in rabbits, but before giving it to people they decided to see if it had any unpleasant effects on themselves. Both men found no ill effects unless they had drunk alcohol, when they felt very ill, with headaches, nausea, and vomiting. The drug was disulfiram, and its development as an antiparasite drug was taken no further, as it was believed that patients would not tolerate the interaction with alcohol. It was several years later, in 1947 that the idea arose of using the drug to help alcoholics give up the demon drink. It is still available under its trade name of Antabuse®.

We now know that disulfiram inhibits aldehyde dehydrogenase, so that the acetaldehyde produced from alcohol in the liver cannot be destroyed. As the amount of acetaldehyde accumulates in the blood, the patient experiences severe headaches, nausea, and vomiting. He or she rapidly learns that any alcohol intake results in these very unpleasant symptoms and drinking soon loses its appeal. Treatment with disulfiram is very dependent on the patient's having a strong desire to break his or her addiction and sometimes it may be necessary to treat in hospital for a week or two.

Dr W M Keung at the Chinese University of Hong Kong has noticed that about half of the Asian population inherits an inactive form of alcohol dehydrogenase. These people rarely become alcoholics, presumably because any intake of alcohol will lead to the same array of unpleasant effects experienced by patients taking disulfiram.

Clomethiazole

An alternative treatment, which is not associated with the same unpleasant effects as disulfiram, is to wean addicts from alcohol by treating with clomethiazole, diazepam, or the recently introduced drug acamprosate. The former drugs have been used mainly for their antiepileptic and sedative effects, but they also reduce the need and craving for alcohol in addicts. All three drugs work by increasing the actions of the brain transmitter GABA, inhibiting the activity of nerve cells. This compensates for the increased activity of the cells which occurs when alcohol is withdrawn and is no longer blocking the effects of glutamate at the NMDA receptors.

Nicotine

The tobacco plant and several varieties of it grow readily in South America and it has been cultivated in many other parts of the world. Some of the first European explorers to reach the Americas observed the natives smoking rolled-up leaves called 'tobago'. One of the first people to send back to Europe some seeds of the plant used by the natives was Jean Nicot de Villemain and the plant was named *Nicotiana tabacum* to recognize the contribution of both Nicot and tobago to its popularity. From about 1570 the practice of smoking tobacco leaves spread throughout Europe. When the main chemical component of the leaves was isolated by the chemists Posselt and Reiman in 1828, it was natural to call it 'nicotine'.

Tobacco smoke contains at least 3000 chemicals, many of them poisonous such as carbon monoxide and cyanide, and several of them, such as nitrosamines being very powerful cancer-producing agents. Nicotine is one component of tobacco smoke, and is mainly responsible for the addiction to tobacco, a condition known as tabagism.

Nicotine acts primarily on the nicotinic receptors for acetylcholine described in Chapter 1. These are found on voluntary muscles so that, in new smokers, nicotine may produce muscle twitching and even experienced smokers will show a tremor in the hands. Nicotinic receptors also occur in the autonomic nerves (*see* Chapter 1) and stimulation of them increases activity of the sympathetic nerves. This in turn leads to an increase of blood pressure. As nicotine passes into the brain it also stimulates nicotinic receptors, causing an initial stimulation, alertness, decreased irritability or aggression, and a reduction of anxiety. In higher doses, the receptors for nicotine become saturated and cause depression of the brain.

With repeated smoking the muscle cells and their receptors become less sensitive to nicotine and the body destroys nicotine more readily so that the effect on muscles disappears. The receptors in the brain, however, are slightly different from those in muscle and are much more sensitive to nicotine, so that repeated smoking is, for a while, still able to cause stimulation. With time, tolerance develops as even these receptors become less sensitive and the amount of nicotine required to achieve the same degree of mental stimulation gradually increases.

Nicotine and addiction

Activation of nicotinic receptors in the brain increases the release of dopamine from nerve cells in the VTA and other areas. The repeated use of nicotine also reduces, to about half, the amount of the MAO enzyme in the brain. As we saw in Chapter 1, MAO destroys dopamine, so a loss of this enzyme would further increase the amount of dopamine in the brain. Together these effects probably account for smokers becoming addicted. It is likely that the addiction to smoking is due to the nicotine rather than a different constituent of tobacco smoke, as animals can become dependent on pure nicotine.

As discussed at the start of this chapter, the addictive properties of many drugs can be traced to their ability to increase the amount of dopamine in the brain. If this is indeed a common pathway to dependence, there arises a strong possibility that all such drugs may make it easier to become dependent on other drugs. This could mean that smokers might be more easily drawn into the use of progressively 'harder' and more dangerous drugs such as cocaine and heroin, a view that lends urgency to attempts to eliminate smoking among the young.

Treatment

Helping people to stop smoking, of course, is valuable not only because of the risk of progression to other drugs, but also because of the strong link between tobacco smoking, heart disease, and lung cancer. The association with lung cancer has been known since the first report of a correlation by Franz Muller in 1939 and has been confirmed many times since, most notably in the definitive report by Sir William Richard Doll and Sir Austin Bradford Hill in England in 1949.

The usual form of treatment is to withdraw smokers gradually from their habit so that they do not experience serious withdrawal symptoms. This is achieved in many cases by using nicotine-containing patches which are placed on the skin, allowing nicotine to be absorbed slowly and continuously. This treatment allows the smoker to break the habitual and ritual aspects of smoking, while still preventing withdrawal. The dose of nicotine administered via the patches can then slowly be reduced.

Recently bupropion has been introduced. This drug has been used to reduce anxiety, a common feature of withdrawal from nicotine, but it also seems to control the craving for nicotine directly. This is probably the result of an action of bupropion on the brain cells which contain dopamine and norepinephrine, reducing the changes in their activity during withdrawal.

As to the future, Michael Pianezza and his colleagues at the Addiction Research Foundation in Ontario recently discovered that people who smoke heavily have a defect in an enzyme which converts nicotine into another chemical, cotinine. This discovery fits in with research suggesting that cotinine may be more important than nicotine in producing addiction to cigarettes. A drug which inhibited the enzyme in smokers would be expected to suppress the formation of cotinine, lower the addictive drive, and reduce the number of cigarettes smoked.

Nicotine as a useful drug?

Smoking has been claimed to reduce the incidence of Alzheimer's disease and research in animals over many years has shown that stimulation of nicotinic receptors for acetylcholine (*see* Chapter 1) can improve learning and memory. This is the basis on which nicotine patches have been introduced for the treatment of Alzheimer's disease, as the beneficial effects of the drug can be obtained without the many dangers, (and irritation to others) of smoking. As we saw in Chapter 10, drugs are being developed which act on a type of nicotinic receptor which is found only in the brain. Such drugs should have much less effect than nicotine itself on the intestine, blood pressure, and heart rate, and should be much more valuable for patients with Alzheimer's disease than a nicotine patch.

There are other intriguing associations between smoking and disease. Patients with schizophrenia, for example, are much more likely to smoke tobacco than other people. There are many possible reasons for this, but one is that smoking helps patients unconsciously to control their symptoms. Research in animals supports this idea, since activating nicotinic receptors in the brain can reverse some of the schizophrenic-like effects of amphetamine and similar drugs. Some companies are investigating the possibility of nicotinic drugs, again acting only on the brain and not the heart or intestine, to treat schizophrenia.

Caffeine

Caffeine is present in the seeds of *Coffea arabica*, a shrub cultivated in Africa, South America, and Arabia. It is also found in tea (from *Thea sinensis*) and cola nuts (from *Cola acuminata*), the latter being used in the manufacture of cola drinks. It is probable that drinks made from coffee plants were used long ago in South America, but its use in Europe and Asia is said to date from around 1500BC when a shepherd tending his sheep in Ethiopia noticed that they were more active and slept less when they had eaten the berries of a local plant. He told this to a local monk, who began making drinks from the berries to help him stay awake when praying through the night.

With the development of trading routes, the use of coffee eventually spread to Europe, the first record of the purchase of coffee being in Venice in 1640. Its popularity waxed and waned several times over the succeeding centuries, partly due to differing views as to its effects on sexual activity. In about 1670, for example, a 'women's petition against coffee' was presented to King Charles II of England, complaining of the sexual inactivity of their menfolk who spent too much time in coffee-houses. Their plea that the 'entire race is in danger of extinction' led Charles to close down all the coffee houses in 1675, only to reopen them ten days later in the face of an avalanche of opposition.

How does caffeine work?

Most of the effects of caffeine are due to its blocking the receptors for a natural hormone, adenosine. This is produced by all organs and tissues whenever they are active and its effects tend to oppose that activity. In other words, adenosine is part of the body's mechanisms for controlling tissue activity. Since caffeine prevents the effects of adenosine, these two substances usually have opposite effects.

There is little doubt that caffeine stimulates the brain, increasing wakefulness, reducing fatigue and tiredness. It also increases the heart rate and makes the heart muscle more excitable with the result that some people experience palpitations and changes in the rhythm of the heartbeat (*see* Chapter 16). Blood pressure usually rises due to the increased heart rate and contraction of the muscle in blood vessels.

In the airways of normal people, adenosine has little effect. In those with asthma, however, it contracts the muscles and can trigger or worsen an asthma attack. Since caffeine blocks the adenosine receptors, it relaxes the airways in asthma. Theophylline, which is used medically to treat asthma (*see* Chapter 2), acts in the same way.

Most of the effects of coffee are due to its content of caffeine, but some are not. In the stomach, for example, drinking coffee increases the secretion of acid and digestive enzymes such as pepsin. These effects are also produced to the same extent by decaffeinated coffee, so they are probably caused by one or more of the other 3000 chemicals in coffee. The stimulation of acid production involves the release of histamine from cells in the stomach wall, and histamine H2 antagonists (*see* Chapter 4) prevent this effect.

In most tissues adenosine relaxes the muscle cells in the walls of blood vessels, and caffeine, by blocking adenosine receptors, causes contraction and raises blood pressure. In the kidney, adenosine contracts the blood vessels so that caffeine here relaxes them. As they relax, more blood flows through the kidney and more urine is produced. Caffeine also acts like some of the diuretic drugs (*see* Chapter 5) and slows the reabsorption of sodium from the kidney tubules. The combination of these effects results in the well-known diuresis—an increased production of urine—which follows a drink of coffee or tea.

Is caffeine addictive?

Most coffee and tea drinkers would agree that they need an early morning 'fix' of caffeine to get themselves going in a morning. When coffee is withheld from regular coffee drinkers or they are given decaffeinated coffee without their knowledge, there is a very well-recognized set of withdrawal symptoms. About 20–30 hours after the last cup of coffee, the subject begins to become irritable and to feel worried and anxious. They develop a headache which becomes progressively worse over about 5–10 hours and is accompanied by a feeling of laziness, great difficulty concentrating, and mental confusion.

These symptoms subside over the next 24–36 hours and are a sign of withdrawal from caffeine. Most coffee drinkers need to top up their caffeine levels during the day so that they remain free from them. After being withdrawn from caffeine for about 8 hours during sleep, however, the coffee addict wakens eager for his morning fix. Consciously or not, he is beginning to feel the approach of the confusion and tiredness of withdrawal which can be staved off only by taking more caffeine.

Cocaine

Cocaine is the main active chemical in the leaves of *Erythroxylon coca*, a shrub which grows in South America and South-East Asia. Some of the indigenous tribes of South America are known from cave paintings to have chewed coca leaves at least 3000 years ago. This practice reduced fatigue, allowing more work to be accomplished, and reduced the need and desire for food. Later cocaine became important in religious rites and festivals and its use was controlled by, and often restricted to, holy men. After the Spanish conquests of South America the use of coca leaves was again liberalized in order to increase the work capacity of the natives.

The introduction of cocaine into European medicine dates from the early

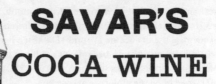

SAVAR'S
COCA WINE

The restorative and tonic properties of Coca are well exhibited in wine, but most Coca Wines are weak in Cocaine.

SAVAR'S COCA WINE, manufactured in our own laboratories, is standardised to contain half-grain Pure Cocaine per fluid ounce, and being of this strength it is classed as a true medicated wine.

N.B.—A 4s. 6d. bottle contains ten fluid ounces; in 2 drachm doses, this would last a patient about a fortnight; a 7s. bottle contains 20 ounces.

EVANS SONS LESCHER & WEBB,
LIMITED,
60, BARTHOLOMEW CLOSE, LONDON
AND
56, HANOVER STREET, LIVERPOOL.

Fig. 24.1 This advert from the British Medical Journal in 1906, for a wine containing cocaine, shows how little was known of the dangers of the drug at that time. (Wellcome Institute Library)

nineteenth century, when a French doctor, Angelo Mariani, began prescribing and selling medicines (such as 'marian powder') which included a generous helping of coca leaves. His happy patients spread the word and these medicines were soon being prescribed by doctors throughout Europe for most of the ills of mankind (Fig. 24.1). Mariani became very rich and was even honoured by one of his most famous customers—Pope Leo XIII.

A local anaesthetic
A German chemist, Albert Nieman, was the first to purify cocaine from the coca plant, in 1860. Nieman, as was the habit of many early chemists, tasted his new

chemical and found that his tongue became numb. This observation led a young Austrian eye surgeon, Karl Koller, at the University of Vienna, to the first serious medical use of cocaine around 1880 when he tried it as a local anaesthetic for eye surgery. It soon became invaluable in many surgical operations, for which general anaesthetics were not available. Most local anaesthetics in use today are based upon the molecule of cocaine.

Coca-Cola®

In 1886 John Pemberton, a pharmacist in Atlanta, adopted Mariani's idea and produced a medicine called 'Pemberton's French wine coca' which contained cocaine and extracts of cola nuts. Although this was used initially as a medicine on prescription, Pemberton later diluted it with carbonated water and saw its popularity soar with the general public as a refreshing, invigorating drink. In 1904, cocaine was removed from Coca-Cola and replaced by caffeine because of concerns for public safety.

Cocaine and the brain

The ability of cocaine to stimulate the brain—the reason for its use in South America—is responsible for its misuse today. Cocaine is available illegally in many different forms, known as coke, snow, gold dust, lady, and crack.* When sniffed or injected it rapidly penetrates into the brain and causes the release of dopamine and 5HT from cells in the brain. This effect is mainly due to the ability of cocaine to stop the uptake of these amines into the nerves once they have been released. The amounts reaching the receptors are, therefore, much higher than in a normal brain and are probably the basis of dependence on the drug. The same effects occur in animals and humans—rats and monkeys will choose cocaine rather than food when given free access to both.

The effect of cocaine is to induce pleasant feelings of euphoria, but these last only a few minutes and become less with successive doses. The subject feels confident, optimistic, and energetic, with increased self-esteem and sex drive. He or she needs progressively larger doses to achieve the same degree of euphoria, and the higher doses bring toxic side-effects. These include feelings of paranoia and of being watched, hallucinations (especially touch hallucinations of insects crawling along the skin and visual hallucinations of snow), and disordered thought patterns in which subjects become obsessed with apparently deep, philosophical issues. Adolf Hitler is reputed to have rinsed his sinuses repeatedly with cocaine and increased the dose of his cocaine-containing eye drops.†

Since cocaine contracts blood vessels, its repeated use can reduce the blood

---

* 'Crack' is so-called because of the noise made by exploding impurities in a burning cigarette.
† Reported by R Gordon in *Ailments through the ages*.

supply to tissues such as heart, lungs, and nose. The result can be severe chest pains, asthma, and collapse of the nasal tissues. Cocaine taken by pregnant women can affect the blood vessels of the embryo and cause seriously under-nourished or damaged babies.

If a subject is withdrawn from cocaine rapidly, he or she will develop intense feelings of desire, or craving, for more drug and will become extremely tired, apathetic, and depressed, with a marked increase of appetite.

Can cocaine addiction be treated?
A great deal of research is being carried out into methods of breaking the cocaine habit and curing addiction. One method involves the administration of a 'vaccine' against cocaine. This can be produced by stimulating the immune system of an animal to recognize cocaine as a foreign molecule and so produce antibodies which combine with the cocaine molecules. These can then be used to treat human addicts, mopping up any cocaine in the blood.

Another approach may be to use drugs which act on receptors for 5-hydroxytryptamine (5HT) in the brain. Rene Hene at Columbia University in New York has found that mice which do not have 5HT-1B receptors in the brain are more likely to become addicted to cocaine. Conversely, drugs which stimulate 5HT-1B receptors might be able to reduce the likelihood of becoming addicted, or at least to reduce the frequency of drug-taking or the doses needed to produce a satisfying 'high'.

Another recent discovery by Maria Pilla and her colleagues at the University of Cambridge and several research institutes in France has been that drugs which block D3 receptors for dopamine can prevent animals from becoming addicted to cocaine. It will be interesting to see whether a similar effect can be shown in humans.

Cannabis

Cannabis is believed to have been used as long ago as 2000BC and there is written evidence in Assyrian documents from 600BC of a preparation called 'qunnabu', a word that means 'the drug that takes away the mind'. Preparations of cannabis are known by a variety of names in different parts of the world depending on how they are made, and include ganja, bhang, hashish, hemp, and marijuana. All are made from the plants *Cannabis sativa* or *Cannabis indica*. The preparation known as hashish, for example, is made from the resin of the *Cannabis* flowers.

The uses of cannabis cover an enormous range. From ancient Persia there come tales of groups of men smoking hashish to excess and committing appalling acts of violence and murder. The word 'assassin' is derived from an Arabic word meaning 'hashish-eaters'.

In ancient Egypt, the dried seed and flowers of cannabis were thrown onto the funeral pyres at burial ceremonies, the vapours being inhaled by those present and, presumably, lessening the sadness of the bereaved families.

In the Dark Ages, however, the first records appear of a truly medical use for cannabis. Ointments were made from the dried flowers and used to cover burns and painful muscles and joints. Later, the practice of smoking cannabis was spread widely throughout Europe by the armies of Napoleon, who presumably found that its use reduced both the fear of battle and the pain of injury.

The modern use of cannabis dates from about 1850 when it was used to reduce pain in patients with severe arthritis. However, the doses needed for this were such that the patients spent most of their time in a stuporous sleep. Nevertheless, by 1860, cannabis had become one of the most popular pain-killing preparations, rivalling opium (Fig. 24.2).

The use of cannabis in Europe declined at the beginning of the 1900s, partly as a result of the increasing emphasis on using pure chemicals rather than crude powders made from whole plants, and partly because the medical establishment

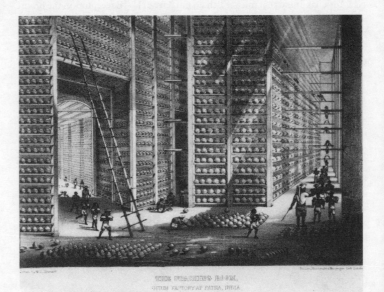

Fig. 24.2 An etching by W.S. Sherwill from around 1880, showing stocks of opium. When collected from poppies, opium was rolled into balls (opium balls) for storage. The illustration shows rows of shelves, full of opium balls awaiting shipment to China. (Wellcome Institute Library)

was beginning to realise that cannabis had properties which made people less interested in work and the harsh realities of life. In a climate which saw the introduction of laws to control drinking, it was natural that there should also be laws to limit the supply and use of cannabis. Its general use was outlawed in 1928, although it remained available for use by psychiatrists until 1973. Its main psychiatric use was to help reduce the hallucinations experienced by schizophrenic patients. The general climate has changed, however, and in 1995 it was estimated that 20 per cent of adults in the UK and 35 per cent of those in the USA had tried cannabis.

Effects of cannabis

Despite the legal restrictions still in force in most countries, many people use cannabis occasionally and believe that there is less danger to health and society than from smoking cigarettes or drinking alcohol. When smoked, cannabis induces pleasant feelings of happiness and exhilaration, well being, and self-confidence. There is usually relief from anxiety and tension, coupled with a mild aphrodisiac effect. Ordinary statements or events may seem hilariously funny, sensations are heightened, and time seems to pass very slowly. Under the influence of cannabis, users often believe their behaviour is quite normal and their state is not obvious to others; the phenomenon is similar to the effect of alcohol.

Unfortunately, however, cannabis reduces motivation and slows the processes of thinking clearly or rationally. It produces marked difficulties in decision-making and reduces both the ability to co-ordinate movements and the perception of sensation such as vision, hearing, and touch. Cannabis also strongly inhibits short-term memory, making it very difficult to remember recent events. Taken together, all these effects make complex tasks, such as driving, extremely hazardous. The great worry is that these changes in muscle co-ordination and mental ability last much longer than the inital, pleasant euphoric effects so that, after eight or ten hours, users of the drug may not be aware that their performance is still impaired. In fact, the depression of memory may last for several weeks.

Some of these effects of cannabis, of course, are similar to those of alcohol. Where cannabis differs most is in the production of mild hallucinations—objects around the drug-user may change shape or colour and inanimate objects may take on a life of their own. Changes in the perception of time are common, with minutes seeming to stretch to hours, or hours passing in what feels like minutes. Even with the use of small amounts of cannabis, therefore, there is a much greater danger to people driving, operating machinery, or using complicated equipment than with alcohol.

In addition, cannabis brings several long-term dangers. There is a danger of lung cancer from smoking marijuana which appears to be as great as that from smoking tobacco. Cannabis also depresses the immune system, increasing the risk of contracting infections, and lowers the production of the male hormone testosterone. Apart from these risks, cannabis is probably safer than alcohol or nicotine and seems to cause no lasting harm in most users. The jazz musician Milton Mezzrow was so well known for his repeated, chronic use of cannabis that the marijuana cigarette was once known as a 'mezz', yet he died only in 1972 at the very respectable age of 73. The report on cannabis prepared by Baroness Wootton in 1968, concluded that '... the long-term consumption in moderation has no harmful effects' with no evidence that cannabis use led inevitably to dangerous drugs such as cocaine and heroin. The reports of a Canadian commission led by Le Dain in 1972 and by the Royal College of Psychiatrists in the UK in 1987 came to similar conclusions.

What causes these effects?

As with most crude plant preparations, cannabis contains thousands of chemicals, but only a handful of these seem to be responsible for its effects. The most important chemical is abbreviated to THC* and the effects of the pure compound have now been studied intensively in animals and humans.

When given to subjects who are not used to using cannabis, THC makes them anxious and may even cause panic. Smoking cannabis does not usually cause panic, because the effect of THC is prevented by another chemical, cannabidiol. Even regular users can experience panic, however, if large doses of cannabis are smoked, because of the different rates of action of THC and cannabidiol.

THC also reduces inflammation. It works in a similar way to aspirin (*see* Chapter 6), preventing the production of prostaglandins in injured tissues. However, it is about twenty times more active than aspirin, which no doubt accounts for its early use to reduce the inflammation associated with burns and arthritis. As well as reducing the formation of prostaglandins, THC lowers the production of similar hormones called leukotrienes, some of which produce a very powerful contraction of the airways and are involved in asthma. THC could, therefore, represent a new type of anti-asthma drug.

Glaucoma is a condition in which the pressure inside the eyeball increases, causing visual changes and, unless treated, blindness. In 1971, doctors began receiving comments from patients being treated for glaucoma, that their visual problems were less after smoking cannabis. This led to the discovery that smoking cannabis reduced the pressure of fluid within the eye. Cannabis reduces the rate at which the fluid is produced and secreted, allowing more time for it to drain away. It has since been shown that THC is responsible for this activity and so could be of value in treating glaucoma. At least one drug has

* THC is an abbreviation for delta-9-fetrahydrocannabinol.

been developed from THC and is now undergoing clinical trials for the treatment of glaucoma.

Patients with serious cancers have often turned to unorthodox methods to cope with the pain which can occur in some cases and with the despair felt if the condition cannot be cured. Some patients may take to alcohol, others to cannabis. One of the unpleasant side-effects of some of the drugs used to treat cancer is intense nausea and vomiting, and in the early 1970s a number of cancer patients being treated with such drugs noticed that if they smoked cannabis they experienced far less of this problem.

This accidental observation has again led drug companies to produce chemicals derived from cannabis, or similar to them. Several, including nabilone, nabitan, levonantrodol, and dronabinol can prevent the severe nausea and vomiting associated with anti-cancer drugs such as cisplatin (see Chapter 18). These are the most effective drugs to treat this problem.

Two of these drugs have also been found to be powerful painkillers. Nabitan and levonantrodol can be used to treat the pain of cancer and post-operative pain after surgery. They do not act at the same receptors as the opiate drugs such as morphine. A major advantage of the cannabis-derived drugs is that they do not produce the dangerous depression of breathing which morphine does, and they are not addictive.

Thus, THC is responsible not only for most of the beneficial, potential medical uses of cannabis, but also for the psychotropic, or 'mind-altering' effects which people find so pleasant and which lead them to misuse cannabis. Some pharmaceutical companies have set out to try to separate these effects by identifying which parts of the THC molecule cause which effects, and then to produce new chemicals which retain the medical activity but lack the addictive properties.

The chemicals in cannabis have other effects too, such as reducing anxiety, stopping convulsions, and suppressing the activity of the cells responsible for our immune responses. Multiple sclerosis sufferers have smoked cannabis to reduce muscle cramps and relax tight sphincters. Further research on these chemicals is continuing and should eventually yield more new substances of use as anti-anxiety, anti-epileptic, and immunosuppressant drugs.

Are there 'receptors' for cannabis? If so, why?

When a group of chemicals produce marked effects in the body, two questions always arise. Is there a specific receptor responsible for those effects and if so, is there a natural chemical in the body which normally acts on those receptors? In the case of cannabis, the answer is 'yes' to both questions.

In the mid-1990s two receptors were found, one existing throughout the body including the brain (the cannabinoid-1 or CB1 receptor) and one existing only outside the brain, primarily in the immune system (CB2). The first of these is certainly responsible for the effects of cannabis on mental function—the hallucinations, confusion, and memory loss. The second receptor modifies the ability of the immune system to combat infections, though different chemicals in the cannabis mixture have opposite effects, some increasing and some decreasing our resistance to infection.

Following the discovery of cannabis receptors, scientists soon found chemicals occurring naturally in the body which act on those receptors. At least one of these substances (called anandamide from the Sanskrit word *ananda*, meaning bliss), has molecules similar to the prostaglandins and fatty acids. These natural substances are shedding new light on the biology of cannabis, and are already beginning to lead to an entirely new family of drugs.

Drugs from cannabis?

From what has been said of the historical uses of cannabis, it is apparent that drugs produced from cannabis could be of use in the treatment of disorders as diverse as asthma, strokes, epilepsy, multiple sclerosis, vomiting, and immune dysfunction.

Pharmacologists have begun to harness the potential medical benefits of cannabis by separating and purifying many of the individual chemicals. It is then possible for chemists to produce similar molecules with which to activate or block the cannabis receptors. Using such compounds scientists have discovered that the cannabis receptors are present on nerve cells in the brain which regulate the response to pain. Ian Meng and colleagues at the University of California and Antonio Calignano in Italy have found that anandamide or its synthetic analogues can activate CB1 receptors to produce a powerful analgesic effect, reducing the responses of animals to pain. The nerve cells involved are the same as those required for morphine to produce its analgesic effects. If new compounds can be produced to activate these receptors without causing the hallucinations and other mental symptoms of cannabis, they could become the non-addictive painkillers of the future.

In Chapter 4 we saw how one new drug, nabilone, has been produced as an anti-emetic. This drug is not entirely free from the mental effects of the cannabis mixture and has to be used under supervision, but its use is vital to those people with some forms of nausea and vomiting which cannot be controlled by any other drugs. The same seems to apply to the analgesic actions—some forms of pain which are quite resistant to conventional drugs can be reduced by cannabis compounds.

Fortunately for the individuals afflicted by some of these conditions, pure components of cannabis are becoming available legally—THC itself is marketed as dronabinol in the USA. Until we have more specific drugs for mutiple sclerosis or chronic pain, however, those patients who suffer from such conditions have a strong case for making cannabis itself legally available on prescription.

Tolerance and dependence

Regular users of cannabis may become tolerant to its effects, so that they have to use more to induce the same intensity of effect. Fortunately, however, cannabis does not produce dependence to the same extent as opiates. This is partly because the chemicals from cannabis remain in the blood for several days after smoking, so that the body has time to adjust as the drug is slowly eliminated. As a result, experimental subjects asked to smoke cannabis for 3–4 hours per day for 4 weeks suffered only some restlessness, irritability, sweating, and nausea when the drug was stopped. Such mild withdrawal symptoms reflect the fact that cannabis does not seem to be highly addictive.

What about chocolate?

Daniele Piomelli and his team at the University of California in San Diego have found that chocolate contains anandamide. Normally, it is broken down very rapidly in the body by enzymes to inactive substances, so that the anandamide by itself would not have much effect on the brain. However, chocolate also contains two other chemicals, related to anandamide, which inhibit the enzymes and slow down the rate at which this destruction occurs. The combination of these chemicals means that the amount of anandamide is more likely to rise in the brain and may in some people reach levels sufficient to activate cannabis receptors there. Dark chocolate and cocoa contain more of these substances than milk chocolate and their presence may help explain the gently stimulant, attractive properties of these foods. However, the amounts present in chocolate are far too small to have any major effect on people's behaviour. What some would claim to be the addictive nature of chocolate probably owes more to the presence of amines such as tyramine and phenyl-ethylamine, which have effects on the brain similar to amphetamine. They promote the release of amines such as dopamine which, as we have seen, seems to be involved in the 'rewarding' and addictive effects of drugs, and so may be responsible for the pleasure many people derive from eating chocolate. There are probably also chemicals in chocolate, as there are in coffee, which can stimulate opiate (morphine) receptors (*see* Chapter 6), because the preference which animals show for chocolate can be prevented by drugs which block morphine receptors.

Hallucinogenic drugs

Drugs have been used to induce hallucinations and mystical states of mind for centuries. Women who indulged in witchcraft and wished to go for a spin on their broomsticks would smear their hands and feet with a 'flying ointment' which contained the powdered roots of monkshood, or wolf's bane. The root in turn contains a chemical, aconite, which has a local anaesthetic action, producing a feeling of numbness in the hands and feet which gave the sensation of losing contact with the ground—of flying.

A different kind of hallucination was probably responsible for the wild, erratic, and often violent behaviour of the Vikings who invaded Britain (the 'beserkers') after eating the hallucinogenic mushroom *Amanita muscaria*, a mushroom with a prominent bright red cap with white spots. Eating a single whole mushroom can provide enough of the active chemical, muscarine (*see* Chapter 1), to kill an adult by dropping the blood pressure and stopping the heart.

It may be difficult to avoid hallucinogenic chemicals. Nutmeg, for example, was the subject of the second quotation at the head of this chapter, which reminds us that even a humble spice can contain mind-altering chemicals. Nutmeg contains myristicin, whose molecules are very similar to mescaline and which can produce hallucinations. It has been used for this purpose mainly by prisoners unable to obtain more effective drugs, but it is not a pleasant way to obtain mental stimulation. To achieve a marked hallucinogenic effect the user needs to stir five or six tablespoons full of the spice into a cup of hot water. The result is a thick, muddy and intensely bitter concoction which is as likely to produce vomiting as hallucinations. It may be reassuring to know that the amounts normally used in cooking would probably have less effect on the brain than eating a bar of dark chocolate.

Drugs which induce hallucinations have often been misused. They include mescaline, from the cactus *Anhalonium lewinii*, and bufotenine from the skin secretions of some toads (*see* Chapter 25). Chemicals such as these have been used for centuries to induce religious or trance-like states in native users. Modern scientists have been fascinated by these drugs since their effects were first reported carefully by the pharmacologist Karl Heffter in 1898 after eating dried slices of *Anhalonium* cactus prepared for him by local Mexicans. One of the best-known hallucinogenic drugs is LSD.

Lysergic acid diethylamide (LSD)

Lysergic acid diethylamide is related to compounds found in a fungus, *Claviceps purpurea*, also known as ergot (*see* Chapter 7). Extracts of ergot have many actions in the body, including the ability to contract the uterus, thus speeding up parturition if labour proves too lengthy, and reducing the loss of blood at the time of birth. Albert Hofmann, a Swiss scientist born in 1906, was asked to produce chemicals similar to, and related to, those in ergot to find more selective uterine stimulants which lacked some of the side-effects. One compound he produced was LSD, but soon after purifying it he reported that he felt dizzy and went home. There, he experienced 'an uninterrupted stream of fantastic images of extraordinary vividness and accompanied by an intense kaleidoscope of colours'. Hofmann found it difficult to believe that his limited contact with the new drug could be responsible for these effects so he experimented on himself, deliberately swallowing a tiny amount—250 micrograms (10 millionths of an ounce). Over the next few hours he experienced dramatic, vivid, visual and other sensory hallucinations. The amounts taken by addicts are normally less than 50 micrograms. Hofmann, therefore, unwittingly subjected himself to an extremely severe demonstration of the powerful hallucinogenic effects of the drug.

How does LSD work?

In normal people, the various pathways which connect different parts of the brain and different aspects of our mental behaviour, function independently. The pathways from our eyes affect those parts of the brain concerned with vision, pathways from our ears induce responses in our 'auditory cortex', projections from the spinal cord up to the brain allow us to feel touch and temperature changes in the skin, and pathways from the brain out to the muscles allow us to move.

Nevertheless, each of these pathways can send branches to parts of the brain which seem to act as co-ordinating centres. These determine which of the sensory inputs will be allowed to reach consciousness. As we shift our attention from looking at an object to listening intently to a sound, for example, these brain areas help to switch the corresponding sensory information into those areas responsible for attention and consciousness. One of the neurotransmitters involved in controlling this complex flow of information is 5HT.

LSD can act on the receptors for 5HT, either activating them or blocking them in different parts of the brain. As a result, LSD confuses the information pathways so that normal everyday objects may become disturbingly distorted images. People using the drug may claim that they can 'hear colours' or 'see sounds'. There are disturbances of thinking and understanding. One subject, whom we may call Sheila, reported the following experiences under the influence of LSD taken under controlled, medical supervision:*

> On one occasion the nurse assumed the appearance of an animal, then on looking away from her and at my knees, I too seemed to turn into another animal with whiskers growing out of my mouth. This terrified me and I seemed to be wandering around lost in a tunnel through which the wind was howling. I felt this lasted an eternity when in reality [according to the tape recording] it lasted less than a minute.

* Reported by Hoffer and Osmond in *The hallucinogens*, pp. 169–172.

> I was asked to look into a mirror and I saw my image change gradually to that of an older and older 'me', until eventually I seemed to get right into the mirror and look out from there. When I looked at paintings of people they got older, then younger. Occasionally I was completely engulfed by the portrait. I found paintings fascinating and landscapes as well were beautiful beyond description, very much alive. I travelled in space to various parts of the world, to other planets, and to the bottom of the sea.

Many of the effects of LSD resemble the hallucinations reported by patients with schizophrenia (*see* Chapter 9), giving rise to the idea that schizophrenia might be due to an LSD-like chemical produced by the brain. There is, however, a crucial difference. Subjects taking LSD normally remain aware of their situation, as in the report by Sheila:

> At no time did I lose sight of the fact that I had taken a drug which had induced this amazing experience. I was able to communicate freely to those present what I saw and felt.

Patients with schizophrenia do not have this luxury; they are convinced that their experiences are very real, a conviction which can make them dangerous to themselves and those around them (*see* Chapter 9).

MDMA (Ecstasy)

One of the drugs to have become very popular among the young in the 1990s is Ecstasy, or MDMA.* This is one of the amphetamine drugs and, like amphetamine itself, it produces feelings of self-confidence and great energy and drive. Part of the behaviour patterns of Adolf Hitler was due to amphetamine, as Richard Gordon has noted:†

> After 1943, every second afternoon the Fuhrer dropped his brown trousers for Morell to inject into his gluteal muscles a mixture of vitamins—to which he had had the clinical inspiration of adding the addictive stimulant amphetamine.

MDMA is said to increase the 'open-ness' and empathy between people at first meetings. It was first produced by the pharmaceutical company Merck in 1912, but found no medical use until psychiatrists began to use it in the 1970s. One therapist, Leo Zeff, found that it made communication with patients easier and removed some of the inhibitions they felt about revealing their innermost thoughts and fears. Other doctors said that it was useful in helping people to give up drug and alcohol abuse. It was made illegal for non-clinicians to possess

---

* The scientific name for MDMA, the most important chemical in Ecstasy is 3,4-methylene-dioxy-methamphetamine. Many samples of Ecstasy contain other, similar substances such as MDA, MDEA, and MBDM.

† Reported by R. Gordon in *Ailments through the ages*.

MDMA in 1977 in the UK, and 1985 in the USA by which time almost half of American University students admitted to trying the drug at least once.

Nowadays, it is used primarily by young people at all-night parties and dances to allow them to remain physically and mentally active throughout the night, increase feelings of mutual warmth between individuals, and increase sensitivity to sensations such as touch and sounds. Like amphetamine itself, it does so by increasing the release of amines in the brain, mainly 5HT, a transmitter which plays a major role in determining whether we feel depressed or euphoric, isolated or gregarious (*see* Chapter 11). Descriptions of their feelings by people taking MDMA vary enormously, but usually include greater intimacy, greater sensitivity, enhanced appreciation of art and music, euphoria, reduced fear and anxiety, and reduced feelings of aggression.

MDMA can also increase the desire for sexual activity, probably as a result of the increased physical and emotional sensitivity. At the same time, however, its activation of receptors for 5HT and norepinephrine on blood vessels can cause impotence and a failure of orgasm in both sexes.

There are other minor side-effects, too. The muscles are tense and ache for a day or two after the drug, especially around the mouth, since it causes some people to grind their teeth for hours on end. It can make some people clumsy and lose concentration easily—a recipe for accidents at home or on the road.

For some people the effects of MDMA seem to be over in a few hours, but for many there are periods of irritability, tiredness, and depression which last several days and produce difficulty performing physical and mental tasks at school or at work. Repeated users are prone to depression, panic attacks, hallucinations, and serious psychiatric disorders. For some people there is a real threat of greater danger, even to those taking the drug in small quantities.

The danger which has attracted most public and media attention is that of death. It has been known since about 1920 that the effects of amphetamines in animals are far greater when they are kept in crowded conditions and when the room temperature is increased. Under these conditions, doses of amphetamine which are normally harmless can kill.

As would be expected of an amphetamine-like drug, the effects of MDMA are also strongly dependent on the ambient conditions. In most subjects it will, for example, produce a small fall in body temperature when taken in a room at normal temperatures of around 20 °C. If the room temperature is increased to nearer 25 or 30 °C, as can easily happen in a crowded dance hall, the drug tends to produce a large rise in body temperature. This effect, which still remains unexplained, is made much worse when the drug is taken in crowded conditions and in people who are somewhat dehydrated as a result of drinking alcohol or strenuous physical activity such as dancing. The rise in body temperature can soon be enough to disrupt the normal functioning of the heart and brain, resulting in death in a few hours. Most of the people who have died after taking Ecstasy have collapsed with a body temperature of 40–43 °C (compared with the normal 37 °C).

Paradoxically, the recommendation to drink lots of fluids can also be dangerous. MDMA reduces the secretion of antidiuretic hormone (ADH, Chapter 5) which slows the production of urine by the kidney. If revellers drink lots of plain water which is not then excreted in the urine, the blood can become so diluted that blood cells swell and die. The result is called 'water intoxication' and several people have died from this cause. The mechanism of death is the same as that after drowning, in which water passes rapidly through the lungs into the blood, diluting the blood, killing the cells, and starving the body of oxygen.

The second danger with MDMA, which many people do not yet seem to appreciate, is one which may take many years to become apparent. When given to rats or monkeys, MDMA produces the same release of 5HT from nerve cells that probably occurs in humans. The animals then recover to normal over several hours, just as do the humans. However, if they are examined at different times after their dose of MDMA, they show a delayed, slowly developing destruction of the 5HT nerve cells in the brain. In humans this is likely to result in serious disturbances of thought patterns, mental confusion similar to that in Alzheimer's disease, and changes in sensory perception. If the ages of affected rats are translated into human terms, we may not see the full effects of this brain damage for twenty or thirty years in people taking the drug today.

At least one study* has confirmed that these effects are not limited to animals and that brain scans show damage to the 5HT cells in the human brain. If recent estimates are correct that more than a quarter of teenagers have taken MDMA at some time, future generations may be faced with a major social disaster.

Other drugs of misuse

There are many drugs which can be, and often are, misused. They include morphine and the opiates which were described in detail in Chapter 6, and drugs which produce a calming or sedative effect, helping to remove some of the anxieties of life (*see* Chapter 13). One of the targets of the pharmaceutical industry is the development of drugs which lack those properties which can lead to abuse. It is a target which, for some types of drug, is proving difficult to attain.

---

* McCann et al. (1998) *The Lancet*, vol. 352, pages 1433–1437.

Summary

- *Some chemicals are used for their ability to relax or improve people's mood. These include drugs such as alcohol, caffeine, and cannabis. Only a fraction of users become dependent (addicted) on them.*
- *Other drugs such as cocaine and heroin produce addiction in most users. They activate the 'reward' pathways of the brain which release dopamine as their transmitter. Rats stimulated in this way will die rather than stop the stimulation of these pathways.*
- *Alcohol activates GABA receptors and blocks glutamate receptors, producing sedation and impairing memory.*
- *Dependence on alcohol can be controlled using diazepam, disulfiram, or clomethiazole.*
- *Nicotine activates nicotinic receptors for acetylcholine in the brain, increasing alertness and concentration. Nicotine patches have been introduced for the treatment of Alzheimer's disease.*
- *Caffeine blocks receptors for adenosine, a molecule within the brain which inhibits nerve cells. Caffeine stimulates the brain.*
- *Cocaine was discovered as a local anaesthetic, but it also releases dopamine and other amines from nerve cells in the brain. This activates the 'reward' systems, leading to pleasurable feelings of euphoria but also causing dependence.*
- *Cannabis contains several chemicals which produce euphoria and increase social confidence. Some of these act on receptors in the brain for natural brain hormones such as anandamide. These same chemicals occur in chocolate and may explain some of its attraction.*
- *Many natural chemicals induce hallucinations. LSD and related drugs activate receptors for 5HT in the brain.*
- *Ecstasy (MDMA) increases the release of 5HT in the brain, producing euphoria and increasing self-confidence. Even a single dose, however, can slowly destroy the 5HT nerve cells over several years, potentially leading to serious mental disorders.*

CHAPTER 25

Poisons

The definition of a poison in the Encyclopaedia Britannica is 'a substance which, by its direct action on the mucous membrane, tissue or skin, or after absorption into the circulatory system can, in the way in which it is administered, injuriously affect health or destroy life'.

Although this book has largely been concerned with medicines—chemicals which bring benefit and relief to ailing people—the world has its share of poisonous chemicals too. Some of these, such as arsenic and mercury have been used as medicines in the past, before the safety of drugs became a paramount consideration. Others are chemicals consumed accidentally, such as MPTP (*see* Chapter 8) while some, such as certain insecticides and sheep dip may be encountered while performing a job. There are also many poisonous substances which are the products of nature—snake venoms, spider and fish toxins, plant chemicals, and arrow poisons. This chapter will try to explain how a few of the world's poisons exert their unpleasant and sometimes fatal effects on the human body.

Sheep dip, Gulf War protection, and lice lotions

This may seem a strange combination of factors, but in fact they have one thing in common. They all involve a group of chemicals known as organophosphorus compounds.

An organophosphate compound was first produced in 1854 by the chemist Clermont, a remarkably fortunate man since he actually tasted his new chemical and survived. Many years later it was realized that similar compounds were effective insecticides and several, such as parathion, were developed specifically for this purpose. It was also realized that these same compounds were very poisonous to humans and, since they are—or readily become gases—that they could be used as agents of chemical warfare, spreading rapidly to affect large numbers of people. The organophosphates, therefore, became the first 'nerve gases'. Compounds such as tabun, sarin, and soman are among the most poisonous chemicals to have been created by man, hence Clermont's lucky escape.

Gulf War protection

At the start of the Gulf War, there were real fears of chemical warfare being waged using organophosphate chemicals. The nerve gases are so dangerous because they are rapidly absorbed into the body either through the lungs or after contact with the skin. They bind to and block the enzyme, acetylcholinesterase. This enzyme destroys the transmitter acetylcholine (*see* Chapter 1) after it has been released by nerve cells onto muscles and in the brain. Inhibition of the enzyme results in the accumulation of acetylcholine, which continues to act on its receptors in muscles. In the airways, the accumulation of acetylcholine contracts the muscle cells and increases secretion of mucus, together resulting in choking and difficulty in breathing. The secretion of epinephrine increases blood pressure and heart rate. Activation of glands causes salivation, diarrhoea, and the production of tears. In the brain, the overactivation of nerve cells causes severe confusion, dizziness, and convulsions, and reduces both sensitivity to stimuli and the brain's ability to process sensory information.

The organophosphates inactivate cholinesterase permanently so that the muscles become paralysed and cannot function correctly again until the cells have made new enzyme, a process that takes days or weeks. In most cases death would occur long before that time because the muscles of breathing would become paralysed.

To protect soldiers against the threat of nerve gas attack during the Gulf War, many were instructed to take drugs which inhibited cholinesterase, but did so reversibly. The theory was that the reversible drug would protect some of the cholinesterase from attack by the nerve gas. If administration of the drug was then stopped, its inhibitory effect would reverse and some functioning cholinesterase would become available on the muscles.

Although nerve gases do not seem to have been employed in the war, some soldiers seem to have been sensitive to the protective drugs used (mainly pyridostigmine) and experienced nausea, fatigue, weakness or paralysis, insomnia, frequent urination, and abdominal pain. The effects of pyridostigmine are thought to have been worsened by the fact that stressful situations, such as war, increase the ability of drugs to pass into the brain.

Some of these symptoms were considered to constitute a new disease—'Gulf War syndrome'. As more soldiers are studied, however, many indeed suffering from some forms of post-war illnesses, there is now real doubt that any of these constitute a specific disorder unique to the conditions experienced in that conflict or to the use of anticholinesterase protective drugs.*

* According to the most recent report by W J Coker and colleagues published in the *British Medical Journal*, 1999, vol. 318, 290–294.

Insecticides and sheep dip

The most common use of organophosphates is as insecticides, but sheep are dipped in solutions of them in order to control and prevent infections by parasites. Unfortunately the farmers who use such dips tend to be splashed and may breathe in tiny droplets of solution or dust particles covered in them. There is, as a result, a real problem of poisoning by organophosphates. Most effects are seen only in the short-term, but there are some long-term effects on the nervous system, mainly a reduced sensitivity to stimuli, poor attention, and a reduced ability of the brain to process sensory information.

Lice

Malathion is an organophosphorus insecticide. It has been used as an aerial spray to eliminate mosquitoes in infested regions but it is also the main in-gredient of some preparations, rubbed into the scalp, used to eliminate head lice (nits).* However, many doctors and pharmacologists have doubts about its effectiveness against the lice, and many patients, especially children, often use far too much in an effort to rid themselves of the pests as thoroughly and quickly as possible. Head louse potions should always be used as part of a concerted effort to remove the lice by frequent washing and combing with a lice comb.

Malathion is absorbed through the skin, and using too much can result in levels in the blood much higher than the recommended limits. There have been few cases of actual poisoning from these preparations, but the long-term effects of relatively high levels on the developing nervous system of young children is difficult to assess.

Overall, the organophosphates are a rather unpleasant group of drugs which are gradually being replaced by safer, although often less effective, drugs as insecticides. Nevertheless, many cases of accidental poisoning occur every year.

Heavy metals

Humans and other animals consume heavy metals in their food and water, but the amounts entering the body are usually excreted rapidly and never reach levels which cause any harm. In a few cases, however, the presence of par-ticularly large amounts of metals can cause them to accumulate in the body and produce signs of poisoning. Two of the most important of these metals are arsenic and lead.

---

* A louse is a small, 6-legged insect about 3 millimetres long which infest head hair and feed off blood from the scalp. They can affect anyone, but are particularly common in small children, who may infect their friends or family by prolonged close contact.

Arsenic

Arsenic and its chemical compounds have been used both as medicines and as poisons from the time of the ancients Greeks until the middle of the twentieth century.

As we have seen in Chapter 17, some of the first pure drugs produced in the early 1900s by Paul Ehrlich contained arsenic. These 'arsenicals' such as arsphenamine were found to be very effective in killing the micro-organisms responsible for diseases such as syphilis and were used for many years for this purpose. The difference between the doses needed for such chemotherapy and those causing signs of poisoning was not large, and some patients suffered from arsenic poisoning.

On 5th May, 1821, after a four-year illness involving nausea, vomiting, shortness of breath, and an irregular pulse, Napoleon died on the Island of St Helena. Seven British doctors all agreed that he had died of stomach cancer. One hundred and fifty years later researchers discovered that a specimen of Napoleon's hair contained sixty times the normal amount of arsenic. Furthermore, in 1980 a scrap of wallpaper from Napoleon's bedroom was found which, in damp conditions, emitted enough arsenic gas to give symptoms of poisoning. Napoleon always believed that he was being poisoned, but perhaps it was by his wallpaper, not a human assassin.*

Small amounts of arsenic are normally present in water and food, especially fish and shellfish, and often occur in insecticides, herbicides, and wood preservatives. Arsenic is also used in the manufacture of glass.

The signs of poisoning include flushing of the skin which, with prolonged or repeated exposure, becomes thickened and leathery before starting to die or develop cancer. There is serious and irreversible damage to the kidneys and liver, and the brain is often affected. This may cause severe headaches, drowsiness, confusion, weakness and paralysis, and a loss of sensitivity in the hands and feet. In the worst cases, these symptoms will lead eventually to coma and death.

How does arsenic work?

The poisonous effects of arsenic chemicals are due to two actions. Firstly, arsenate can fool the body into using it instead of phosphate in biochemical reactions. When this happens, however, the natural sequence of biochemical reactions cannot occur at the correct speed, so the delicate molecular machinery of the cells is disrupted and tissues cannot perform their normal functions.

The second action of arsenic is to interact with molecules which contain sulphur atoms in the form of sulphydryl groups. These are essential components of many large proteins and enzymes as they determine their structure

* Adapted from *Ailments through the ages* by Richard Gordon.

and reactiveness with other molecules. Arsenic compounds bind tightly to these sulphur groups and disrupt their function, ultimately causing serious damage to cells or killing them.

Lead

The dangers of lead were known to Marcus Vitruvius, one of the architects of ancient Rome living in the first century BC, who cautioned against the use of lead pipes for carrying drinking water and lead utensils for cooking. Despite this ancient knowledge, lead has become an important metal in modern society, including its use in water pipes.

According to Nick Kollerstrom,* four million tons of lead are mined every year and in a few years the Earth's supply will be exhausted. 'The Earth's entire stock of this most toxic element will by then have been distributed over its surface, and concentrated around areas of human habitation'.

Lead can be toxic in amounts not much greater than those to which most of us are exposed, and may easily reach toxic levels in people living near main roads or airports or exposed to lead in occupations dealing with munitions, batteries, or solder. Until recently most people in 'motorized' countries were being exposed to lead daily as it left petrol-driven motor vehicles in the exhaust fumes. For several decades lead had been added to petrol as an 'antiknocking' agent and the levels in the environment were slowly increasing in parallel with the number of motor vehicles. The amount of lead in leaded petrol is about one thousand times higher than that which is dangerous to humans. In the 1980s, lead levels in city centres were found to be 50 000 times higher than in rural areas.†

People, especially children, have become seriously ill and even died as a result of drinking acidic beverages (colas, fruit juices) from cans in which the sealing lead-containing solder was not properly covered, or as a result of eating fragments of coloured lead-containing paints flaking from walls and windows. Lead in toys and water pipes is also potentially dangerous. Now, the move to lead-free petrol and paints in many countries, the replacement of lead water pipes and the production of safer toys without lead is reversing the trend towards higher environmental lead levels and the incidence of poisoning is falling.

Why is lead dangerous?

Lead can cause excruciating abdominal pain, vomiting, and diarrhoea with weakness and eventually paralysis and kidney damage. The brain is also

---

* The author of a book on lead. See the lists of additional reading.
† Micrograms per cubic metre compared with 0.0001 (R W Elias, 1985, *In dietary and environmental lead*, edited by K R Mahaffey, Elsevier, Amsterdam).

affected, with adults showing clumsiness, dizziness, insomnia, restlessness, and hallucinations. Most of the concern about lead, however, has been directed at children, as long-term exposure to lead can slow the development of the brain in babies and young children, causing a loss of small movement skills and of the ability to talk, coupled with poor learning, restlessness, and aggression. Several research studies have shown a very good correlation between the amounts of lead in the blood of children and adolescents, and their antisocial and aggressive behaviour, as well as an inverse correlation with a poor IQ. Several cases of mental retardation have been ascribed to the high levels of lead in the bodies of infants. The ability of lead to cause such changes has been supported by experiments with rats, which developed learning problems after exposure to lead. Most worrying of all was the fact that when their exposure was stopped completely, these animals never recovered the learning ability of normal rats.

Some of the varied effects of lead are due to its interfering with the actions of other metal ions in the body, especially calcium. Lead interacts with reactive sulphur atoms in enzymes, reducing the formation of haemoglobin and essential proteins. It also causes red blood cells to become very fragile so that they are destroyed prematurely by the liver, causing anaemia.

Treatment

Arsenic and lead poisoning are treated by removing as much as possible from the body, as quickly as possible. Calcium edetate, penicillamine, and dimercaprol are three drugs known as 'chelators'. They bind tightly to metal ions and the complex of drug and metal is then excreted. Using the correct dose of these drugs is important because too high a dose will also remove some of the valuable metal ions which the body needs to function healthily.

Cyanide

Perhaps the best known of all poisons is cyanide. Tablets of cyanide have been used for a variety of nefarious purposes through the ages from murder to suicide. Cyanide-containing gases are often used to fumigate large buildings and ships. Cyanide also occurs in some insecticides, rodenticides, and silver polish, and is produced when some plastic materials are burnt. There are many recorded cases of human deaths from cyanide poisoning following fires involving plastics made of nitrogen-containing substances. Burning wool, silk, nylon, and rubber produce cyanide. Almonds and the seeds of some fruits, especially apricots, peaches, and plums contain amygdalin which can be converted into cyanide by enzymes and bacteria in the intestine. Several cases are known of poisoning from these sources.

How does cyanide work?

Oxygen is essential for life, but to be of use in cells it must be processed by a series of enzymes known as the cytochromes, the 'respiratory chain'. Cyanide combines with one of these enzymes very readily, preventing cells from using oxygen. Paradoxically, the inhibition of oxygen use results in the blood in the veins remaining as bright red as in the arteries, so that the patient does not appear to be suffering from a lack of oxygen. But within minutes of consuming cyanide, the cells of the body are indeed starved of oxygen because they are unable to use the oxygen they have. The patient may then have convulsions and die unless treated rapidly.

Treatment

Cyanide poisoning can be treated by administering drugs such as amyl nitrite and sodium nitrite. These oxidize some haemoglobin in the blood into methaemoglobin, which binds cyanide more tightly than the cytochrome chain enzymes. Sodium thiosulphate is also given to patients as it helps to convert cyanide into the much less toxic thiocyanate which is then soon excreted in the urine.

Carbon monoxide

Carbon monoxide is best known as one of the main constituents of vehicle exhaust fumes. It is so toxic that laws to reduce its emission have been introduced, making it illegal for a vehicle to be stationary with its engine running. There are also laws to promote the installation of catalytic converters which convert exhaust gases, including carbon monoxide, into less toxic chemicals. However, carbon monoxide is present whenever carbon-containing materials are burned, so that fires and smoking cigarettes also produce carbon monoxide which will be inhaled by anyone in the vicinity. Carbon monoxide passes easily across the placenta and the developing foetus is very sensitive to the gas. Smoking during pregnancy is, therefore, very likely to produce abnormalities in the baby.

Carbon monoxide* is a colourless, odourless, and tasteless gas, but it is highly toxic because of its ability to react with haemoglobin in the blood. Haemoglobin is the molecule in red blood cells with the vital function of combining with oxygen (*see* Chapter 14). Oxygen from the air in the lungs combines with haemoglobin and is carried around the body in the bloodstream until it reaches the tissues. There it is exchanged for carbon dioxide† which is carried back to the lungs to be excreted into the atmosphere. Oxygen is absolutely essential for

* The chemical formula for carbon monoxide is CO.
† The chemical formula for carbon dioxide is CO_2.

life and anything which compromises the ability of haemoglobin to carry oxygen is dangerous.

Carbon monoxide is such a compound. It binds to haemoglobin 220 times more strongly than oxygen, so that exposure to quite small quantities reduce considerably the ability of the blood to carry oxygen.

As the amount of carbon monoxide in the blood rises, the symptoms experienced progress from slight to very severe, throbbing headache, with flushing of the skin, nausea and vomiting, increased rate and depth of breathing, convulsions, coma, and death. The only treatment for carbon monoxide poisoning is to remove the source of the gas and substitute pure oxygen as quickly as possible.

Strychnine

The crushed seeds of *Strychnos nux vomica*, a tree found in parts of India, were introduced into Germany in the sixteenth century as a rat poison. The chemical responsible for the poisoning was later isolated and called strychnine. It is still used as a rodenticide today in many parts of the world and its accidental (or occasionally deliberate) consumption can cause fatalities.

Despite this potential for toxicity, strychnine was also introduced into medicine and was available until the 1970s as a component of some 'nerve tonic' preparations which could be purchased in pharmacies.

How does strychnine work?

The activity of the brain and spinal cord depends on a fine balance between nerve cells producing excitatory effects and those producing inhibition. In several sections of this book we have met one of the major inhibitory amino acids, GABA,* but there is another related one, glycine.

The nerves which pass from the spinal cord to the muscles send branches back into the cord, where they excite small nerve cells called interneurons. These release glycine as their inhibitory transmitter onto the nerve cells which project to the muscles. This arrangement is designed to prevent the nerves to the muscles from firing too rapidly, as this might produce a convulsion. As these nerves become more active, they activate the interneurons and the glycine produced by them suppresses the activity of the motor nerves.

Strychnine is an antagonist at the receptors for glycine. In the presence of strychnine, glycine can no longer suppress the activity of the motor nerves, which become more and more active until a convulsion occurs. If the convulsions are sufficiently prolonged the patient may die from exhaustion and because the nerves controlling the muscles of breathing fire out of control.

* GABA is gamma-amino-butyric acid.

Treatment

The only form of treatment for victims of strychnine poisoning is to stop the convulsions before they exhaust the muscles and paralyse breathing. Diazepam (Valium®) is the most effective drug. Described in Chapters 12 and 13, it suppresses strychnine convulsions by increasing the effects of the inhibitory substance GABA in the brain and spinal cord.

In the most serious cases of strychnine poisoning it may be necessary to anaesthetize the patient completely and to use drugs such as pancuronium which block the effects of acetylcholine on the muscles, stopping all movement and convulsions.

Animal toxins

Some of the most poisonous substances known to man are present in the stings and venoms of animals. The range of toxins already known to science is large and probably represents only the tip of a poisonous iceberg.

Molluscs

Cone snails (*Conus*) are molluscs which produce powerful poisons called conotoxins. These, and a related toxin, agatoxin from *Agelenopsis,* block sodium, calcium, or potassium channels in nerve and muscle cells. Ion channels are essential for nerves to function correctly and to release their neurotransmitters, since the movement of sodium and potassium through cell membranes is needed for nerve impulses and calcium is needed for transmitter release. They are also essential in muscle cells, since it is an increase in the amount of calcium in the cells which triggers contraction. The blockade of these channels, therefore, may lead to paralysis, cessation of the heartbeat, and cessation of breathing.

Scorpions

Potassium channels are critical for the normal functioning of nerve and muscle cells as well as for the secretion of hormones and the regulation of fluid balance in the body. The venoms of several species of scorpions contain toxic chemicals (Fig. 25.1) which block different types of potassium channel, causing widespread disruption of physiological processes and rapidly causing death unless treated. These scorpion toxins include a series of dendrotoxins from *Dendroaspis*, charybdotoxin from *Leiurus,* pandinotoxin from *Pandinus*, and tityustoxin from *Tityus*.

The scorpion *Centruroides*, found in the Southern USA, produces a toxin which causes the sodium channels in nerve membranes to remain open much longer than normal. This make the cells fire more impulses, giving rise to pain

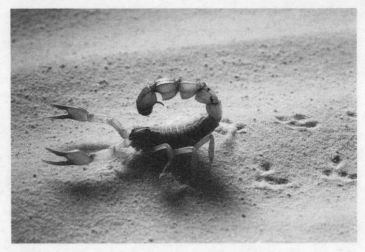

Fig. 25.1 One of many species of scorpion, the yellow fat tail scorpion, *Androctonus australis*.

and a loss of the ability to control muscle function. The patient experiences uncontrollable movements of the eyes, mouth, throat, and limbs, eventually leading to a cessation of breathing. The venoms of these creatures also contain margatoxin and noxiustoxin which block potassium channels and increase the effects of opening the sodium channels.

Scorpions do not have a monopoly on potassium channel blockers. The sting of the bee *Apis mellifera* contains at least one toxin able to block potassium channels. This is a protein called apamin. The block of potassium channels in humans causes nerve cells to fire impulses more rapidly in the pain-sensitive nerves near the sting site. The increased firing of these nerves is partly responsible for the pain felt at the site of the sting.

Amphibians
Although they do not bite, some frogs and toads produce toxic secretions from their skin which can provoke severe reactions in animals or people (usually children) who touch them and then lick their paws or hands. Frogs of the Dendrobatid family such as the tree frog *Phyllobates* secrete a variety of substances including the very poisonous batrachotoxin (from the Greek *batrachos*, meaning 'frog'). This opens ion channels in nerve endings, allowing a large number of ions into the cells. This results in muscle cramps and paralysis. The increased ion flow into the heart causes an irregular heart rhythm and can stop the heart from pumping blood efficiently, leading rapidly to death.

Toads belong to the animal family *Bufonidae*. As a result, chemicals secreted from their skin have been given names such as bufotenin. This is a hallucinogenic compound with effects similar to LSD. Another chemical from toad skin is bufotalin. It has effects similar to ouabain and digoxin, disrupting the balance of ions in cells and rapidly leading to abnormal heart rhythms and death. Many cases of poisoning are known to have resulted from people or animals handling these animals.

A special study of Australian frogs and toads has shown that many secrete poisons of one kind or another onto the skin. Most of these are produced in large quantities (several hundreds of millgrams per day) by the salivary glands or specialized glands in the skin itself, so that researchers do not need to harm the animals to study their secretions. Members of the *Uperoleia* species secrete a peptide poison called uperolein. This causes localized inflammation of the skin of a predator by dilating blood vessels and making them very fragile. It also causes a large fall in blood pressure and contractions of smooth muscles, giving rise to diarrhoea, pain, and breathing problems.

Snakes

Snake venoms, like those of scorpions are often a serious danger to human life. Several species of viper, such as the pit vipers (*Bothrops* and *Lachesis*) in South America and the scaled viper (*Echis*) in West Africa are capable of causing serious illness or death.

The toxins of several families of snake including the rattlesnakes (*Crotalus*) contain chemicals which prevent blood clotting. The venom of these creatures contains a cocktail of enzymes. There is an enzyme similar to thrombin (Chapter 14) which promotes blood clotting, and another chemical which promotes the aggregation of platelets in the blood. Together these form tiny clots in the bloodstream. However, as soon as the clots form, they are broken up by another enzyme in the venom. The overall effect is to remove the fibrin and fibrinogen proteins from the blood so that clotting cannot occur. Various other enzymes and small compounds such as histamine increase the movement of blood through the walls of the blood vessels. The victim of a bite then effectively bleeds to death, with haemorrhaging into the internal organs, unless treated urgently.

Several snake toxins contain enzymes* which damage the tissues around the bite site and allow the venom to spread to other parts of the body. These enzymes also damage the red cells in the blood, causing them to burst and leading to anaemia.

Most of these venoms contain enzymes called phospholipases which disrupt

---

* For example phospholipase A2, hyaluronidase, and collagenase.

cell membranes and thus the normal balance of ion movements through them so that enzymes cannot function properly. There are dozens of phospholipases, some of them unique to particular species of snake. They are mainly responsible for destroying red blood cells, stopping the clotting ability of blood and exerting a direct depressant action on vital organs such as the heart and brain.

Venoms may be used in defence, but also are used to kill or immobilize prey and to begin digestion. The venoms therefore contain enzymes which initiate the process of killing and breaking up cells ready for absorption by the predator.

The death adder (*Acanthophis*) is typical of many species of snake whose venom has several different pharmacological effects. It contains toxins with three distinct actions—decreasing the ability of the blood to clot, breaking down muscle cells, and inactivating nerves. The anticoagulant activity assists the spread of toxin away from the site of injection.

Some snake toxins have very specific effects on nerves. The α-toxins, for example, block the receptors for acetylcholine on muscles, while the β-toxins, such as β-bungarotoxin from the Taiwanese krait *Bungarus*, destroy the nerve stores of acetylcholine or prevent the nerves from releasing their transmitter. In either case the result for anyone bitten may be paralysis and death from respiratory failure.

Some components of animal poisons have been subverted to medicinal use. The venom of the Malayan pit viper, for example, contains a toxin which causes small clots to form in the blood. These are then removed by white cells, gradually depleting the blood of its fibrin, a protein essential for clotting. The toxin has been purified and marketed as Arvin®, for the treatment of disorders in which the blood tends to clot too readily.

Treatment

Many cases of envenomation can now be treated with antivenoms. These are made by injecting animals, usually horses or rabbits, with very low and non-poisonous doses of the venom. The animal's immune system then reacts to the toxins in the venom by producing antibodies. After a few days or weeks, blood is taken from the animal and the antibodies are separated from the rest of the blood proteins so that they can be injected into a poisoned subject. The antibodies combine with the various components of the venom in the person's blood, preventing it from acting. These procedures do not harm the animal used to make the antibody.

The biggest problem, however, is that the combination of toxins in a venom can be quite different in animals of the same species obtained from different regions of a country. The composition even seems to vary dramatically with the age of the animal. An antivenom prepared using the venom of one snake may, therefore, be quite useless against a bite from another snake of the same type.

Poisoning by toxins such as those of the death adder, which inactivate nerves, can partly be reversed by drugs such as the anticholinesterases (*see* Chapter 1). These inhibit the enzyme which breaks down acetylcholine after its release from nerves. The small amount of acetylcholine still released by nerves after poisoning is allowed to act for much longer than normal, partly compensating for the loss of nerve function.

Marine toxins

The puffer fish (Fig. 25.2),* fugu, is considered a delicacy in Japan, but is among the most hazardous of foods. The liver and ovaries contain high concentrations of tetrodotoxin, a poisonous agent which can be fatal if consumed in significant quantity. Restaurants in Japan are permitted to serve puffer fish only if prepared by specialized chefs with the knowledge and ability to remove all the toxin-containing parts. However, even with this official safeguard, several people die every year as a result of eating poorly prepared puffers. The same toxin occurs in other marine animals too such as the porcupine fish (*Diodon*) which has also been responsible for several deaths.

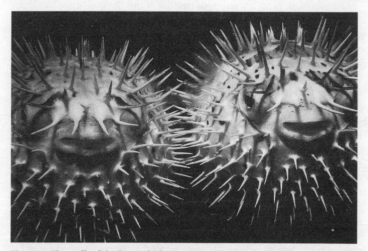

Fig. 25.2 The puffer fish, *Fugu*, which contain tetrodotoxin in the liver and ovaries in amounts which are potentially lethal to human diners.

* Also known as globefish or blowfish.

How do they work?

Tetrodotoxin and the related chemical saxitoxin block sodium channels in the membranes of nerve and muscle cells. A nerve impulse is a change in the voltage across the nerve cell wall caused by the opening of sodium channels. The impulse travels along the nerve because the sodium channels open one after the other along the nerve, in a 'domino effect'. If the sodium channels are blocked by tetrodotoxin, the nerves cannot work. The first signs of poisoning are a growing numbness in the mouth, arms, and legs, followed by weakness and paralysis. Death occurs from paralysis of the muscles of breathing.

Plankton

One of the most common sources of marine poisoning is from fish which have consumed deep-sea plankton* containing the toxins ciguatoxin and maitotoxin. These small organisms, Ciguatera, are usually associated with coral reefs. Ciguatoxic fish can be of any type and cannot be distinguished by sight, smell, or taste from non-toxic specimens. Ciguatoxin affects the sodium and calcium channels in nerve and muscle cells, causing pain, weakness, hallucinations, clumsiness, and an increase in blood pressure. Maitotoxin is especially danger-ous, causing depression of the heart and death after the consumption of as little as 1 part in 1 billion (1 microgram per kilogram).

Some shellfish become poisonous because of the plankton on which they feed. The 'red tide' plankton, (*Gonyaulax*) for example, which can bloom under certain conditions to cover vast areas of ocean, are eaten by a number of shellfish. The organisms produce several toxins, the most dangerous of which is saxitoxin. This works in much the same way as tetrodotoxin, blocking sodium channels in nerve and muscle cells leading to paralysis and death due to the cessation of breathing. The condition has become known as 'paralytic shellfish poisoning'.

In the 1980s, several people died on the West coast of North America after eating shellfish which had eaten an algal toxin called domoic acid. This toxin is unusual in that it acts directly on receptors in the brain which normally respond to the transmitter glutamate. Domoic acid activates those receptors far more effectively than glutamate itself, causing confusion, loss of motor control, convulsions, and eventually death.

The most potent animal toxin known is palytoxin from the coral *Palythoa*. It can kill mammals at a dose of less than 1 part in 1 billion (1 microgram per kilogram of body weight). Palytoxin increases the movements of ions into nerve cells, causing them to become far more active than normal and resulting in vomiting, muscle cramp, and respiratory arrest.

* These are known as dinoflagellates.

Bacterial toxins

The injurious effects of bacterial infection are often not due to the presence of the bacteria themselves, but to the toxins which they produce. The most common bacteria causing food poisoning, for example, are *Campylobacter*, *Staphylococcus aureus*, *Clostridium perfringens*, and *Escherichia coli (E. coli)*.* In each of these cases the cause of symptoms is the chemical toxin produced by the bacteria. These toxins all slow the absorption of water from the intestine, leading to diarrhoea, increased intestinal activity, and abdominal pain, often associated with nausea and vomiting. Cholera, due to infection by *Vibrio cholerae*, is due both to a cessation of fluid absorption and an active stimulation of fluid secretion into the intestine caused by the very dangerous cholera toxin. The loss of fluid is so dramatic in cholera that death can occur rapidly from dehydration.

Botulinum toxin

One of the most feared of bacterial poisons is botulinum toxin, a highly specialized product of evolution. It is produced by *Clostridium botulinum* and is occasionally responsible for extremely serious cases of food poisoning known as botulism. People affected by this bacterium experience blurred vision followed by difficulty in swallowing and muscle weakness. Unless treated, this may progress to paralysis and death from the paralysis of breathing.

Botulinum toxin attacks the nerves which control the contraction of muscles, preventing the release of the transmitter acetylcholine. The nerves can then no longer contract the muscles, causing paralysis.

Botulinum toxin consists of two connected molecules, one of which is responsible for attaching tightly to molecules present in the walls of nerve cells. Following this binding, the nerve cell transports the toxin into its interior, where the second component blocks transmitter release. Nerve cells store the transmitter in small packets called 'vesicles' and the release of transmitter from these is controlled by several proteins, one of which is called synaptobrevin. Botulinum toxin destroys this protein, so that the vesicles cannot be released.

Despite the serious health hazard presented by botulinum toxin when produced in an out-of-control fashion by bacteria in the body, it has been possible to harness small quantities of the purified toxin for a range of medical uses. In 1983, Dr. Alan Scott was the first to realize that a chemical as powerful as botulinum toxin might be of use in patients who had disorders of muscle control. His interest was in patients with squint, a disorder in which one or more of the eye muscles contract uncontrollably so that the patient cannot move both eyes to look in the same direction. Scott injected a tiny amount of

* Only some strains of *E. coli* produce toxins. Most strains are quite harmless.

botulinum toxin into the overactive muscles and found that the paralysis of those muscles afforded the subject much better control over the movement of his eye.

Since this work by Scott, many other disorders have been treated with botulinum toxin. For example, in cerebral palsy or following a severe stroke, the brain may not control correctly the movements of muscles, some being almost permanently contracted. This may be extremely painful and make movement extremely difficult for the patients, a condition known as spasticity. A localized injection of botulinum toxin in the contracted muscle blocks the release of acetylcholine from the overactive nerve and relaxes the muscle, allowing the patient much more freedom to move around at will.

These and other 'dystonias' (abnormal movements which the patient is unable to control) are now being treated with botulinum toxin. Fortunately, there are several different forms of toxin so that even if a patient develops antibodies to one type, they can still be treated with another.

Insect toxins

The stings of bees and wasps contain a mixture of chemicals, including melittin and apamin. Melittin induces cells of the victims body to secret histamine, which causes local itching and pain, inflammation, and contraction of muscles in the blood vessels, intestine, and airways. It also induces the formation of ion channels in the membranes of nerve cells near the site of the sting, increasing the activity of the nerves and contributing to the pain. Other components include the enzyme hyaluronidase which digests the material holding cells together, allowing the pain-producing chemicals to travel further from the sting area and affect a larger area of skin.

Apamin is a small peptide molecule which blocks potassium channels, further increasing nervous excitation and causing pain.

Spider toxins

The female black widow spider (*Latrodectus mactans*), found throughout the USA and Australasia, is one of the most poisonous spiders on the planet. One of the major components of its venom is known as latrotoxin. This acts on the walls of nerve endings to open pores or channels which allow ions to pass into the interior. One of the ions is calcium and the increased level of calcium inside the nerve triggers the release of acetylcholine. This relaxes blood vessels so that the skin flushes but it also causes increased sweating, painful muscle cramps, and difficulty in breathing.

The best treatment for latrotoxin poisoning is to administer large amounts of calcium ions, as these block the ion channels opened by the toxin.

Food toxins

The relationship between normal nutrition, toxins, drugs, and health is enough to fill a volume by itself. Here it is only possible to mention the existence of lectins in food. These chemicals occur in most plant foods but are usually destroyed by cooking. The increasing trend to consume raw or lightly cooked vegetables in order to provide roughage and reduce the incidence of colon cancers, also increases the consumption of lectins.

Lectins bind tightly to the cells lining the intestine and stop the absorption of important amino acids, fats, and vitamins. The vegetables which contain most lectins of danger to animals are black beans and red kidney beans, although almost all raw fruits and vegetables contain some lectins. Kidney beans contain enough lectins and other toxic substances that they can cause severe food poisoning unless thoroughly soaked overnight, washed, and cooked well.

Plant poisons

Many plants produce chemicals which can be either harmful or beneficial depending on dose and circumstance. In North West Africa the Calabar bean was used up to the mid-1800s in ordeals and trials. The accused person had to chew the beans and then march before the king until symptoms appeared—intense thirst, profuse salivation, and secretions in the intestine and lungs. Death usually followed in about half an hour. It is said that the guilty tended to eat the bean slowly, giving time for its poisons to work, whereas the innocent ate the beans with confidence and relish, causing them to vomit and survive.

The main active substance of the Calabar bean, physostigmine (from *Physostigma venenosum*) was isolated by the chemists Jobst and Hesse in 1864. It is now one of the most effective drugs for improving the cognitive functioning (memory and thinking) in patients with Alzheimer's disease (*see* Chapter 10).

In areas around Sierra Leone an ordeal trial used to be held every year to eliminate sorcerers believed responsible for all the bad events in the preceding year. Everyone consumed a preparation of the plant *Erythrophloeum guineense*, known as Tali. The plants contain a chemical similar to digitoxin (*see* Chapter 16) which stimulated the heart to a level at which the heartbeat became irregular and the heart was no longer able to pump blood efficiently around the body. Although there are few western witnesses or records to such events, it is known that about 2000 people died in this way in 1912.

Poisons in the environment

MPTP and paraquat

In California in 1982, Dr Jim Langston was called to examine a series of young patients who had been brought into hospital suffering from a combination of symptoms which no-one had previously encountered. A day or two earlier these patients had been relatively normal, apparently healthy adults, mostly in their early twenties. Now they had the appearance of zombies. They were lying in bed, immobile, not showing any response to questions or commands and with stiff muscles which made it difficult for the doctors to move their limbs. The doctors were baffled, until it occurred to Langston that these symptoms were very similar to those of patients with advanced Parkinson's disease.

Despite the fact that Parkinson's disease was only known to occur in much older, usually elderly, patients and that it was a degenerative disorder which only developed slowly over several years, Langston decided to give some of his new patients the antiParkinson drug, levodopa. The effects were astonishing. Within half an hour or so, the patients were able to move around and to walk normally, and could answer questions. It was then that the sad background to these patients was revealed.

Almost all these patients had been drug addicts and had bought what they believed to be samples of pethidine on the street. Analysis of the remaining samples showed that they contained very little pethidine. Later investigations revealed that they had been produced by a back-street chemist who had made, not pethidine, but a related chemical called MPTP. Research in animals then showed that this chemical acts directly on the same nerve cells which are damaged in Parkinson's disease but that it kills them, not over 20 years, but over 20 hours.

The use of MPTP in animals has allowed new drugs to be developed for Parkinson's disease, as we discussed in Chapter 8, but it has also raised questions about the existence of other, MPTP-like chemicals in the environment. In particular, the structure of the molecules of MPTP and herbicides such as paraquat and rotenone are very similar and the incidence of Parkinson's disease is higher in agricultural communities using large amounts of herbicides. It is possible, therefore, that we are all being exposed to small amounts of some chemicals like MPTP and that Parkinson's disease develops in a few people who are particularly sensitive to their effects.

Arrow poisons

Some of the oldest poisons known to man were probably those used as arrow poisons. Poison arrows were widely used by humans to kill prey and in tribal conflicts. In the latter case, some tribes developed sophisticated, brittle arrow-heads which would shatter if they missed their human target, so they could not be reused against them. Our word 'toxic', which means poisonous or causing harm, comes from the Greek word *toxon* which meant 'arrow'. The Greek *toxikon* meant 'the poison into which arrows are dipped'.

The substances used as arrow poisons have varied enormously. The ancient Celts used the juice produced by squeezing hellebore plants, which would contain protoanemonin. This poisonous substance rapidly causes inflammation and breakdown of the cells around the site of an injury, induces the formation of ulcers and causes haemorrhage. Similar effects, mainly in the intestine, occur when humans or cattle eat these plants. Death can occur in a few hours. Another plant poison is the extract of the tree *Acokanthera ouabai*. Sir Morton Stanley saw humans die in Africa soon after a slight, needle-point injury with an arrow smeared with this extract. The active substance in the extract is ouabain, which increases the activity of the heart and induces an irregular heartbeat to the point at which it can no longer pump blood around the body.

Animal poisons have also been used on arrows including, according to Ovid, the blood of vipers. The secretion from the skin of the tree frog *Phyllobates* in Columbia contains batrachotoxin (*see below*) and is among the most powerful of poisons, capable of killing even large mammals.

Curare

One of the best understood arrow poisons is curare. Many early explorers travelling along the Amazon river in the sixteenth century reported that native tribes used an arrow poison, now known often to be a complex mixture made from extracts of *Strychnos, Erythrina*, and *Chondrodendron* plants. Similar poisons were used in other parts of the world too, and in 1584 Sir Walter Raleigh brought samples of curare to England. In the nineteenth century the French biologist Claude Bernard showed that curare acted by antagonizing the action of acetylcholine on nicotinic receptors on muscle, blocking the transmission of nerve impulses to muscles, so that animals receiving the poison collapsed from paralysis of the muscles and then died as the muscles of breathing were affected.

By 1930 scientists had managed to bring back to Europe and America enough curare to begin the task of identifying the active ingredients. Harold King, working at the National Institute for Medical Research at Mill Hill in London in 1935, isolated the most active chemical. He called it tubocurarine because he had extracted it from a sample of curare stored in a tube similar to that used by the native Indians. This drug was introduced into western medicine in the 1940s as its carefully controlled administration relaxed muscles sufficiently for surgeons to carry out complex surgery. Until then, the only method for relaxing muscles during surgery was to increase the depth of anaesthesia, a practice which also increased the chances of death from overdosage.

Since the 1940s, many drugs have been developed which are easier to use and safer than tubocurarine. Tubocurarine itself causes mast cells in the body to release histamine and it blocks nervous transmission at synapses in the sympathetic nervous system. This causes a fall in blood pressure, which is already low during anaesthesia, and contraction of the airways. Such effects can be dangerous in patients under deep anaesthesia or with asthma. The newer drugs including gallamine, pancuronium, vecuronium, and atracurium do not have these dangerous side-effects and they are now almost always used in preference to tubocurarine.

The benefits of poisons

This chapter has introduced only a few of the many poisonous chemicals which exist in nature, but hopefully it will also have served a second purpose. That is to illustrate how many of those natural poisons have provided us with crucial insights into the workings of our own bodies. Without the many toxins which block different channels in the membranes of cells, for example, we would understand far less than we do today because we would not have the chemical tools with which to separate the different components of the complex behaviour of cells.

Drugs of the future

We have also tried to illustrate how even some of the most powerful and feared toxins, such as botulinum toxin, can be harnessed to provide drugs for distressing conditions which otherwise might remain untreatable. There are far more examples of beneficial animal and plant chemicals which may prove to be valuable. The *Litoria* species of tree frogs, for example, secrete the peptide chemical caerulein, which is several thousand times more potent than morphine as an analgesic, as well as chemicals which kill bacteria on the frogs' skin. Drugs derived from these may be developed in the future to treat humans and other animals. There is often a fine line to be drawn between benefit and injury.

Summary

- *Organophosphates are chemicals developed as nerve gases in the two World Wars, but they are in use to kill parasites in farm animals and head lice in children in addition to remaining possible threats during times of war. By inhibiting cholinesterase, the enzyme which destroys acetylcholine, they interfere with the transmission of signals between nerves and muscles and cause severe distress, even death.*

- *Arsenic and lead are around us in the environment and inhibit the actions of enzymes and metal ions, leading to chronic ill-health and lowered intelligence.*

- *Cyanide damages the enzymes which cells need to make use of oxygen. This can rapidly kill the cells.*

- *Carbon monoxide combines with haemoglobin and prevents oxygen from doing so. As the supply of oxygen to cells decreases, they may die.*

- *Strychnine is still present in some rat poisons. It blocks receptors for the inhibitory transmitter glycine, leading to increased nerve cell activity and convulsions.*

- *An impressive range of toxins are produced by bacteria and by animals and plants in their attempts to kill or paralyse prey or predators. Some of these natural toxins are among the most poisonous chemicals on the planet. They may cause the blood to clot within a few minutes, or may stop it from clotting to the extent that the animal bitten dies from multiple haemorrhages. Some toxins prevent transmitter release or cause it all to be released, in either case leading to paralysis and death. Yet other toxins activate or block the channels or pores which are essential to allow ions to move in and out of cells. The result is a complete disruption of tissue function.*

- *Out of the misery of such powerful poisons, medicine is beginning to reap benefit. Some of the toxins can be used in tiny amounts to treat patients with muscular or nervous disorders which cannot be treated by any other drugs.*

CHAPTER 26

The development of new drugs

In 1881 Thomas Huxley foresaw a time when pharmacologists would be able to produce drugs with very specific actions against individual diseases, which he described as working rather like 'a very cunningly contrived torpedo'. The same concept was pursued later by Paul Ehrlich who believed it should be possible to produce drugs which affected only bacteria without harming the cells of the host organism. These drugs, he suggested, would be like 'magic bullets which seek their target of their own accord'.

The pages of this book have introduced many drugs, some old, some new, some still being developed. It is certainly true that about one in four of the drugs available today had its origin in an ancient remedy such as opium (morphine and many of the newer opiate analgesics) or willow bark (aspirin, *see* Chapter 6). Many of these drugs have been available as pure chemicals only since the beginning of the twentieth century, when the concept of using any pure chemicals in medicine was itself revolutionary; these drugs represent the founding of the pharmaceutical industry.

Other drugs, such as penicillin (*see* Chapter 17) and warfarin (*see* Chapter 14), have been discovered by accident. Others, such as chlorpromazine (*see* Chapter 9), iproniazid (*see* Chapter 11), and Viagra® (*see* Chapter 23) were developed for one disorder and found to be far more effective in another.

Modern pharmacology and drug development are less dependent on accidental observations. Scientists can now isolate from cells the receptors with which drugs interact (*see* Chapter 1), and determine their molecular structure, even though many of them consist of around 20 000 atoms. These structures can then be programmed into computers, which can calculate the ways in which drugs could interact with them. This information can then be used to design new drug molecules which interact more powerfully, or more quickly, or in a slightly different fashion, with the receptor.

These are the first stages in drug development. In a typical pharmaceutical company, the first step is to find a starting, or 'lead' compound. Many years and vast amounts of money may be required to understand the causes of a disease and possible ways of producing specific molecules to prevent, stop, or reverse its progress. Much of this fundamental research work is also carried out in university laboratories.

The next step is for chemists to produce new molecules based on the arrangement of atoms in the starting molecule. This usually means making hundreds or even thousands of new chemicals, each of which may take weeks or months to make. Most clinically useful drugs are made of molecules composed of between 10 and 100 atoms, but the number of ways in which these atoms can be combined is astronomical. A molecule composed of 100 atoms could be rearranged into at least 1 million million different molecules. The job of the medicinal chemist is to work out which hundred or so of these are most likely to have the desired biological activity.

These new substances are then passed on to biologists who test, or 'screen' these chemicals to find out which (if any) are active. Many of the new molecules will in fact have little or no activity because biological tissues are very selective (*see below*). Even those molecules which have the same or better activity than the original 'lead' compound will sometimes have undesirable properties (for example being poisonous, or toxic). These initial screens are usually carried out on isolated cells, tissues, membrane fragments, or even on solutions of proteins such as enzymes and receptors in test tubes. These tests, which were once carried out individually in test tubes are nowadays performed by robotic, automated machines which can carry out thousands of tests per day.

Only a handful out of every thousand new substances shows enough promise at this stage to go further. This usually means testing in animals. The point of this is several-fold. Firstly, it is obviously important to ensure that effects seen in the test-tube occur in a living animal. There might, for example, be enzymes in the whole animal which destroy the new molecules in seconds or minutes, rendering the drug useless. The new molecule may also have a totally novel spectrum of effects so that, whereas the pharmacologist may be seeking a drug to lower blood pressure, the new compound may also disturb liver function, or may decrease acid secretion in the stomach, or may affect amines in the brain. (The new molecule may, of course, then become a new lead compound in another research programme, such as one designed to develop a new anti-ulcer drug by reducing acid secretion.)

Two or three new compounds may pass all these tests. The third stage is to increase the dose of drug in mice or rats, or to administer it daily for several weeks to see if it is likely to have any harmful effects after prolonged treatment, or in patients who take an overdose. If luck is still on the side of the scientists, one out of an original 1000 compounds may pass all these activity, selectivity, and toxicity tests.

The final stage of drug development is to test it in man. The drug passes from the scientists to the clinicians who select a small number of volunteer patients who are carefully asked whether they wish to take part in the clinical trial of the new drug. If they agree, the doctors will then monitor as many aspects as possible of their subjects' bodily functions, just as in the case of the rats earlier. If the drug produces no untoward reactions in about 20 healthy volunteers (a 'phase 1' trial) it will subsequently be tried, again only with informed consent, in patients suffering from the relevant disease (a 'phase 2' trial). If the new drug is effective in treating the illness in around a hundred patients with different disease severity, it will progress to phase 3 trials in which it will be tested by several clinicians in hospitals around the world on a thousand or more patients.

If the drug still performs better than the drugs currently available, and shows no serious undesirable side-effects, the pharmaceutical company gathers together all the basic and clinical data it has and applies to a regulatory body for a licence to release and market the drug for medical use. This body is the Committee on the Safety of Medicines (CSM) in the UK and the Food and Drugs Administration (FDA) in the USA. After considering all the accumulated evidence for the drug, these bodies can approve it for general medical use. Even after approval, however, they continue to monitor the effects and side-effects of all drugs (phase 4) by asking doctors to report any unusual or unexpected effects in patients. The regulatory authorities can, and do, force the withdrawal of any drug considered to be unsafe.

Animals and drug development

Most of the tests used in the early stages of safety testing involve animals. These tests are required by law before a company can even consider a new drug for testing in humans. Although many people regret the need for animals in medical research, few would want an untested drug to be used first on them or on their children. The vast majority of safety tests are on mice and rats, which over the last one hundred years have proved to be excellent predictors of activity and toxicity in humans. Arguments that this is not so are based on exceptional drugs such as thalidomide. This was tested in pregnant animals of nine different species, including primates, before being approved for use in humans. However, it turned out that the disastrous effects of thalidomide on embryonic development occur only in humans. This degree of selectivity is unusual and the overwhelming majority of tests on rodents do predict how chemicals will affect human beings.

There are, indeed, few alternatives to using animals that would be acceptable to regulatory authorities such as the FDA and CSM or, for that matter, to most ordinary people likely to take the new drugs. At one extreme, some groups acclaim the use of cell cultures (isolated cells growing in laboratory flasks), which can be kept alive for many months in the laboratory. Unfortunately, such cells have two major disadvantages. Firstly, in the absence of other types of cell from the same tissue, they usually regress to an earlier, less well-developed and less specialized cell, so that their biological properties change substantially from those in the living organism. Most cells in culture age and die after a few (around fifty) generations. The usual way of circumventing this problem is to use cells from cancers, which will continue to grow and divide forever (though scientists are still trying to find out why). However, while cancer cells may be ideal for testing new anticancer drugs, they are not so useful for testing drugs developed for high blood pressure or schizophrenia.

Secondly, the behaviour of cells in a dish cannot realistically reflect that of a tissue or organ in the body, where there is a continuous supply of blood, and hormones, nutrients, and other factors whose levels vary from minute to minute. Also in the body, cells are surrounded by different types of cell which interact intimately with each other both biologically and chemically. This situation can never be reproduced in a test tube.

The danger of testing a new drug only on isolated cells before administering it to humans is, therefore, that the results are likely to be very misleading. They may even produce consequences no less tragic for the families involved than were the effects of thalidomide.

Despite all these reasons for testing drugs on animals, scientists avoid causing unnecessary injury and discomfort to animals. All research is strictly controlled by laws in the USA and Europe. In the UK, for example, every scientist wishing to work with animals must undertake a course in the proper handling and treatment of animals and must then apply for a special licence after discussions with local vets and interviews with National Inspectors. There is a continuing ethic amongst scientists of three R's—reduction (of animal use for research), refinement (of experimental design so that fewer animals are needed), and replacement (of animals by cell cultures, enzymes in test tubes, or computers when these can provide the level of information needed for drug use by humans). Many scientists are devoting themselves entirely to developing these and other new methods of reducing the use of animals.

The costs of drug development

Many of the drugs being developed today are, therefore, the product of years of intensive research and the expenditure of huge amounts of time, effort, and money. In 1995 it was estimated that the cost of developing a new drug to the point of launching it into clinical practice was £250 million ($340 million).*

One reason for this enormous cost is that companies see little point in

* Gambardella, A (1995). See additional reading list.

producing new drugs which are very similar to those of their competitors ('me-too' drugs). Most companies nowadays try to find a completely different type of drug: a different chemical type which may not have the same side-effects as those produced by other companies, or one which acts in an entirely new way to treat a particular disorder. Producing such a new drug increases the possibility that it will be better than those already available. Even if it is not, it may be sufficiently different in its actions that it can be taken by patients who, for one reason or another (such as an allergy), cannot take the existing drugs.

The frustration of 'non-compliance'

After so much time, effort, and money has been spent on developing drugs, it seems tragic that patients fail to take up to one half of all the drugs prescribed—an enormous waste of scientific and health service resources. Those patients with long-lasting, chronic disorders such as asthma, high blood pressure and diabetes are often the worst at taking their drugs. In part this is because patients are afraid of side-effects and in part also because they do not wish to spend the rest of their lives depending on drugs for their health and perhaps survival. Many disorders which cannot be cured by drugs at present can nonetheless be *controlled* by drugs, and patients who stop taking their medication run the serious risk of greater damage to their bodies, and a shorter lifespan, than if they had taken them. Examples include the increased likelihood of heart disease and strokes if high blood pressure is not controlled, and the development of nerve damage, impotence, strokes, and blindness if diabetes is not controlled.

Side-effects: real or imagined?

Throughout this book we have placed far more emphasis on understanding how drugs produce their intended effects than on listing their unwanted side-effects. This may seem strange to someone who opens a bottle of medicine and reads the manufacturer's information sheet, which may list twenty or thirty possible side-effects. We have not detailed these partly because 25 out of 30 side-effects will be experienced only very rarely and will not be of general interest and partly because many side-effects will be very minor symptoms such as tiredness or headache. It should be remembered that patients treated with dummy 'placebo' preparations often show the same 'side-effect' symptoms. Many of the 'side-effects', therefore, appear to be in the mind of the patient, possibly arising from anxiety and concern about taking any medication.

Patients' anxieties are perhaps heightened by the requirement that they be told about all the side-effects attributed to a drug. This is partly an attempt by the drug companies to avoid litigation by patients claiming that they were not given all the available information. Doctors need to make clear that not every-one suffers from side-effects and that most drugs give overall far greater benefits than risk. Such communication between doctors and patients is essential if patients are to feel sufficiently confident to take their prescribed medications.

Do we need new drugs?

The fact that 4999 out of every 5000 new potential drugs are simply thrown away sounds like an astonishing and perhaps unacceptable waste of time and money. Indeed, some critics of the pharmaceutical industry argue that most new drug development should be stopped, since it is this degree of wastage which contributes to the high cost of putting many new drugs on the market.

The unfortunate truth is, however, that serious drug development is a very young science, less than a hundred years old, and there are many illnesses for which we need to find better and more effective treatments. They include muscular dystrophy, some cancers, multiple sclerosis, motoneurone disease (amyotrophic lateral sclerosis in the USA), Crohn's disease, arthritis, Alzheimer's disease, Parkinson's disease, schizophrenia, strokes, malaria, and many others). Finally, there is the continuing worldwide problem of bacteria, viruses, and parasites becoming resistant to drugs, raising the need to maintain a continuing programme of new drug and vaccine development if terrifying diseases such as leprosy, bubonic plague, tuberculosis, malaria, etc. are to be controlled. Tens of millions of people around the world die from these diseases every year and, as resistance increases, that number will rise and affect the more developed countries of the world in addition to those of the Third World.

Are we being too cautious?

Perhaps part of the answer to these problems is not to stop developing new drugs altogether, but to place the beneficial effects of drugs and their side-effects into better perspective.

The word 'pharmacology', meaning the study of drugs, is derived from the Greek word *pharmakon* which means medicine or poison. All people (except identical twins) are slightly different biologically and in their responses to drugs, just as our faces and fingerprints all differ slightly. This means that the side-effects of a drug will, in a few people, be worse than in others.

This problem raises an ethical and logical dilemma. Suppose a million people are suffering persistent, severe pain, as in the case of arthritis, with the greatest difficulty in moving and tending to their bodily needs such as eating, washing, bathing, and toilet. Then suppose that a new drug is produced which relieves those patients of most of their pain, and gives them back the freedom to move and to live a normal life. The prevalence of side-effects of most drugs, around 5 per cent, would mean that 950 000 of those people would suffer no side-effects at all. The other 50 000 might expect mild effects such as feeling sick, headaches, or slight dizziness but those people would always have the option of not taking the drug if they found these effects too unpleasant. Suppose, also, that 5 people died because they reacted to the drug. What action should we take as a society? There would seem to be at least two main options.

The first would be to argue that no death is worth the risk and that the drug should be withdrawn. This action denies 999 995 people in every million of the opportunity to live a normal life.

The second option is to leave the drug on the market, but to make clear to patients that there is a tiny risk of 5 in a million, of serious side-effects or death. The patient is then allowed to make his or her informed choice on how they would prefer to live the remaining years of their troubled lives.

Perhaps the saddest reflection on those involved in making decisions on these matters is that a sense of perspective is often completely lost. The occurrence of 5 deaths per million caused by a drug with tremendous benefits to 999 995 needs to be compared with the fact that of every million people in the USA and Europe over 100 will die each year in road accidents and of every million people who choose to smoke, 200 000 will die from the effects of smoking (mainly heart disease and cancer). Yet smokers and drivers are allowed a free choice of whether they accept these far, far higher risks of death, as are skiiers, climbers, and pot-holers. Why not give the same informed choice to the ill and disabled when the benefits are greater and the dangers less?

Specific examples

If the numbers quoted in these paragraphs seem difficult to believe, let us use a specific example. A few years ago a new drug (benoxaprofen) was produced with the trade name of Opren. It was an NSAID (see Chapter 6) and was used to reduce the pain for thousands of patients with arthritis. It was a much better drug than aspirin because it did not cause as much irritation and bleeding from the stomach. Unfortunately, the incidence of serious side-effects led to the withdrawal of Opren from patients. The risks were not considered to justify its use, partly because other drugs were available at the time, even though Opren was safer in many patients.

A greater ethical dilemma has emerged more recently. Patients suffering from Parkinson's disease derive benefit from several drugs (see Chapter 8) but these are not ideal. In 1997 a new drug, tolcapone, was introduced. This increases the effects of L-dopa in Parkinson's disease, allowing a lower dose of this drug, fewer side-effects, and better control of the disease symptoms. Unfortunately it was withdrawn worldwide in November 1998 following several cases of liver damage. This problem affected less than 1 patient in every 25 000, yet the sometimes dramatic benefit to the other 24 999 has had to be abandoned.

In the light of these facts, why then do we as a society press for the withdrawal of tolcapone and many other drugs which offer real hope to the overwhelming majority of patients. Why do we not provide patients with the figures and let them make their own choice?

The answer is, of course, complicated. Doctors always work on the basis of the old Latin saying *primum non nocere* (first, do no harm). There is always a wish that patients should not be damaged by what doctors have done to them, even when the doctors were trying to prevent inevitable damage to the patient caused by the disease itself.

Secondly, the problem of litigation complicates the subject since drug companies and Government departments are always keen to protect themselves against being sued.

Furthermore, 'giving people the facts and allowing them to make their own choice' assumes that doctors are going to communicate the facts sufficiently well and that patients are going to understand and to have the intelligence, judgement, and indeed, the desire, to make such decisions for themselves. While some may wish to do so, many will simply wish to feel that someone with more knowledge and experience has made the decision for them. It should not be impossible, however, to find a compromise solution which gives freedom of choice to those who want it and reassurance to those who do not.

The need for communication

In the meantime, however, what is certainly necessary is for doctors to spend more time and effort in communicating with their patients to explain the probable benefit and possible risks involved in taking any drug. If a doctor cannot convince a patient that a drug is safe and valuable for his or her long-term health, it is unlikely that the patient will take it.

It is this thought—the need for communication of information about drugs—that is one of the reasons why this book has been written. We hope that, in understanding why they should take a drug for their own benefit, patients will do so with less anxiety and with greater confidence.

Glossary

*Words in **bold** type have their own definition*

accommodation   adjustment of the lens of the eye to focus on near objects

ACE   angiotensin converting **enzyme**: the **enzyme** which produces angiotensin

acetylcholine   a chemical released from nerve endings as a **transmitter**, passing signals onto other nerve cells, causing **muscles** to contract and glands to secrete

acetylcholinesterase   the **enzyme** which destroys **acetylcholine**

acid   a chemical which produces hydrogen ions (protons)

agonist   a drug, **hormone**, or **transmitter** which activates a **receptor** to produce an effect

AIDS   the Acquired ImmunoDeficiency Syndrome, a depression of the immune system caused by **HIV** (Human Immunodeficiency Virus)

alkaline   not **acid**

allergens   **molecules** which provoke an allergic reaction (antigens)

allergic rhinitis   the medical term for hay fever

alpha-receptors   receptors for **epinephrine** and **norepinephrine** which cause contraction of blood vessels and other effects (Table 1.1)

alveoli   the tiny air sacs which make up the lungs

androgens   male sex **hormones**

amines   a class of chemicals which contain a nitrogen atom in the **molecule**

amino acid   a class of chemicals which contain both an amine (nitrogen) group and acid group of atoms in the **molecule**

amygdala   part of the brain concerned with fear, sex drive, and feeding behaviour

anabolic   increasing tissue growth

anaemia   lack of red cells and haemoglobin in the blood

analgesic   drug producing a reduction of pain

androgens   the male sex hormones

angiotensin   a **hormone** which raises blood pressure by contracting blood vessels and reducing the loss of water in the urine

antagonist   a chemical which blocks the effect of a drug, hormone or **transmitter**

antibody   a molecule produced by some **white blood cells** which sticks to bacteria and damaged cells, prompting their attack and removal by other white cells

anticholinergic drugs   drugs which reduce the activity of nerves releasing **acetylcholine**, or which block the effects of acetylcholine

antidiuretic hormone   a hormone which reduces the loss of water in the urine

antidysrhythmic drugs   drugs which reduce abnormal contractions of parts of the heart and restore the normal heart rhythm

antigens   molecules which provoke an allergic reaction (allergens)

antihistamine   drug which blocks the receptors for histamine

antimetabolites   drugs which have **molecules** similar to natural chemicals and which fool **enzymes** into reacting with them instead of the natural substance

antioxidants   chemicals which prevent cell damage caused by **free radicals**

antipsychotic drugs   drugs used in the treatment of psychotic disorders such as schizophrenia

antipyretic   reducing the high body temperature seen in fever

antitussives   drugs reducing coughing

arteriosclerosis   'hardening of the arteries'; narrowing of the arteries caused by fatty deposits on their inner walls

atherosclerosis   'hardening of the arteries'; narrowing of the arteries caused by fatty deposits on their inner walls

athlete's foot   fungal infection of the feet

atrial fibrillation and flutter   conditions in which the atria of the heart beat at a higher rate than the ventricles, resulting in poor performance of the heart in pumping blood

atrium   one of the two upper chambers of the heart which receive blood and push it into the ventricles (plural: atria)

baroreceptors   sensory receptors in the blood vessels which respond to changes of blood pressure and trigger reflexes trying to keep the pressure constant

beta-blocker   drugs which block **beta-receptors**

beta-receptors   receptors for **epinephrine** and **norepinephrine** (see Table 1.1 for a list of effects)

bronchi   the airways

carbon dioxide   the gas produced by cells as a waste product of their activity

cardiac   of the heart

cardiac muscle   specialized muscle cells found only in the heart
cardiac glcycosides   drugs which act on the heart to increase the strength of contraction
catalysts   substances which speed up a chemical reaction without becoming changed themselves
cerebral cortex   part of the brain most highly developed in primates and responsible for thinking and reasoning in addition to processing information
channels   pores or holes in the walls of cells allowing atoms, ions, and molecules into or out of the cell
chemical   every molecule is a chemical, whether it is oxygen, water, cyanide, aspirin, or strychnine
cholesterol   a steroid molecule used in the manufacture of cell walls and steroid hormones
cholinesterase   the enzyme which destroys acetylcholine
chromosomes   the sets of genes in a cell
cirrhosis   degeneration, usually of the liver
cofactors   chemicals needed in small amounts for the activity of enzymes
collagen   the proteins which form the basic material of cartilage and bone
compound   another word for a chemical substance
coronary   of the heart

dementia   disorder of thinking and reasoning, usually with loss of memory
dependence   addiction; the need for continued use of a drug
dermatitis   inflammation of the skin
diastolic pressure   the lowest value of blood pressure, obtained when between contractions of the heart
diuresis   production of urine
diuretic drugs   drugs which increase the formation of urine
DNA   the molecules which make up the genes
dopamine   a neurotransmitter in the brain
dropsy   an old word for oedema: swelling of the tissues to the accumulation of fluid
dyskinesias   abnormal movements
dysrhythmia   abnormal rhythm of the heartbeat
dystonias   abnormal movements

embolism   blockage of a blood vessel by part of a blood clot
endothelial cells   the cells which line the inside of blood vessels
enkephalins   peptide hormones involved in the control of pain

enzymes **protein molecules** which carry out the chemical reactions in cells. They act like catalysts – they are not themselves changed during the reactions

erythrocytes red blood cells

fibrinolytic destroying and removing the fibrin components of blood clots

free radicals highly reactive **molecules** which cause widespread damage to other molecules and cells

GABA an inhibitory **transmitter** in the brain which decreases the activity of nerve cells

gene a portion of DNA

glaucoma increased pressure of the fluid in the eye

glutamate an excitatory **transmitter** in the brain, increasing the activity of nerve cells

glycogen a storage form of glucose sugar

heart attack blockage of blood vessels supplying blood to part of the heart, leading to pain and decreased pumping effectiveness

heart failure decreased strength of contraction of the heart

HIV or human immuno deficiency virus the virus which causes **AIDS** (acquired immuno deficiency syndrome)

hormone chemical secreted by a gland and usually acting on cells in other parts of the body

HRT hormone replacement therapy: the use of **hormones** to replace those lost by removal of an **organ** such as the ovaries, or lost after the menopause

hypertension raised blood pressure

hypoglycaemia lowered amount of glucose sugar in the blood

intrinsic factor a substance produced by cells in the stomach which is needed for the absorption of vitamin B_{12}

involuntary movements movements which the person cannot stop or control

ions one of the forms of an atom when it combines with another atom

leucocytes white blood cells

leukaemia a form of cancer in which the **white blood cells** multiply far beyond their normal numbers

leukotrienes hormones important, for example, in contracting the airways in asthma

levodopa L-dopa; a drug used in the treatment of Parkinson's disease

limbic system parts of the brain concerned with emotions, feelings, and mood

lipases enzymes which break down fats into smaller **molecules** for absorption in the gut

lipids fats

loop diuretics drugs which act on the 'loop' part of the kidney tubules to increase urine formation

mania excitable behaviour

MAO monoamine oxidase; the **enzyme** which destroys **amine transmitters** such as norepinephrine, dopamine, and 5HT

mast cells cells present throughout the body which have similar effects to the **white blood cells**

mediators chemicals produced by cells during an inflammatory response to damage or invasion by bacteria

metabolism the chemical reactions carried out by a cell

metabolites the substances produced by the chemical reactions of the cell

molecules groups of atoms

monoamine oxidase the **enzyme** which destroys **amine transmitters** such as **norepinephrine**, dopamine, and 5HT

motor nerves nerves which cause contraction of **muscles** or secretion of glands

mucus a secretion of sticky substances which form a layer lining **organs** such as the stomach and airways

muscarinic receptors receptors for **acetylcholine** which are also activated by muscarine, a chemical from the mushroom *Amanita*

muscle cells which can contract when stimulated by nerves. Muscle cells can be either **skeletal, smooth, or cardiac**

myocardial infarction damage to the heart resulting from a heart attack

narcotic analgesics pain-killing drugs which can produce sleep in high doses; 'narcotic' can be a general term for drugs which produce addiction

neurotransmitter (or transmitter) a substance which carries signals between nerve cells, or between nerves and **muscles** or glands

NGF nerve growth factor; a hormone needed for the survival of **sympathetic** nerves and some cells in the brain

nicotinic receptors   receptors for **acetylcholine** which are also activated by nicotine

nigrostriatal pathway   the nerve fibres which release dopamine and which degenerate in Parkinson's disease

noradrenaline (norepinephrine)   a transmitter produced by sympathetic nerves and some nerve cells in the brain

norepinephrine (noradrenaline)   a transmitter produced by **sympathetic** nerves and some nerve cells in the brain

NSAIDs   Non-Steroidal Anti-Inflammatory Drugs; drugs which reduce inflammation such as aspirin but which have very different molecules from the **steroids**

nucleic acids   the molecules of DNA which make up the genes, and RNA which are used to 'translate' the DNA in the manufacture of **proteins**

oedema   swelling of the tissues due to the accumulation of fluid

oestrogens   female sex hormones

oncogenes   genes which can increase the rate of cell division and cause cancer

opiates   drugs similar to morphine

organs   collections of cells, such as the heart, stomach, liver, and kidney

pancreas   a gland associated with the intestine and which secretes insulin

parasympathetic nerves   nerves which release **acetylcholine** as their transmitter (see Table 1.1 for a list of effects)

parietal cells   cells in the stomach wall which secrete **acid**

peptide   a small **protein**, made up of between 3 and about 100 amino acids

placebo   chemical with no effect on the body, used to compare with a drug being tested to examine the psychological effects of care and treatment

plasma   blood without the red and **white cells**

platelets   cell fragments in the blood, important in clotting

polysaccharide   a chain of sugar **molecules**

prostacyclin   a **hormone** involved in reducing blood clotting

prostaglandins   **hormones** manufactured from the fatty acid arachidonic acid

prostate gland   gland involved in the secretion of seminal fluid during ejaculation

protein   large **molecule** made up of **amino acids,** usually more than 100

proton pump   an **enzyme** which secretes **acid**

psychosis   any psychiatric disorder in which the patient is unaware he/she is ill

psychotropic drugs   drugs which affect the mind or behaviour

receptors molecules in the walls of cells which respond to drugs, **hormones**, and **transmitters**

reflex an automatic response

RNA the **molecules** which are used to 'translate' the DNA in the manufacture of proteins

selective toxicity toxicity to cells of bacteria or cancers with less effect on normal cells

sensory nerves nerves which carry information about touch, temperature, vision, hearing etc. to the brain

serotonin 5-hydroxytryptamine (5HT)

serum the liquid remaining after blood has clotted

sex hormone hormones responsible for maintaining the sex organs and behaviour

skeletal muscles the **muscles** which move the skeleton; the main, voluntary muscles of the body

smooth muscle the muscles that make up the **organs** such as the stomach, bladder, intestine, and airways

spasticity inability to control movements

SSRIs selective serotonin reuptake inhibitors, a group of antidepressant drugs which slow the removal of **serotonin** (5HT) from its receptors

steroid hormones a class of **hormones** that have **molecules** with a similar basic structure

steroids a class of **molecules** with a similar atomic structure

sympathetic nerves nerves which release **norepinephrine** as their **transmitter** (see Table 1.1 for a list of effects)

tachycardia increased heart rate

testosterone the male sex hormone

thrombosis a blood clot

tissues collections of cells with a similar function, such as **muscle**, blood, skin

tolerance decreasing response to a drug with repeated administration; this requires increasing the dose of drug

toxin poisonous substance

transmitter (or neurotransmitter) a substance which carries signals between nerve cells, or between nerves and muscles or glands

triglycerides fatty substances which have **molecules** made of one molecule of glycerol combined with 3 molecules of fatty acids

tubule the hollow structures which make up the kidney and are responsible for the formation of urine

tumour a solid cancer

vascular of blood vessels

vasodilators compounds (hormones or drugs) which dilate blood vessels, increasing their diameter

vertigo dizziness, usually associated with middle ear infections or Meniere's disease

viruses infectious agents consisting only of **nucleic acid** and **proteins**; they must enter a living cell to reproduce

voluntary muscles the **muscles** which move the skeleton; the main, voluntary muscles of the body

white blood cells the leucocytes and other cells which remove bacteria and viruses and produce **antibodies**

withdrawal symptoms the symptoms seen in a person addicted to a drug when the drug is stopped

Further reading

Ajanki, T. (1995). *Medicinal reading*. Swedish Pharmaceutical Press, Stockholm.

Allardice, P. (1989). *Aphrodisiacs and love magic*. The mystic lure of love charms. Prism Press, Dorset, UK.

Baldry, P.E. (1976). *The battle against bacteria—a fresh look*. Cambridge University Press.

Ban, T.A. *et al*. (1998). *The rise of psychopharmacology*. Animula, Budapest.

Barnes, N. (1997). Leukotriene receptor antagonists: clinical effects. *Journal of the Royal Society of Medicine*, **90**, 200–204.

Benjamin, D.R. (1995). *Mushrooms: poisons and panaceas*. Freeman, London.

British Medical Association (1987). *Living with risk*. Wiley & Sons, Chichester.

British Medical Association (1997). *The therapeutic uses of cannabis*. Harwood Publishers, Amsterdam.

British National Formulary (BNF) (1998). British Medical Association and Royal Pharmaceutical Society, London.

Bucherl, W. (ed.) (1968).*Venomous animals and their venoms*. Academic press, NY.

Challand, R. and Young, R.J. (1997). *Antiviral chemotherapy*. Oxford University Press.

Charlish, A. and Gazzard, B. (1988). *How to cure your ulcer*. Sheldon Press, London.

DiPiro, J.T. *et al*. (1997). *Pharmacotherapy: a pathophysiologic approach*. Prentice-Hall, London.

Dixon, B. (1994). *Power unseen: how microbes rule the world*. Spektrum/ Oxford University Press.

Edstrom, A. (1992). *Venomous and poisonous animals*. Krieger, Florida.

Eley, A.R. (1996). *Microbial food poisoning*. Chapman & Hall, London.

Gambardella, A. (1995). *Science and innovation: the US pharmaceutical industry during the 1980s*. Cambridge University Press.

Godwin-Austen, R. (1993). *The Parkinson's disease handbook*. Sheldon Press, London.

Golding, A.M.B. (1993). Two hundred years of drug abuse. *Journal of the Royal Society of Medicine*, 86, 282–6.

Goodwin, D.W. (1986). *Anxiety*. Oxford University Press.

Greer, J. (1937). *A history of pharmacy*. Pharmaceutical Press, London.

Hampl, J.S. and Hampl, W.S. (1997). Pellagra and the origin of a myth: evidence from European literature and folklore. *Journal of the Royal Society of Medicine*, 90, 636–8.

Hardman, J.G. *et al.* (eds.) (1996). *The pharmacological basis of therapeutics*. McGraw-Hill, New York.

Harris, J.B. (1986). *Natural toxins: animal, plant, and microbial*. Clarendon Press, Oxford.

Hoffer, A. and Osmond, H. (1967). *The hallucinogens*. Academic Press.

Holland, B.K. (1996). *Prospecting for drugs in ancient and mediaeval European texts: a scientific approach*. Harwood, Amsterdam.

Inglis, B. (1975). *The forbidden game: a social history of drugs*. Hodder & Stoughton, London.

Jorgensen, C.D. and Lewis, J.E. (1981). *ABC of diabetes*. New English Library, London.

Kendall, M.D. (1998). *Dying to live*. Cambridge University Press.

Kollerstrom, N. (1982). *Lead on the brain*. Wildwood House, London.

Krieg, M. (1966). *Green medicine: the search for plants that heal*. Bantam Books, N.Y.

Lazell, H.G. (1975). *From pills to penicillin*. Heinemann, London.

Leake, C.D. (1975). *An historical account of pharmacology to the twentieth century*. C.C. Thomas, Springfield, Illinois.

Lockley, K. (1994). *Headaches*. Parragon Press, London.

Lucia, S.P. (1963). *A history of wine as therapy*. Lippincott, Philadelphia.

Mann, J. and Crabbe, J.C. (1996). *Bacteria and antibacterial agents*. Oxford University Press.

Mann, J. (1994). *Murder, magic and medicine*. Oxford University Press.

Mann, R.D. (1984). *Modern drug use*. MTP/Kluwer Press, Dordrecht.

Martindale (1996). *The extra pharmacopoeia*. Royal Pharmaceutical Society, London. 1996.

Melzack, R. (1977). *The puzzle of pain*. Penguin Books.

Milroy, C.M. (1999). Ten years of 'ecstasy'. *Journal of the Royal Society of Medicine* 92, 68–72.

MIMS: *Monthly index of medical specialties*. Haymarket Publishing, London.

Nesse, R.M. and Williams, G.C. (1995). *Evolution and healing*. Weidenfeld & Nicholson, London.

Nestler, E.J. and Aghajanian, G.K. (1997). Molecular and cellular basis of addiction. *Science* 278, 58–63.

Pasternak, C.A. (1998). *The molecules within us*. Plenum Press, New York.

Po, A.L.W. and Po, G.L.W. (1992). *OTC medications*. Blackwell, Oxford.

Pond, C.M. (1998). *The fats of life*. Cambridge University Press.

Porter, R. and Teich, M. (eds.) (1996). *Drugs and narcotics in history*. Cambridge University Press.

Pratt, J.A. (1991). *The biological bases of drug tolerance and dependence*. Academic Press, London.

Rees, J. (1988). *Asthma*. British Medical Association, London.

Robson, P. (1994). *Forbidden drugs*. Oxford University Press.

Sack, O.W. (1976). *Awakenings*. Penguin Books.

Sakula, A. (1988). A history of asthma. *Journal of the Royal College of Physicians* 22, 36–43.

Samuelson, G. (1992). *Drugs of natural origin*. Swedish Pharmaceutical Press.

Sneader, W. (1985). *Drug discovery: the evolution of modern medicines*. Wiley & Sons, Chichester.

Stone, T.W. (1995). *Neuropharmacology*. Oxford University Press.

Taberner, P.V. (1985). *Aphrodisiacs—the science and the myth*. Croom Helm, London.

Tsuang, M.T. (1982). *Schizophrenia—the facts*. Oxford University Press.

Wainwright, M. (1990). *Miracle cure. The story of penicillin and the golden age of antibiotics*. Blackwell, Oxford.

Wardlaw, A.J. (1990). *Asthma*. Bios Scientific publishers, Oxford.

Watts, G. (1990). *Irritable bowel syndrome*. Octopus Publishing, London.

Weatherall, M. (1990). *In search of a cure; a history of pharmaceutical discovery*. Oxford University Press.

Wolf, S. and Wolff, H.G. (1943). *Human gastric function*. Oxford University Press.

Zanca, A. (1989). *Pharmacy through the ages: from the laboratory to industry*. Farmitalia Carlo Erba, Astrea, Parma.

Index

mood 155, 156
moracizine 248
morning-after pill 310
morning sickness 63, 66
morphine 58, 67, 94, 370, 380, 386, 401, 431
  antagonists 98
  and asthma 98
  and breathing 97
  and constipation 98
  discovery 93
  for diarrhoea 98
  and intestinal movement 98
  receptors 100
mosquitoes 274
motion sickness 63, 64
moulds 251, 254
mouth movements 136
movement and its control 118, 169, 236
  involuntary 123–36
  and Parkinson's disease 118
MPTP 119, 425
mucolytic 20, 21
mucus 8, 16, 20, 21, 23, 51, 54, 55, 410, 443
mulberry 79
multi-infarct dementia 141
multiple sclerosis 399, 400
mumps 269
muscarine 6, 402
muscarinic receptors 6, 8,9, 54, 59, 443
  and Alzheimer's disease 151
muscle 416, 443
  diseases 315–34
muscular dystrophy 301
mustine 294
muzolimine 77
myalgic encephalitis 164
mycobacteria 262
mycoses 266–9, 277
myocardial infarction 238, 443; (see also heart
  attack)
myristicin 402
myrrh 252

nabilone 64, 67, 399
nabitan 399
nabumetone 333
nadolol 113, 115, 222, 248
nadroparin 201
nafarelin 312
nafcillin 276
nail infections 266, 268
nalbuphine 98
nalidixic acid 262, 276
nalmefene 103
naloxone 98, 99, 103
names of drugs xv–xvi
nandrolone 312, 345
naphazoline 32

naproxen 103, 333
naratriptan 112, 115
narcotics 93, 370, 443
narcotic analgesics 91, 93, 443
nasal congestion 15–20
natamycin 277
nausea 63, 146, 181, 272, 274, 309, 310, 351,
  387, 399, 423
nebuliser 27, 29
nedocromil 20, 29, 32, 33
nefazodone 164, 186
nefopam 103
negative symptoms of schizophrenia 128, 137
Neisseria 255, 257, 258
nelfinavir 278
neomycin 276
nephrogenic diabetes 44
nephron 69
nerve cells 5, 141
nerve gases 409
nerve growth factor (NGF) 150, 443
nerves 5
  and pain 80, 81
netilmicin 276
nettles 375
neuralgia 174
neuroleptic drugs 132, 132–9, 371, 440
neuropeptide Y 63, 386
neurotransmitters 2–9, 382, 417, 443
  (see also dopamine, GABA, glutamate,
  hydroxytryptamine,norepinephrine)
nevirapine 278
NGF 150, 443
niacin 348, 349, 350, 351
  sources 349, 350
niacinamide 349
nicardipine 223, 248
nicergoline 148, 151
nicorandil 223, 248
nicotinamide 348–50
nicotine 6, 147, 151, 381, 388–90
nicotinic acid 220, 223, 348, 349, 350
nicotinic receptors 6, 8,9, 388, 389, 443
  and Alzheimer's disease 147, 151, 390
  and schizophrenia 390
nicoumalone 197, 198, 201
nifedipine 114, 115, 217, 223, 233, 248
nigrostriatal pathway 118, 443
nimodipine 149, 247
nisoldipine 223
nitrates 231, 240
nitrazepam 182, 186
nitrendipine 223
nitric oxide 232, 367
  and erection 367
nitrites 231, 240, 371, 415
nitrofurantoin 277
nitroglycerin 223, 232, 243
nitroprusside 223

Oxford Paperback Reference

Concise Medical Dictionary

Over 10,000 clear entries covering all the major medical and surgical specialities make this one of our best-selling dictionaries.

'"No home should be without one" certainly applies to this splendid medical dictionary'

Journal of the Institute of Health Education

'An extraordinary bargain'

New Scientist

'Excellent layout and jargon-free style'

Nursing Times

A Dictionary of Nursing

Comprehensive coverage of the ever-expanding vocabulary of the nursing professions. Features over 10,000 entries written by medical and nursing specialists.

An A-Z of Medicinal Drugs

Over 4,000 entries cover the full range of over-the-counter and prescription medicines available today. An ideal reference source for both the patient and the medical professional.

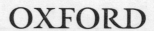
OXFORD

Oxford Paperback Reference

A Dictionary of Chemistry

Over 4,200 entries covering all aspects of chemistry, including physical chemistry and biochemistry.

'It should be in every classroom and library ... the reader is drawn inevitably from one entry to the next merely to satisfy curiosity.'

School Science Review

A Dictionary of Physics

Ranging from crystal defects to the solar system, 3,500 clear and concise entries cover all commonly encountered terms and concepts of physics.

A Dictionary of Biology

The perfect guide for those studying biology – with over 4,700 entries on key terms from biology, biochemistry, medicine, and palaeontology.

'lives up to its expectations; the entries are concise, but explanatory'

Biologist

'ideally suited to students of biology, at either secondary or university level, or as a general reference source for anyone with an interest in the life sciences'

Journal of Anatomy

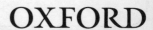

Popular Science from Oxford

Nature's Building Blocks: An A-Z Guide to the Elements
John Emsley

A readable, informative, fascinating entry on each of the chemical elements, arranged alphabetically from actinium to zirconium. A wonderful 'dipping into' source for the family reference shelf and student.

'What for many might be a dry and dusty collection of facts has been turned into an amusing and finely crafted set of mini-biographies . . . . This is a fine, amusing and quirky book that will sit as comfortably on an academic's bookshelf as beside the loo. . . .'

Nature

Molecules at an Exhibition: Portraits of Intriguing Materials in Everyday Life
John Emsley

What is it in chocolate that makes us feel good when we eat it? What's the molecule that turns men on? What's the secret of Coca-Cola? This fascinating book takes us on a guided tour through a rogues' gallery of molecules, from caffeine to teflon, nicotine to zinc.

'A fine example of popular science writing at its best. It is educational, interesting, may prove inspirational and therefore deserves to find a very wide readership.'

Times Higher Education Supplement

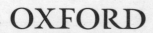

Popular Science from Oxford

Fabulous Science: Fact and Fiction in the History of Scientific Discovery
John Waller

The great biologist Louis Pasteur suppressed data that didn't support the case he was making. Einstein's theory of general relativity was only 'confirmed' in 1919 by an eminent British scientist who massaged his figures. Gregor Mendel never grasped the fundamental principles of 'Mendelian' genetics. Often startling, always enthralling, *Fabulous Science* reveals the truth behind many myths in the history of science.

'Everyone with an interest in science should read this book.'

Focus

Eurekas and Euphorias: The Oxford Book of Scientific Anecdotes
Walter Gratzer

Around 200 anecdotes brilliantly illustrate scientists in all their varieties: the obsessive and the dilettantish, the genial, the envious, the preternaturally brilliant and the slow-witted who sometimes see further in the end, the open-minded and the intolerant, recluses and arrivistes. Told with wit and relish by Walter Gratzer, here are stories to delight, astonish, instruct, and entertain scientist and non-scientist alike.

'There is astonishment and delight on every page . . . a banquet of epiphanies, a reference book which is also a work of art.'

Oliver Sacks, *Nature*

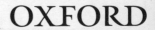